GUT SOLUTIONS

How to Solve Your Digestive Problems Naturally

BRENDA WATSON, C.N.C.

with Leonard Smith, M.D., Suzin Stockton, M.A. and Jamey Jones, B.Sc.

ISBN 9780980216363

Library of Congress Control Number 2011929300

Second Edition

Renew Life Press and Information Services
198 Alt. 19 South
Palm Harbor, FL 34683
1-800-830-4778

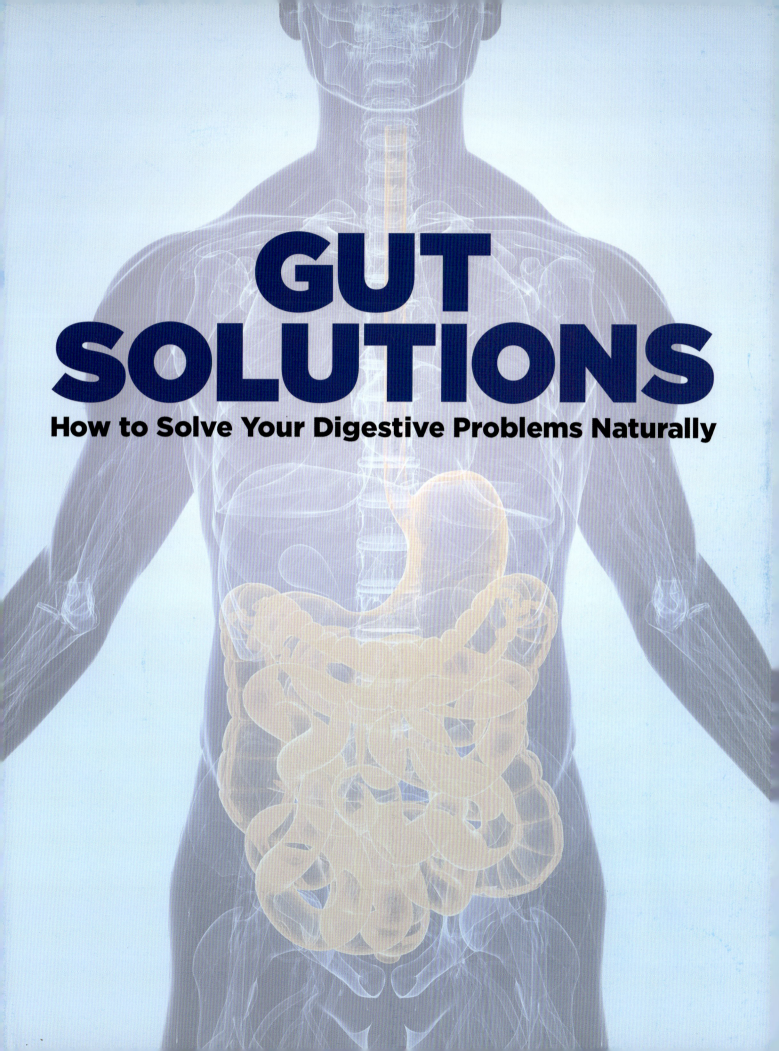

GUT SOLUTIONS

How to Solve Your Digestive Problems Naturally

Acknowledgements

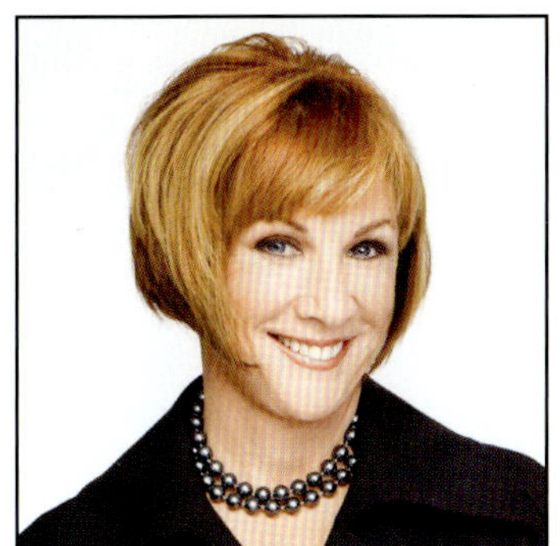

The gratitude I feel for bringing a book of this magnitude to fruition goes not only to the people who have spent countless hours in creating it, but to the thousands of people I have encountered along the way. These people have given me the inspiration to create a book that will help millions more find solutions to not only digestive, but to all health problems.

It is the ongoing crusade to contribute naturally to the digestive health of millions of people that inspired the creation of this 2nd edition of Gut Solutions. Thanks to the tens of thousands of people that purchased the original Gut Solutions, and inspired us to update the book for the 2nd edition.

For the creation of Gut Solutions, we wish to give a special acknowledgement to the following folks, both inside and outside of the Renew Your Life Press family, for their valued contribution to this book. Without the skill, commitment and hard work of the Renew Your Life Press staff, this book would not be a reality. Thanks to:

Suzin Stockton and Jamey Jones for providing research, and guidance in creating this book. Their knowledge of natural digestive care and writing contributed greatly to the completion of this book.

Thank you again Dr. Leonard Smith, my friend and mentor. Dr. Smith has a perspective on health that is both conventional and alternative. With both of these aspects, from a surgeon's perspective and an integrative approach, he contributes to this book with such an amazing level of knowledge.

I want to say a special thank you to Jerry Adams for keeping me on track. This is, to say the least, a very special gift, and not easy. We have brought this project to fruition due to your tenacity.

For the design of the book a special thanks to Paul Pavlovich. Paul brings enthusiasm and passion to any project he is involved in. Also special thanks to Jesse Lockwood for being able to take direction and bring the desired results to this project.

To the special family of ReNew Life and Advanced Naturals: Since the publishing of the first book ReNew Your Life, you have shown me constant love and support. I am so grateful and happy to have watched the growth of a wonderful organization full of passion and desire to help others. I could not have asked for more support through the years.

And last but not least, I thank my husband Stan for his support and guidance in all my endeavors to educate the public on the importance of digestive health. Without him it would not have been possible to bring all my books forward and help so many people have a better life.

Sincerely,

Brenda Watson

Brenda Watson, C.N.C.
Clearwater, FL
2011

Preface

By Brenda Watson, C.N.C. and Dr. Leonard Smith, M.D.

For the purpose of education, this book is divided according to conditions, using both medical and common lay names. These common names have been included because most people, through various media pronouncements, have come to know them to some extent. While these labels—both common and technical—can be useful in identifying different aspects of what can happen to the esophagus, stomach, intestinal tract, liver and gallbladder, it can be even more important to understand the common ground that ties these conditions together. It will become apparent throughout this book that we have the option to focus on labels and details as they relate to symptoms or to see the bigger picture of what is the underlying cause before symptoms manifest. This is essentially the difference between the focus of allopathic medicine (symptom and disease oriented) and naturopathic medicine (primary cause and prevention oriented).

It should be obvious that both the allopathic and naturopathic approaches are of great value. Tumors, bleeding or obstruction in the intestinal tract usually require direct outside intervention to save and or restore health. On the other hand, in our era of skyrocketing health costs (well over a trillion dollars spent annually in the U.S.), prevention through a deeper understanding of cellular function is of paramount importance.

This book has been created in a particular format to help the reader understand what the condition is, what causes it, what are the signs and symptoms, how it is traditionally diagnosed, what are some of the standard medical treatments and, finally, what are some of the nutritional approaches and lifestyle changes that can be implemented to entirely avoid the condition. These same optional nutritional approaches and lifestlyle changes can be profoundly helpful when combined with more invasive allopathic treatments.

A variety of tools are needed in every toolbox to accomplish any task, and so it is with health. The simple principles of drinking pure filtered water; eating more organic vegetables, fruits, seeds and nuts; exercise; high quality sleep; efficient bowel function; stress modification (including psycho-emotional and spiritual rejuvenation) and appropriate dietary supplementation are "tools" that will help maintain or restore lost health.

Too often, health care practitioners give such vague, generalized (and often inaccurate) advice as: "Just eat your standard, balanced diet," and "You can take supplements, but they really don't matter and won't be helpful," or "A bowel movement every two or three days is okay." These are examples of arcane attitudes being espoused by some who are not even reading their own literature. It is statements like these that we would like to address with further clarity and documentation from the medical literature.

Finally, there will be notable repetition in the nutrition and lifestyle section at the conclusion of each condition in the book. This repetition underscores the fact that all of these conditions arise from the common ground of cellular dysfunction. We have even created a simple acronym, which is weaved throughout the book: HOPE. High-fiber diet, Omega Oils (essential fats), Probiotics, and Enzymes. These are the diet and supplement "tools" that, along with lifestyle changes, form a firm foundation of good health. Solid foundations last longer, resist destructive forces and are generally easier to reconstruct in the face of disaster. In the same fashion, humans who maintain a healthy foundation recover and survive stress and illness better than the less healthy. This book is about educating and helping restore foundational health.

Table of Contents

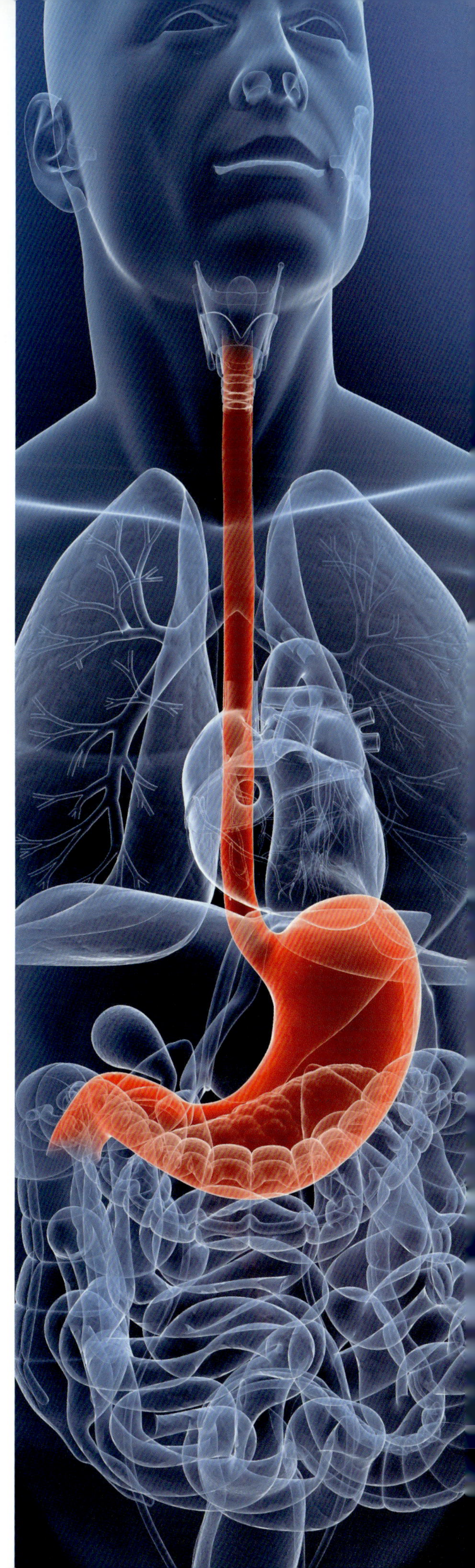

Healthy Digestive System

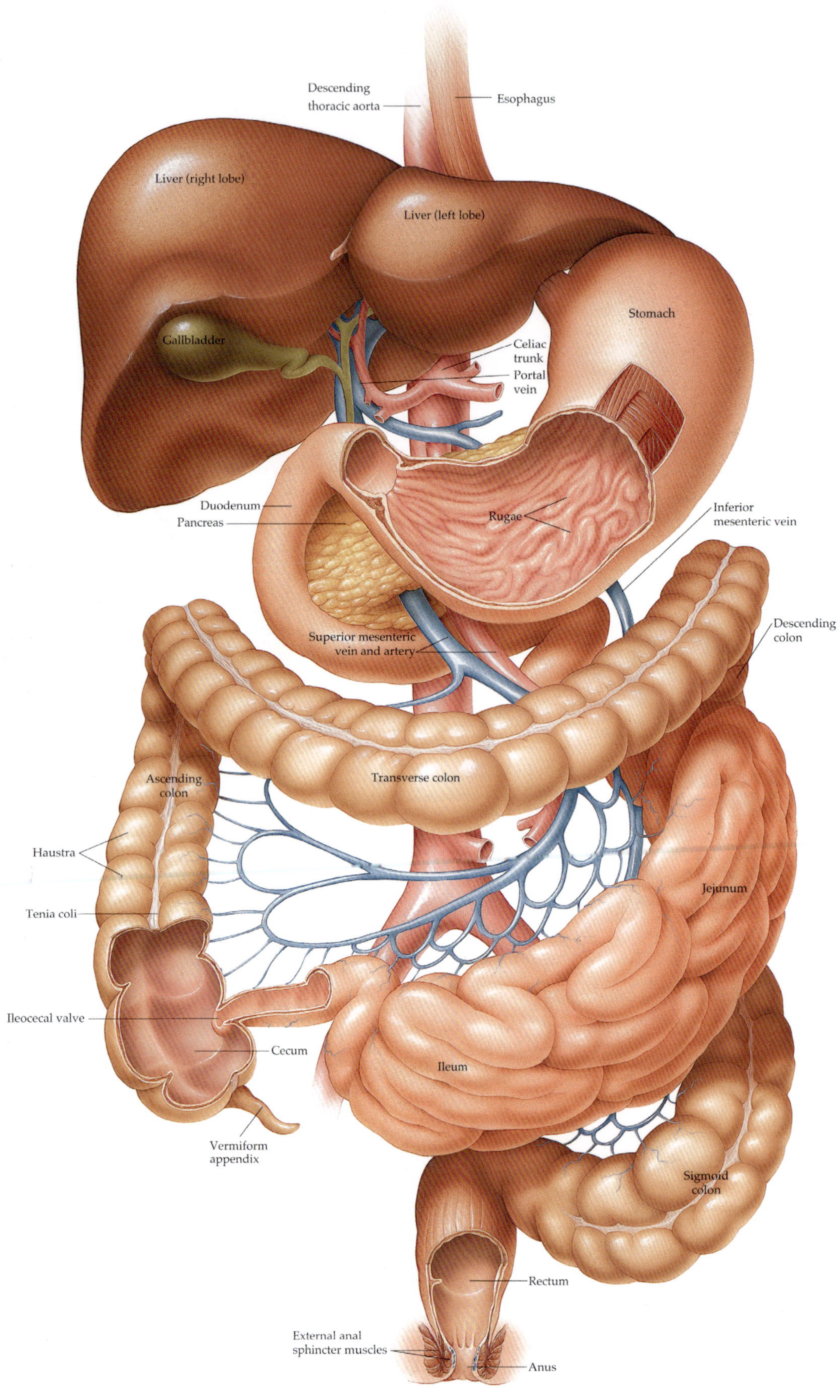

Descending thoracic aorta
Esophagus
Liver (right lobe)
Liver (left lobe)
Stomach
Gallbladder
Celiac trunk
Portal vein
Duodenum
Pancreas
Rugae
Inferior mesenteric vein
Descending colon
Superior mesenteric vein and artery
Transverse colon
Ascending colon
Haustra
Tenia coli
Jejunum
Ileocecal valve
Cecum
Ileum
Vermiform appendix
Sigmoid colon
Rectum
External anal sphincter muscles
Anus

Unhealthy Digestive System

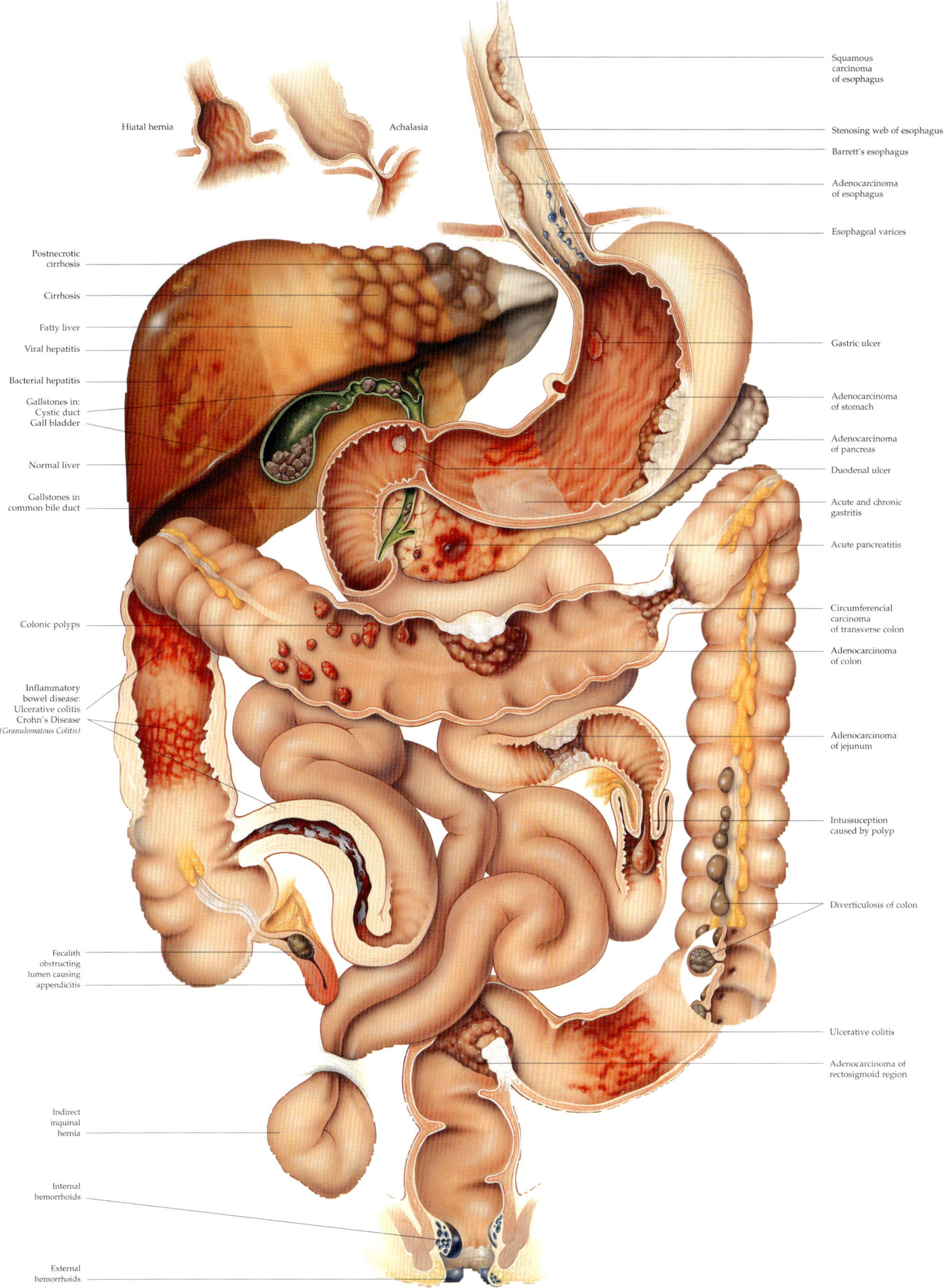

Hiatal hernia
Achalasia
Squamous carcinoma of esophagus
Stenosing web of esophagus
Barrett's esophagus
Adenocarcinoma of esophagus
Esophageal varices
Postnecrotic cirrhosis
Cirrhosis
Fatty liver
Viral hepatitis
Bacterial hepatitis
Gallstones in:
Cystic duct
Gall bladder
Normal liver
Gallstones in common bile duct
Gastric ulcer
Adenocarcinoma of stomach
Adenocarcinoma of pancreas
Duodenal ulcer
Acute and chronic gastritis
Acute pancreatitis
Colonic polyps
Circumferencial carcinoma of transverse colon
Adenocarcinoma of colon
Inflammatory bowel disease:
Ulcerative colitis
Crohn's Disease
(Granulomatous Colitis)
Adenocarcinoma of jejunum
Intussuception caused by polyp
Diverticulosis of colon
Fecalith obstructing lumen causing appendicitis
Ulcerative colitis
Adenocarcinoma of rectosigmoid region
Indirect inquinal hernia
Internal hemorrhoids
External hemorrhoids

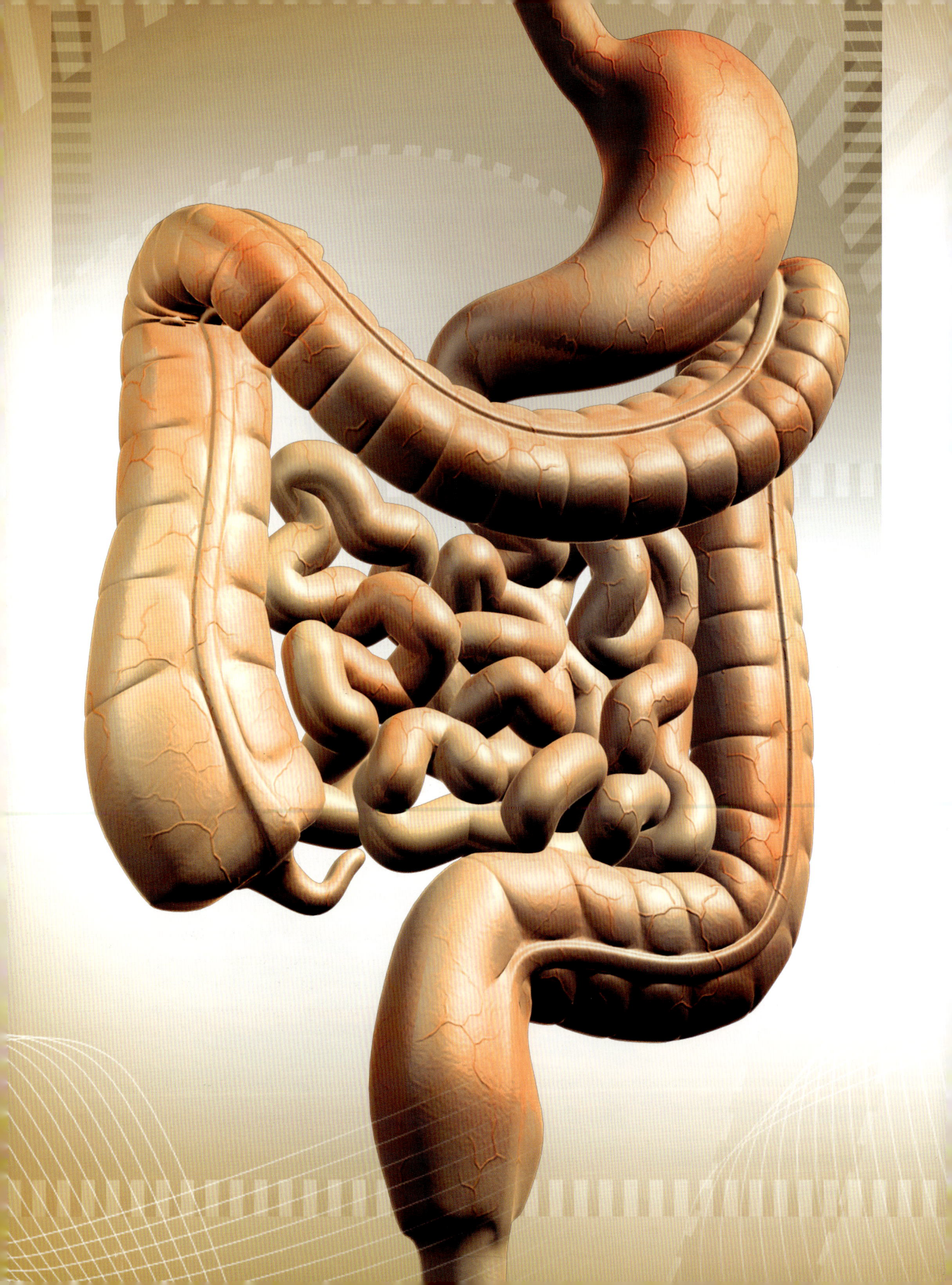

Basics of Digestion

Balance Your Gut, Heal Your Body

It's called "the gut," also known as the gastrointestinal (GI) tract or the digestive tract. It is essentially a long tube made up of layers of muscle lined by cells and glands imbedded in a mucous lining. The job of the gut is to ingest food, digest it, absorb nutrients, and to excrete waste products. The digestive system works hard. It is pressed into service every time we eat. In fact, over the course of a lifetime, it will digest some 23,000 pounds of solid food.[1]

There are numerous organs involved in the digestive process: mouth, esophagus, stomach, small and large intestines, anus, gallbladder, liver and pancreas. These last three organs are located outside the digestive tube or tract, but still play an important role in digestion. Should something go wrong with any of the digestive organs, the process of digestion becomes impaired. Nutritional status and overall health are then adversely affected. This happens more often than we might suspect. More people are hospitalized for GI disorders than for any other,[2] *and more than 100 million Americans are reported to have digestive disorders.*

The health of the digestive system impacts the health of the rest of the body. When digestion is not optimal, whether from a recognized digestive disorder, inadequate diet, or even a silent digestive imbalance, the rest of the body not only misses out on vital nutrients, but it also receives toxins that can adversely affect many different areas of the body. The many gut connections to overall health highlighted in this book illustrate just how important digestive health is.

In the process of digestion, food is converted into fuel, or energy, to run the body. Large pieces of food are broken down physically (through chewing) and chemically (through enzyme activity) into microscopic particles, so that they are small enough to cross the cell membranes of the gut and enter the bloodstream. Any glitch in the digestive conversion process short-circuits the body's energy supply, and can have far-reaching effects on health.

Before looking at what can go wrong in the process, let's look at what a properly functioning system does and how it works.

SOME BASICS OF DIGESTION

Peristalsis

From the time food is put into the mouth until its waste products are excreted, it is propelled through the body by a series of muscular contractions known as peristalsis.

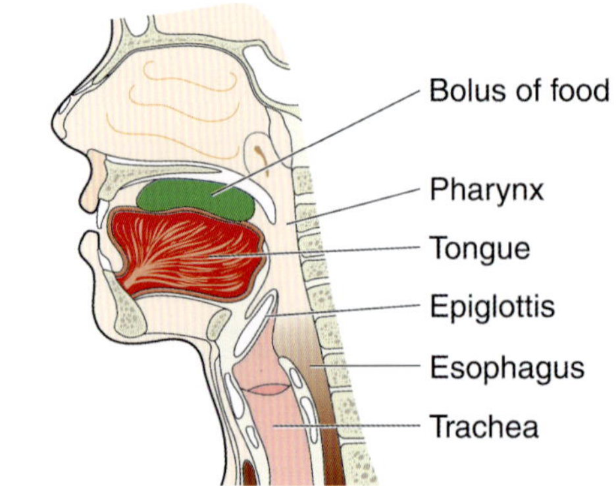

In the mouth, food is pushed by the process of deglutition (swallowing), a voluntary action, which moves the food bolus into the upper esophagus; then, the involuntary contractions (peristalsis) of the esophagus deliver the food into the stomach. When the food reaches the stomach, the lower esophageal sphincter high pressure zone (LES-HPZ), created by the diaphragm and esophagus, normally prevents reflux of food into the esophagus.

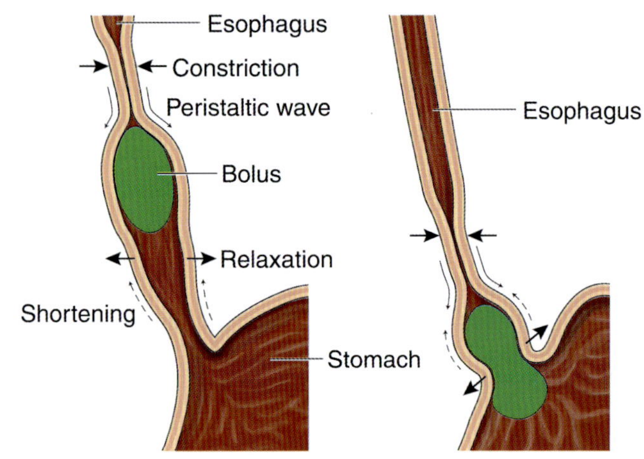

The LES-HPZ is normally closed, but, as food approaches, the surrounding muscles relax allowing a temporary opening through which food may enter the stomach. As the LES-HPZ opens, the muscle of the upper part of the stomach relaxes permitting large volumes of food to enter. Here food is stored and broken down. The stomach acts like a large blender, churning and mixing food and liquid with its own digestive juices.

Finally, the stomach empties its contents into the small intestine. By the time food enters the first section of the small intestine (the duodenum), it has already changed significantly. What enters the duodenum is called chyme, which is a mixture of food, hydrochloric acid (HCl), gastric enzymes and mucus. It is here in the doudenum that the pancreas releases its enzymes and bicarbonate to neutralize the acid, and the liver adds bile at the same time. The food bolus then enters the major part of the small intestine (jejuneum and ileum), which also secretes digestive juices and mucus that act upon and dissolve the food.

The next step is the absorption of digested nutrients through the wall of the small intestine into the bloodstream. The part of the food that is not digestible (fiber), along with worn out cells shed from the mucosa (mucus lining of the GI tract), and some unabsorbed toxins constitute waste products. These products are propelled by peristalsis into the large intestine (colon) where they are dehydrated, turned into stool, mixed with trillions of bacteria and expelled from the body in the form of a bowel movement.

In this sequence of events, we see the importance of peristalsis. The muscles in the GI tract work in harmony with hormones and nerves to control motility (spontaneous movement) throughout the digestive system. Most GI problems are functional, rather than structural, and involve defects in motility, absorption or secretion.[3]

Beneficial Bacteria

Trillions of bacteria, yeasts, parasites and other microbes live in the digestive tract, primarily in the colon. In a healthy person, the bulk of intestinal bacteria will be of the commensal (neutral) or beneficial variety— primarily many species of Lactobacillus and Bifidobacterium— with a minority being potentially pathogenic (disease-causing).

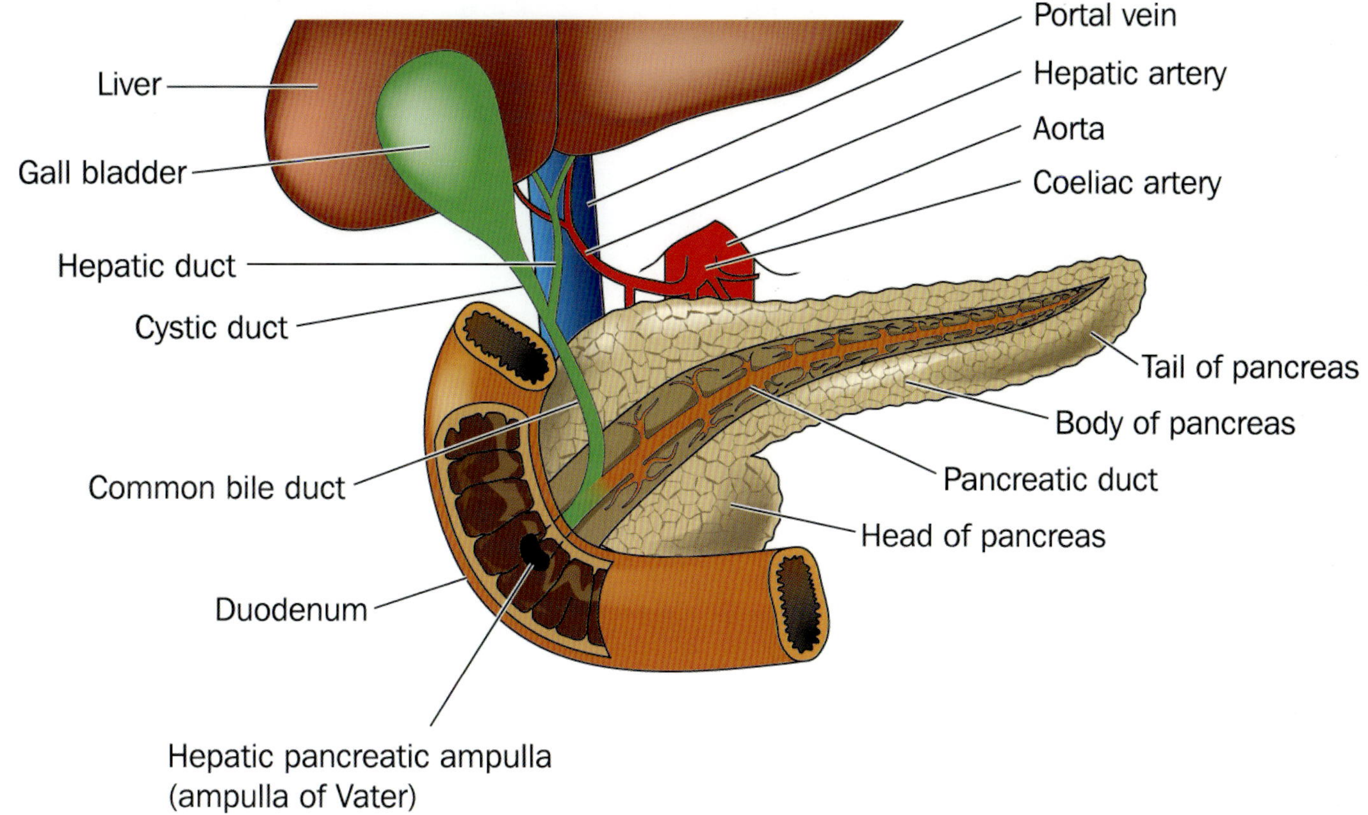

There are now estimated to be between 1,000 and 5,000 different bacterial species of bacteria residing in the gut. Most agree that an ideal ratio of good/neutral to bad bacteria would be approximately 80 percent to 20 percent. In the presence of many digestive disorders, however, a state of dysbiosis exists in which this ratio is distorted, or even reversed. Restoring the optimal bacterial balance in the GI tract is vital to full recovery of health. Dysbiosis also involves other microorganisms like fungi, parasites or viruses.

Beneficial bacteria in the GI tract serve many vital functions. In the colon, they produce certain B vitamins, including B12 and biotin, as well as vitamin K. They also control the growth of harmful microorganisms, break down toxins and stimulate the immune system. Additionally, bacteria ferment dietary fiber into short-chain fatty acids, like butyrate, which is a primary fuel for the colon and protects the colon against cancer.

Secretion

Glands in the GI tract produce digestive juices that break food down into its component parts—fat into fatty acids, protein into amino acids and carbohydrates into simple sugars. These same glands produce hormones that assist in controlling the digestive process. These secretions begin in the mouth where saliva is produced by the salivary glands. These glands contain the enzyme amylase, which begins to break down starch (carbohydrates).

Thus, the digestive process begins in the mouth, before food even enters the mouth. The term "mouth watering" refers to a very real physiological reaction, because the very thought of food is sufficient to trigger salivary gland activity.

Glands in the stomach lining produce hydrochloric acid (HCl) and the enzyme pepsin. Both of these secretions increase when food enters the stomach, and are essential for protein digestion. Pepsin functions to break down proteins. HCl works to denature proteins, making them easier to digest. HCl also plays an important role in killing infectious microorganisms (bacteria, parasites, fungi) that are ingested with food. This is one reason that the stomach is so acidic.

Secretions from the pancreas and the liver act upon ingested food once it enters the duodenal portion of the small intestine. Pancreatic juice contains enzymes

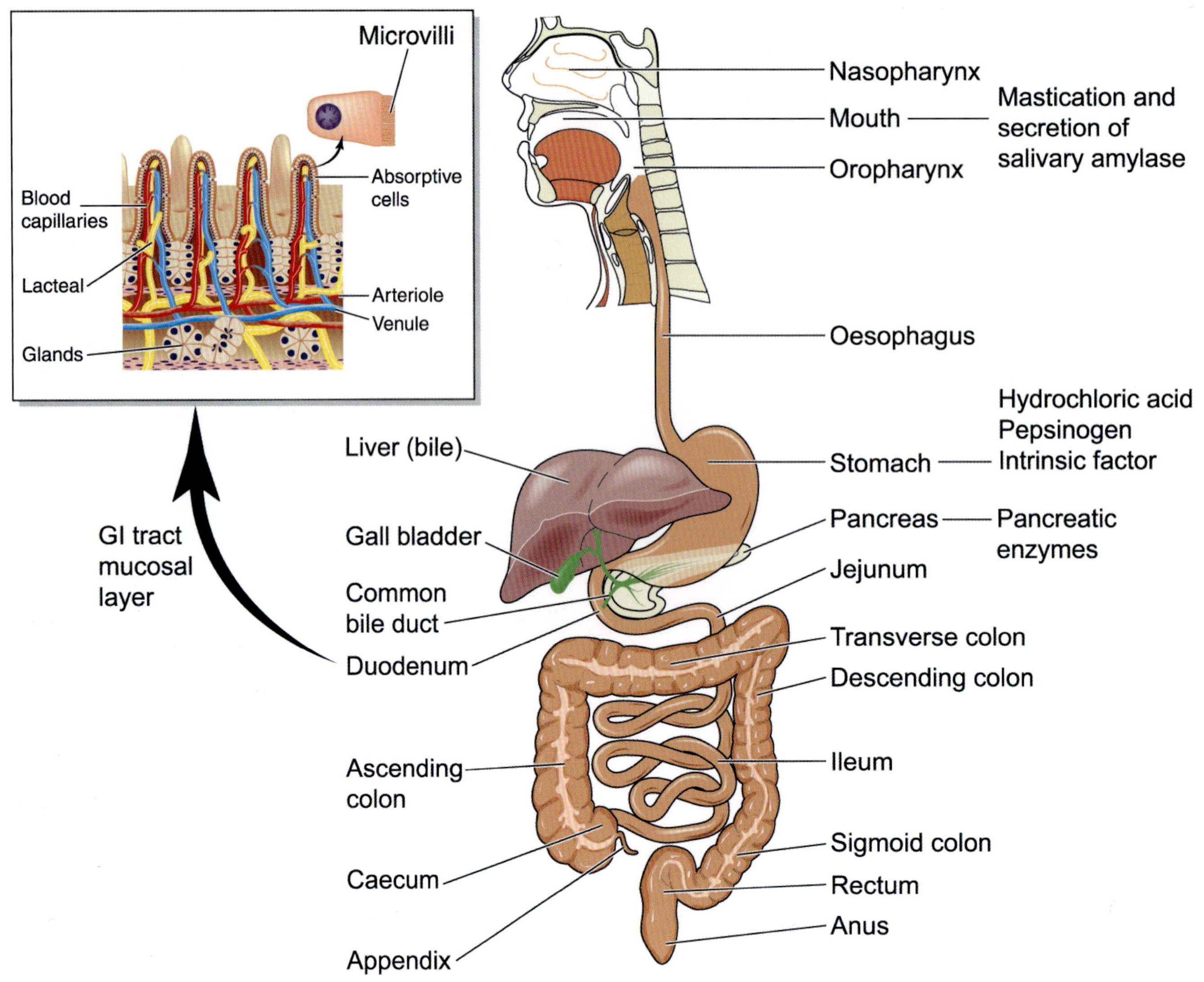

that break down fats (the enzyme lipase), carbohydrates (amylase) and proteins (protease). Also the small intestine itself secretes enzymes: lactase (breaks down milk sugar), DDP IV (dipeptidyl peptidase IV breaks down peptides), disaccharidases (break down starches and sugars) to assist in the digestive process. The pancreas also secretes sodium bicarbonate to neutralize stomach acid. The liver produces bile, a digestive secretion that is stored in the gallbladder. When food is eaten, the bile is released from the gallbladder into the small intestine (via bile ducts) where it emulsifies or dissolves fat. The fat is then digested by pancreatic lipases and enzymes that line the intestine. Bile also contains toxins and hormones that are carried out with feces.

Absorption

Absorption takes place in the small intestine. Here macronutrients (fats, carbohydrates and protein) are broken down into smaller units and absorbed through the wall of the small intestine, and then carried throughout the body along with micronutrients (water, vitamins and minerals) via the bloodstream. These materials will either be stored for later use, or undergo further chemical change for use in the many different processes of the body.

The surface of the duodenum, the first section of the small intestine, is smooth for the first few inches, but quickly changes to a surface with many folds and small, fingerlike projections called villi and microvilli. These threadlike projections cover the surface of the mucous membrane lining the small intestine, and serve as the site of absorption of fluids and nutrients, actually sucking up small particles of digested food. The villi and microvilli greatly increase the surface area of the small intestine maximizing nutrient absorption capabilities.

The walls of the small intestine consist of four layers of muscle. Inside both the small intestine, as well as the

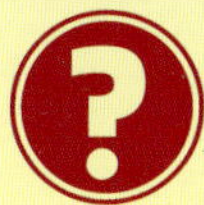

Did You Know

The Human Microbiome Project

The Human Microbiome Project is funded by the National Institutes of Health (NIH), and involves the genetic identification of the microorganisms that live within and on the body. This project will also investigate the influence of these microorganisms on human development, physiology, immunity and nutrition.[4] Using advanced DNA technologies in a field of research known as metagenomics, researchers have determined that the human digestive tract is estimated to house between 1,000 and 5,000 different bacterial phylotypes, or species.[5]

entire digestive and respiratory tracts, is a layer of mucous known as the mucosal layer, or mucosa. This mucous lining serves two vital functions: It allows nutrients of the proper size to pass through and to enter the bloodstream, and it blocks the passage of undigested food particles, pathogens and toxins into the bloodstream. The surface of the mucosa is thick and slippery. Much of the mucus here consists of the amino sugar N-acetyl-glucosamine (NAG), which the body makes from L-glutamine, one of its most abundant amino acids. An adequate amount of glutamine must be present in the body to manufacture NAG (N-acetyl-glucosamine), which is vital to the health of the mucosa.

The mucosa is normally shed and rebuilt every three to five days. In the presence of some inflammatory bowel conditions, however, it appears to be sloughed off at a higher rate possibly due to an inability of the body to convert L-glutamine to NAG or due to the inflammation iteself.

Gut Immunity

The immune system is a complex, multi-level defense system that protects the body from foreign invaders. The digestive system plays a major role in the body's immunity. More than 70 percent of the immune system is located in the gut. This is in reference to the gut-associated lymphoid tissue (GALT) that resides in the gut. The digestive tract is constantly in contact with foreign invaders, also known as antigens. The job of the immune system is to determine which antigens are potentially pathogenic and which are harmless. (For example, food should be seen as harmless.)

Once the immune system determines that an antigen is a potential pathogen or invader, the innate immune system, which is the first part of the immune system to respond, mounts an inflammatory reaction against the invader. It also begins to send messages to the adaptive immune system. This more sophisticated branch of the immune system remembers specific antigens, so that the next time they are encountered, the body is better equipped to respond.

In addition, the fact that the digestive tract itself is a physical barrier separating the rest of the body from the bloodstream makes it an effective blockade against invaders as well. The protective mucous layer makes it difficult for pathogens to come in contact with the epithelial cells that line the intestinal wall. Additionally, the mucosa creates a safe haven for beneficial bacteria, immune cells and other beneficial molecules, which all work together to shield the body from invasion.

Hormones

Hormones within the digestive system control its functions by regulating secretions and movement of digestive organs. Cells within the mucosa of the stomach and small intestine produce and release the major hormones that control GI activity. Some examples of these hormones and their functions are:[6]

Gastrin—released by the antral cells in the stomach:

- Strongly stimulates the stomach to produce HCl (regulates its release from parietal cells in the stomach)
- Strongly stimulates the stomach to produce pepsin
- Weakly stimulates the secretion of pancreatic enzymes
- Weakly stimulates the gallbladder contraction
- Stimulates secretion of histamine by special cells (ECL cells) in the stomach lining
- Controls gastric motility

Secretin—secreted by mucosa in the upper two-thirds of the small intestine in response to the presence of acid chyme:

- Stimulates the secretion of bicarbonate-containing pancreatic juice

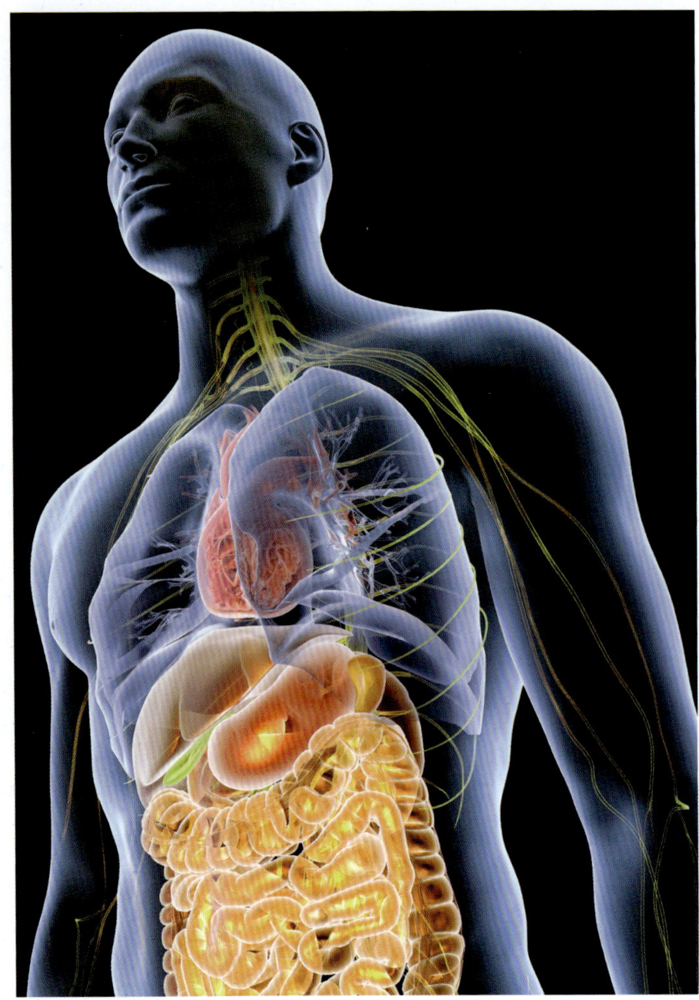

Illustration of the digestive system and its connection to the nervous system

- Stimulates, to a lesser extent, bile and intestinal secretion

Cholecystokinin (CCK)—secreted by the small intestine:
- Creates a feeling of fullness by acting directly on the satiety centers in the brain
- Stimulates gallbladder contraction
- Stimulates secretion of pancreatic enzymes

The Two Nervous Systems

While the digestive process is under the control of the hormonal system, hormone release is under the control of the nervous system. The central nervous system (CNS) is made up of the brain and spinal column. Not as familiar is the enteric nervous system (ENS). The word "enteric" means pertaining to the small intestine. **Half of the body's nerve cells are located in the gut**.[7]

The central nervous system and the enteric nervous system connect directly through the vagus nerve, which is the longest of the cranial nerves. This connection allows for direct communication between the gut and the brain. It is said that the gut has a mind of its own. The ENS is the gut's brain, and it runs the length of the GI tract.

There are two types of nerves that control all activity in the digestive system. They are extrinsic and intrinsic nerves. The extrinsic nerves enter the digestive organs from the outside, from the spinal cord or from the brain, while the intrinsic nerves are embedded in the walls of the digestive organs, and so are inherent within the ENS. The extrinsic nerves release the neurotransmitters acetylcholine and adrenaline that cause the muscles of the digestive organs to contract and relax respectively (peristalsis). The intrinsic nerves go into action when food enters the digestive organs. They release a variety of substances to regulate the speed with which food moves through the system, and the production of digestive juices.

In the 1960's, it was discovered that the neurotransmitter serotonin was produced in and targeting to the ENS. **Today it is known that there is more serotonin in the gut than in the brain.** A neurotransmitter is a chemical substance that facilitates communication among nerve cells, as well as from nerves to muscles, glands and vessels.[8]

It has since been verified that, not only is serotonin found in the ENS, but that every class of neurotransmitter found in the brain is also found in the ENS.[9] All this new information about the gut-brain connection is profoundly altering the understanding of how the digestive system works.

The Gut-Brain Connection

As stated, it is known today that there is a brain, or inherent nervous system, in the bowel. This nervous system is able to mediate reflexes in the digestive system without input from the brain or spinal cord. As a result,

Did You Know

The surface area of the small intestine is greater than 200 square meters. That's about the size of a tennis court. The surface area of the entire digestive tract would cover an area about the size of two football fields!

Brenda's Case Studies

In my work as a colon hydrotherapist with thousands of clients over the years, I found many with emotional/gut issues. It was quite common for people to come for colon therapy, and not be at all in touch with their "gut feelings." After having a few sessions of colon therapy, many would begin to process unpleasant experiences or emotions.

In the following case studies, we'll look at two specific instances of emotional distress impacting digestive health. These represent only a small fraction of the patients I've seen over the years.

John came into the clinic one day to "experience cleansing." He had heard about it, but had never had the opportunity to undergo colon therapy. John wrote on the intake form that he had irritable bowel. As we began the first therapy session, he had a lot of spasms as water was leaving the colon. It was uncomfortable, but he was enthusiastic about coming back for a second treatment. During the second session, John began to talk about his mother. His mother had committed suicide. This had no doubt hurt John immensely, and as he talked during this session and subsequent sessions, he realized that he felt responsible for her actions, and had actually taken on a lot of guilt over the situation. As John went through this cleansing process, the colon therapy treatment ceased to be uncomfortable, and he realized his irritable bowel was due to his emotional state surrounding his mother's suicide. Imagine the breakthrough and healing John experienced by unpacking the emotional baggage that was the cause of most of his bowel problems!

Jill was in her 30s. She had suffered from constipation most of her life. She had a very good job, one that put her on the road a good deal of the time. But Jill could not have a bowel movement unless she was at home. This meant she went for days, and sometimes a week at a time without bowel movements. Jill came in for colon therapy because of her constipation. Over a period of a few months, Jill became more comfortable, and started to talk a lot about her childhood during her sessions. As it unfolded, Jill's mother had an obsession with cleanliness. During Jill's childhood, when the family traveled and stopped to use the restroom at a service station or rest stop, her mother would line the floors and toilet with paper towels. Jill became terrified of germs and, as a result, developed constipation that carried over into adulthood.

Over and over again, I saw real healing take place as people looked beyond diet and supplementation to handle their digestive problems. The truth is, if you are experiencing any of the conditions we address in this book, you must discover the underlying emotional, psychological or spiritual issues. The following affirmations, written by one of my teachers, Bernard Jensen, can help in this regard:

- We are living in a world of cause and effect. I myself set up the causes, by thinking good or bad, for the things that happen to me. The result is that I live in cause and not effect.
- Through negative thinking, I force the power within to work against me; therefore, I will think positively.
- In each different situation, I look for new, positive ideas, constructive possibilities, people who can be helpful and enterprises with new vistas.
- Success, health and happiness lie within me; they do not come from the outside.
- In each situation, I will search for positive thoughts as I would search for the pearls of a broken necklace.
- From now on, I take one step at a time.
- To all difficulties, I respond with impartiality, courage and self-confidence.
- My life is what my thoughts make it.
- When I am kind to others, I am the best to myself.
- I nurture my mind with great thoughts because to believe in the heroic makes heroes.
- I will be true to myself that others may know me just as I am, and know all that it is possible for me to be.
- To love others as myself is to accept them as they are, to receive them without resentment, and to so live in such a way that all my actions reflect harmony, happiness, joy and serenity—in my own body and in everyone I meet.

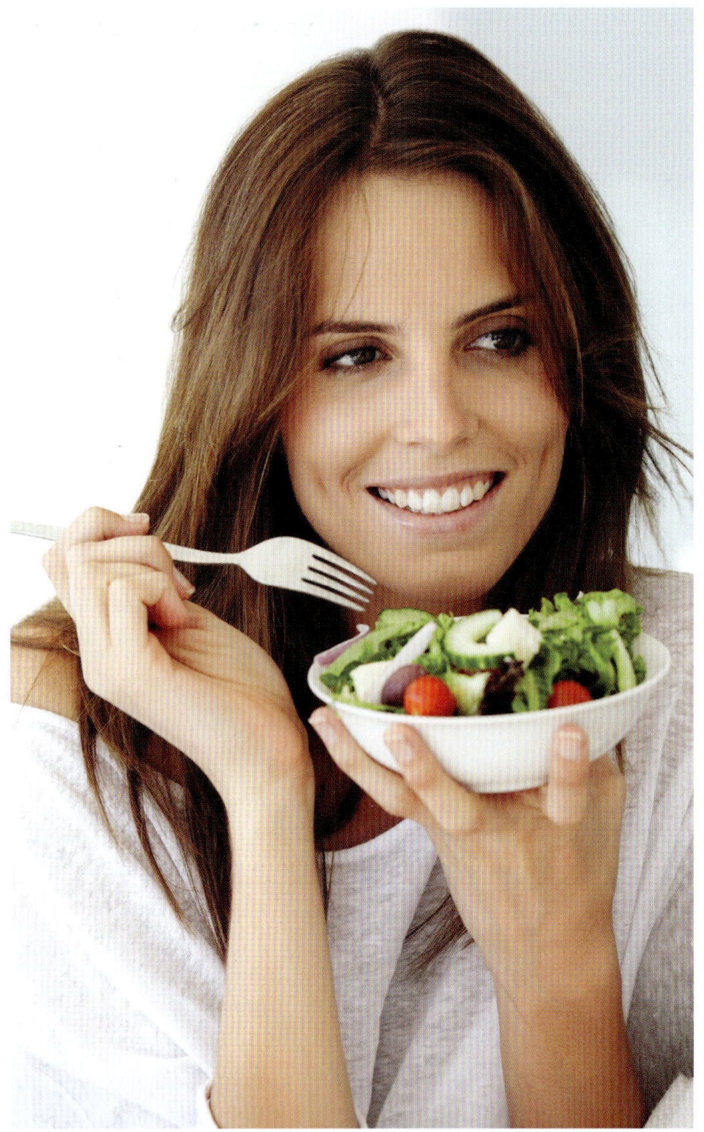

the so called "nervous system in the gut" is able to accomplish some very important jobs without conscious thought. One such job is sending a warning when the digestive system is in trouble. Most people know something is wrong in the gut when they experience pain, heartburn, gas or diarrhea; these symptoms are the gut's way of signaling something is amiss.

As many studies have shown, stress, anger and fear have a profound effect upon the digestive tract—even a greater effect, in fact, than food. It is important to get in touch with these gut feelings, and sort these feelings out as part of the process of healing. If there are unresolved conflicts with relationships, enduring sorrow from loss of loved ones, residual effects of childhood traumas, or an excess of daily stressful situations, these hidden issues can have a negative effect on digestion and, indeed, on the health of the rest of the body.

Conversely, digestive function has an impact on the brain. Digestive imbalance occurs for a number of reasons such as toxin exposure, medications, poor diet, enzyme deficiency and food sensitivities. Dysbiosis creates inflammation in the gut which damages the protective intestinal lining. Toxins, undigested food particles, and potentially pathogenic microorganisms enter the bloodstream triggering yet more inflammation. All this inflammation travels throughout the bloodstream, as well as via the vagus nerve, resulting in negative effects on brain function.

Many people turn to traditional medicine when they begin to experience digestive problems. Unfortunately, traditional medicine is split into specialties. Unlike most holistic practitioners, specialists often do not treat the body as a whole. It is necessary to look at the whole person when dealing with health conditions; this includes consideration of the emotional and mental state of the individual. Many doctors address patients' gut problems by prescribing drugs. Often, these drugs create more problems than they solve. Drugs can serve a constructive purpose when there is an acute problem, but most GI problems are chronic in nature, and can be best solved with a non-drug approach.

In summary, the responsibility resides within each of us to find the right balance and work through our issues, past and present, so that we may experience good health. This requires getting in touch with ourselves, and developing awareness about how stress affects us and how to begin to effectively handle it rather than letting it handle us. We will then listen to our "gut feelings" as a positive guide to lead us through life's many trials and tribulations.

What Can Go Wrong?

With aging there is a tendency for metabolism to slow down, meaning that food is converted to energy more slowly. Enzyme production decreases with age. So does HCl production. This leads to a decrease in digestive efficiency and nutrient absorption, resulting in sluggish body functions, including digestion and elimination.

Apart from the aging process, digestion can become impaired as a result of such factors as stress, processed food consumption (which leads to nutritional deficiency), inadequate chewing, intake of fluids with meals (which dilutes digestive juices), and over-eating. When gut bacteria act upon undigested food that reaches the end of the intestine and colon, toxic chemicals and gases are produced. These internally produced toxins (endotoxins) damage the mucosal lining, increasing gut permeability. Consequently, the gut will leak permitting toxins and undigested food particles to enter the bloodstream. These toxins trigger an inflammatory reaction of the immune system, which circulates throughout the body, settling in organs of greatest weakness, and causing disease. Intestinal toxins also produce renegade chemical fragments known as "free radicals." These molecules containing unpaired electrons can get the upper hand and cause toxic damage if the body is lacking in sufficient antioxidants to buffer them.

The major antioxidant nutrients, vitamins A, C and E, and the minerals selenium and zinc, serve as free radical scavengers. A steady diet of processed foods will create a deficiency of antioxidant (and other) nutrients. Such a diet will also provide inadequate fiber needed by the body to absorb toxins, reduce cholesterol, increase short-chain fatty acid production, and combat constipation by reducing bowel transit time (the amount of time it takes for food to pass through the body).

A toxic environment in the bowel makes it difficult for beneficial bacteria to survive. Dysbiosis sets in when the pathogenic bacteria and other microorganisms gain the upper hand. With this condition, the stage is set for the development of parasite problems and/or proliferation of normally harmless organisms such as the yeast Candida albicans. In its fungal state, Candida grows long roots, known as rhizoids, which can actually puncture the mucous lining of the intestine increasing the leakiness of the gut. A build up of toxicity results in a decrease of enzyme production by the pancreas and intestine, which in turn further impairs digestion. A vicious cycle sets in where toxicity leads to overgrowth of pathogens, and enhances the absorption of yeast toxins, which further increase the leakiness of the gut.

As the body burden of toxins builds up, an increased load is placed on the organs of elimination—the liver, colon, kidneys, lungs and skin. The problem is made worse when processed foods, junk food, alcohol, prescription drugs and over-the-counter medications are ingested, and when exposure to environmental toxins (exotoxins), such as chemicals and heavy metals, is high. Many commonly used household and personal-care items have a high degree of toxicity and will add to the problem.

The bottom line is that many of us unknowingly lead a toxic lifestyle, which makes it very difficult to recover from digestive (and other) disorders that invariably have a strong toxic component to them. Toxicity, from the natural healing perspective, is the basic cause of disease. It makes sense, therefore, that the first step toward wellness is detoxification.

Symptoms of Digestive Dysfunction

It is a tribute to the strength and resiliency of the human body that it can often endure years of toxic abuse before breaking down. Many who consider themselves to be in good health are, in fact, accidents waiting to happen. The deterioration of the digestive system can occur silently for some years, producing no symptoms or only minor, non-specific ones. Headaches, reduced energy, lowered resistance to infections, gas, bloating, constipation and indigestion—these can be a prelude to the onset of chronic degenerative disease, which has its roots in the toxicity produced by digestive dysfunction.

As this dysfunction progresses and the GI tract continues to deteriorate, more serious problems may appear—anything from allergies to cancer. Chronic digestive problems can take the form of irritable bowel syndrome or the more serious inflammatory bowel diseases Crohn's disease and ulcerative colitis. Since the skin is a major organ of elimination, chronic skin conditions like psoriasis

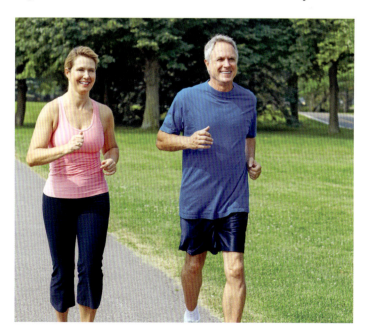

and eczema can result from faulty GI function. In fact, virtually any chronic disease can have its roots in poor digestion and absorption of nutrients, increased intestinal permeability and dysbiosis, the hallmarks of digestive dysfunction. That is the whole premise of this book—to highlight the gut connections that are inherent in so many of today's illnesses.

"Virtually any chronic disease can have its roots in poor digestion and absorption of nutrients, increased intestinal permeability and dysbiosis, the hallmarks of digestive dysfunction."

Restoration of Normal Function

Subsequent chapters will describe specific gastrointestinal disorders in addition to many of today's common health conditions. Natural solutions will be offered at the end of each condition. What is good for one person with one disorder may not be good for another person with another (or even the same) disorder. While it is important to tailor a health regimen to individual needs, there is some degree of generalization possible with regard to digestive health. What follows are some general guidelines for keeping the GI tract in good health or restoring it to good health:

- Eat a well-balanced diet of whole, natural, unprocessed food, preferably organic (grown without chemical fertilizers and pesticides), 80 to 90 percent plant-based, and 10 to 20 percent animal products; some will do well either with vegetarian or vegan diets if done properly.
- Avoid large meals.
- Avoid eating two to three hours before going to bed.
- Identify and eliminate foods to which you're allergic (See the Appendix for information on sources for allergy testing.)
- Exercise on a regular basis.
- Minimize (or eliminate) use of alcohol and caffeine.
- Take prescription drugs only as directed by your physician. Do not discontinue them without his or her consent and supervision.
- Use over-the-counter drugs with care, if at all.
- Chew thoroughly.
- Avoid drinking beverages with meals.
- Avoid carbonated drinks.
- Avoid icy cold beverages. Room temperature water is preferred.
- Avoid eating starchy carbohydrates (like bread and pasta) at the same meal with proteins (like meat and eggs).
- Do not eat fruit at the same time that other foods are eaten.
- Avoid the use of sugar and artificial sweeteners.
- Rest after meals whenever possible (to aid absorption).
- Get adequate rest at night, preferably eight hours of sleep.
- Do not eat when upset.
- Minimize stress.
- Drink 1/2 oz. of water for every pound of body weight. (Divide weight in half, and drink that many ounces of water daily.)
- Use appropriate herbal formulas to cleanse and support digestive organs.
- Take digestive enzymes (and HCl, if stomach acid is low) with each meal to improve digestion.
- For most digestive problems, follow the Candida Diet (see the Appendix) for a minimum of one to three months.
- Reduce or eliminate exposure to environmental toxins.

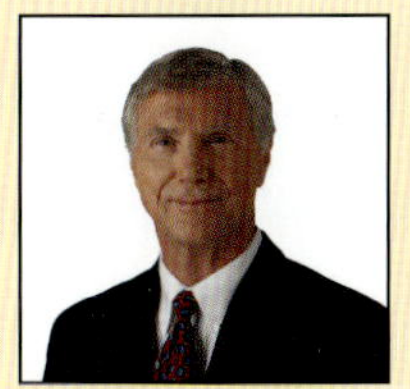

Dr. Smith's Comments

Virtually every illness in the body has some psycho-emotional elements. This certainly includes the intestinal tract, ranging from swallowing difficulties, psychogenic vomiting and abdominal pain, to IBS, diarrhea and hemorrhoids. The treatment for stress of the GI tract is basically the same as for the entire body. It requires employing some new strategies, and having a major shift in how we perceive our world.

One of the past presidents of the Americal Medical Association, in a speech years ago, stated a fundamentally important question for humankind to consider, "Is the Universe a friendly place for us to be or not?" He went on to point out that humans need not have only purpose in life, but a sense of peace, security and order to deal with the challenges and stress of life. Another physician pointed out that time urgency may well be the basis of most, if not all, illnesses.

Living by the clock, meeting deadlines (this word says it all), running out of hours before the tasks are done: these are major causes of underlying chronic stress that ultimately can cause physiologic derangement and earn one a label (disease) that takes him or her into the "healthcare" system. It would be more appropriate to call it a "sickness care" system. Few would question that we have the best sickness care system in the world. However, it is now time for professions dealing with health to learn more about lifestyle changes, diet and nutrition, and stress reduction, and share these concepts with their patients. This is not new. At the turn of the century, Dr. Charles Mayo stated that the physicians' real purpose was to educate their patients about health and how to eliminate the need for doctors!

STRESS

Since stress seems to be the central theme to illness, it is worth pointing out some of the methods of managing it:
- Time management and learning to say "no"
- Eight to nine hours of sleep most nights and catch up on the weekends, if needed
- Exercise—aerobic (30-60 minutes), five days/week; resistence training or Pilates, three times/week
- Yoga, tai chi, progressive muscle relaxation, and swimming or water aerobics to balance the aerobic and resistence training, two to three times per week
- Spiritual rejuvenation of your choice, could include singing and dancing
- Meditation of your choice; according to research, the best physiologic benefits come from spending about 20 minutes twice each day in meditation, and then consciously attempting to hold the feeling of peace and joy throughout the day.

Meditation has been shown to rebalance the autonomic nervous system. With meditation, the over-stimulated life, with attention directed outward, becomes more inwardly centered, coherent, focused and peaceful. There can be an inner body awareness of joy in the midst of outward worldly activity. Various meditation programs have documented significant improvement in many common illnesses with regular practice.

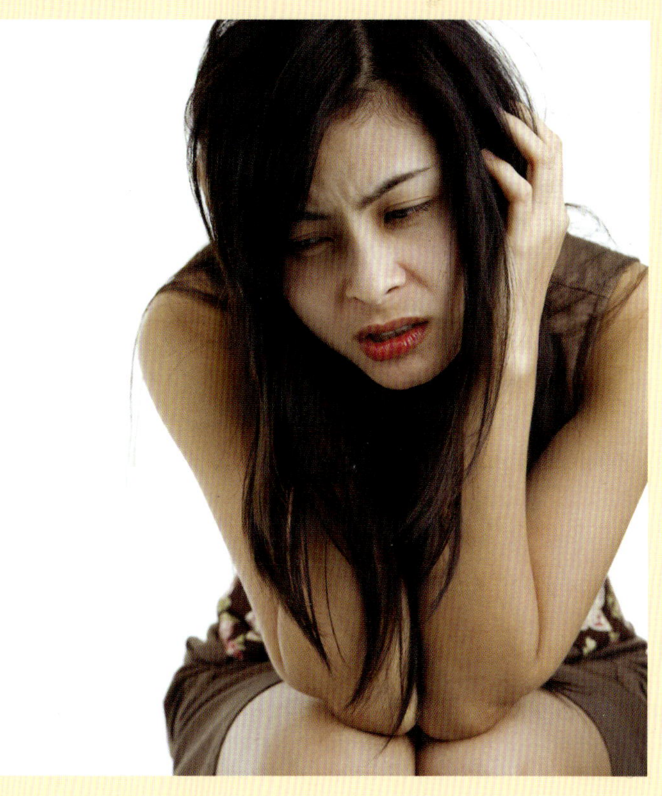

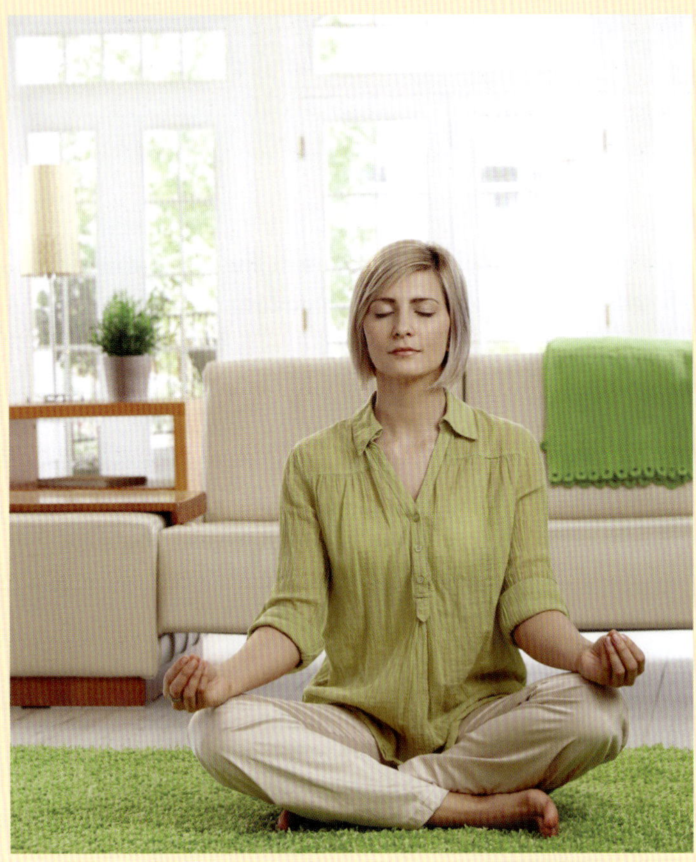

We will mention here some of the salient features found in different meditation programs:

• Sit comfortably in a chair, with your back erect, legs uncrossed and feet flat on the floor. This tends to prevent falling asleep. It is not bad if you fall asleep; we would call that a nap. Attempting to meditate is the major diagnostic test for sleep deprivation. After the nap, if there is time, attempt again to meditate.
• Breathe slowly in through your nostrils into your abdomen (if need be, place your hands over your abdomen to see if it is expanding on inhalation). Take about four seconds to breathe in; hold it for one to two seconds, and let it out for another four seconds; hold it out for one to two seconds, and then start the cycle over. Each in/out cycle takes about 10-12 seconds; this drops your normal unconscious breathing from 12-18 breaths/minute to five to six breaths/minute. Your brain tends to entrain, or fall into step with your slow deep breathing. It shifts from an outward-oriented thinking form of consciousness known as a beta rhythm, which is 13-30 cycles per second (cps), to an inner, still, feeling form of consciousness which is alpha (7-12 cps). In alpha, you can be in the present moment with minimal (if any) thoughts, just observing your breathing pattern.
• Since stopping thought is a challenge, some recommend visualizing light or divine energy coming in on the in breath, and allowing any accumulated negative energy to leave on the outbreath. Alternatively, if thinking comes up, choose to focus on an "attitude of gratitude" for all of your blessings in life.
• As you watch the breath (and/or light) going in and out, become aware of the entire inner energy field of the body. Feel it; don't think about it. This will help reclaim conscious awareness from the always thinking mind. This technique is beautifully described in Eckhart Tolle's book "Practicing the Power of Now," pages 61-64. I highly recommend this to anyone.
• At times, and with practice, as you go deeper into a state of stillness, thought stops, and the perception of time changes radically. You may think you have been sitting still for 20 minutes only to find you have been there for over an hour! Yet, you did not sleep. This is considered by many to be the true state of meditation; you are neither sleeping, dreaming, or thinking. (Some traditions call it Turiya, the fourth state of consciousness.) It is the state of present moment, choiceless awareness, or being. Isn't it strange we call ourselves human beings, and yet spend so little time just being? Often feelings of peace, joy, or even bliss arise from this state of expanded consciousness.

For those who are interested, this type of meditation works well with the Heart Math programs. (See Biofeedback in the Appendix.) It is a nice way to monitor the inner body awareness that arises from this practice. Regularity is the key. With time, most stress-related conditions in the body, including IBS, may improve.

BENEFICIAL BACTERIA

Most people, including healthcare practitioners, are not aware of how critical it is to manage the bacteria living in your intestinal ecosystem. This is definitely not a new concept. Ancient records from Iraq, from 3200 years ago, indicated that fermented milk and cheese were used in the human diet. Dr. Eli Metchnikoff, who won a Nobel Prize in 1908, postulated in 1904 that friendly bacteria may be essential to human health and longevity. Over 100 years later, modern-day research is proving him correct. Throughout the cultures of the world, fermented foods, such as dairy, vegetables and meat, have been a mainstay of the diet. This has largely changed due to refrigeration. Before refrigeration, managing bacteria was a matter of life and death—either put the safe bacteria in the food, or the disease-producing ones could kill you. I actually think this is still true today despite our improved hygiene and refrigeration.

There are major negative effects of not-so-friendly bacteria in the human intestinal tract, which have far-reaching consequences. These effects are largely due to high enzyme activity of the bacteria, 90 percent of which live without much oxygen (anaerobic). Here are some things that parasitic, un-friendly (or pathogenic), bacteria do:

• Deactivate enzymes made in the pancreas, like trypsin and chymotrypsin (needed to digest protein)
• Consume many of the B vitamins that are in our diet
• Produce ammonia, increasing the work load on the liver and kidneys
• Inactivate intestinal brush border enzymes, such as disaccharidases (sugar-digesting enzymes)
• Inactivate dietary antioxidants such as flavonoids
• Destroy essential fatty acids and make them free radicals, so an essential food now becomes a poison
• Degrade the protective mucus of the intestinal lining
• Produce carcinogens (cancer-producing chemicals) from ingested food
• Consume nutrients, and then produce toxins that damage the lining and cause it to leak, which creates immune imbalance leading to autoimmune diseases like lupus and arthritis
• Produce enzymes that affect normal metabolism of hormones like estrogen; this allows estrogen, which was packaged and ready to leave the body, to be resorbed and to create high estrogen levels that can lead to fibrocystic disease and cancer.
• Enter the circulation from the GI tract and travel via the blood to areas that are damaged, such as wounds and injuries; in addition, the bacteria can take up residence in the lungs, urogenital tract and vagina, and cause infections there as well.

These are a just some of the problems created by bad bacteria. Actually, most of this can be prevented by regular use of fermented foods with live cultures of various strains of Lactobacilli and Bifidobacteria.

The following is the **HOPE** we can give people to keep their digestive systems well-functioning. This is recommended as a maintenance protocol for everyone:

High Fiber
Omega-3 Oils
Probiotics
Enzymes

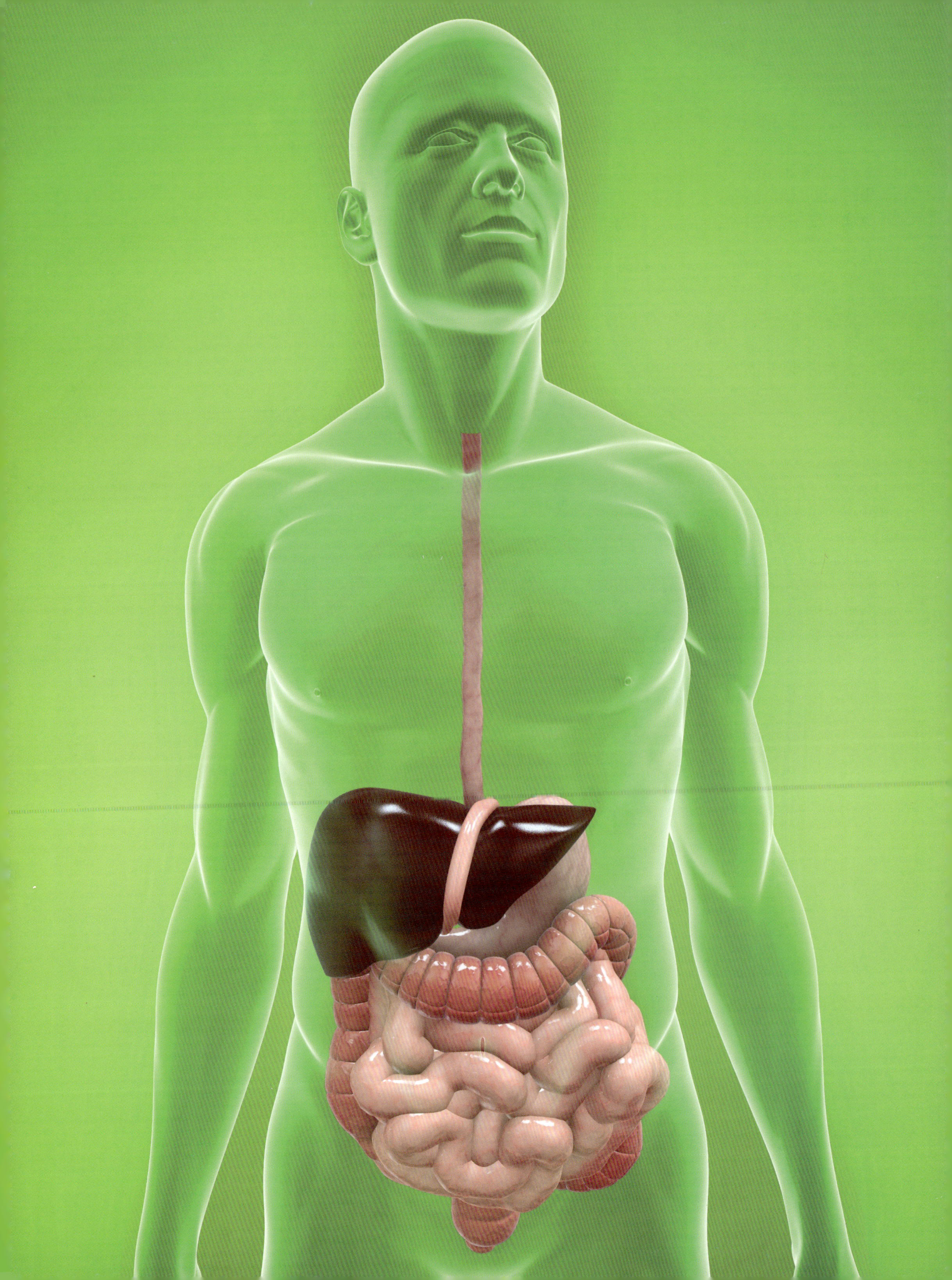

Digestive System

Balance Your Gut, Heal Your Body

The Gut Connection. That says it all. Indeed, the gut is connected to all systems of the body. This connection is sometimes direct, for example the gut connection to the immune system, nervous system and the circulatory system. More than 70 percent of the immune system is located in the gut in the gut-associated lymphoid tissue (GALT). In addition, the microorganisms that reside in the gut (which outnumber the cells in the entire body by 10 times), have a huge influence on the immune system. Digestive health is one of the most important issues surrounding the overall health of the body.

Gut microflora (friendly bacteria) affect the immune system in three ways: they kill pathogenic bacteria, parasites, fungi and viruses that enter the gut, they crowd out the pathogens in terms of space control and, finally, they interact with the immune system, clinging to the endothelial lining of the intestinal tract to keep the pathogens from damaging the mucosal lining and creating a leaky gut (increased intestinal permeability). Gut microflora also influence the nervous system by way of the vagus nerve, a nerve that directly connects the brain to the intestines.

The circulatory system is another important system that links the digestive system with the rest of the body by way of the portal vein. The portal vein transports nutrients and toxins directly to the liver for detoxification.

Sometimes the gut connection is indirect, as with the musculoskeletal system, respiratory system, endocrine system and the urinary system. These systems are all influenced by the digestive system by way of the immune system (lymphatic network), the nervous system (nerve network) and the circulatory system (blood vessel network). When the digestive system suffers, the rest of the body pays the price. When leaky gut is present, toxins enter circulation, and this toxic load ultimately spreads throughout these systems creating inflammation.

This chapter outlines the major health conditions of the digestive tract, and gives guidelines for natural approaches for improving gut health and, thus, the health of the entire body.

Esophageal

Barrett's Esophagus
Esophagitis
GERD
Heartburn
Hiatal Hernia

Stomach

Gastritis
Peptic Ulcers

Intestinal

Appendicitis
Candidiasis
Constipation
Diarrhea
Diverticular Disease
Gas
Hemorrhoids
IBD-Crohn's Disease
IBD-Ulcerative Colitis
IBS
Lactose Intolerance
Leaky Gut Syndrome
Parasitic Disease

Liver, Pancreas & Gallbladder

Cirrhosis
Gallstones
Hepatitis
NASH/NAFLD
Pancreatitis

Barrett's Esophagus

ESOPHAGEAL CONDITIONS

What Is It?

Barrett's esophagus is a condition characterized by abnormal cell growth in the esophagus (the tube connecting the throat to stomach). The lining of the esophagus is normally pinkish-white, but the abnormal cells of Barrett's esophagus are red in color. This red tissue may consist, in part, of normal tissue from the stomach lining that has migrated into the esophagus. Only microscopic analysis can distinguish true Barrett's esophagus tissue from stomach-lining tissue. The abnormal (Barrett's) esophageal tissue (not the displaced stomach lining-tissue) is considered to be pre-malignant—that is, it may develop into cancer.

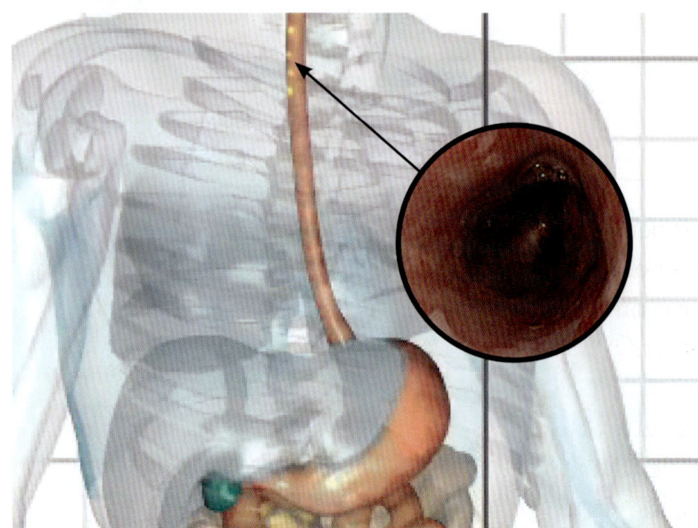

Illustration of the body with a zoomed image of an internal scope of the esophagus that is inflamed and has Barrett's esophagus

While most patients suffering from Barrett's esophagus will not develop cancer, those with Barrett's do have a 30- to 40-fold increased risk of developing esophageal adenocarcinoma (a cancer of the lower esophagus) as compared to the general population.[1] However, autopsies of Barrett's esophagus patients have shown that most never develop cancer and die of other causes.[2]

What Causes It?

The presence of abnormal red tissue (Barrett's tissue) in the lining of the esophagus appears to be largely the result of stomach acid, bile, food and bacteria all rising into the esophagus over a prolonged period of time. This abnormal reflux, or backflow, of corrosive material from the stomach into the esophagus is characteristic of gastroesophageal reflux disease (GERD). The most common symptom of GERD is heartburn or a burning sensation that can extend from the upper abdomen behind the breastbone up into the back of the throat. After years of acid irritation, the injured cells of the esophagus lining can fail to grow back normally. Instead, they are replaced by the abnormal lining known as Barrett's esophagus, which is similar to the lining of the intestine.[3]

Though long-standing acid reflux is the most prevalent cause of Barrett's esophagus, in some rare cases, the disease may be congenital (present at birth).[4] About five to 15 percent of patients with GERD are also found to have Barrett's esophagus.[5] No one knows why some GERD patients develop Barrett's esophagus and others do not. However, it seems likely that healthy functioning esophageal cells are an important factor. Intracellular nutrition, including hydration, pH balance, redox balance (oxidation balance), oxygenation, antioxidant levels, and mitochondrial ATP production (the body's energy source), will help to produce high-quality mucus and optimum cell membrane integrity and function. This intracellular nutrition minimizes cellular transformation.

GERD develops when the valve connecting the stomach to the esophagus (the lower esophageal sphincter or LES) weakens and fails to prevent the backflow of stomach contents. Causes of this weakening are discussed in the GERD section. The presence of stomach-lining tissue, along with Barrett's tissue in the esophagus, appears to serve the purpose of helping to protect the esophagus from ongoing assault from gastric reflux. This may be the reason why GERD symptoms sometimes diminish in Barrett's esophagus patients. This is known as a physiologic adaptation: if the esophagus repeatedly receives stomach contents it will begin to make more mucus, and, thus, in some ways perform as a stomach.

Anyone with a long history of heartburn or GERD is at risk for developing Barrett's esophagus, which has the potential to progress to malignancy. However, as many as

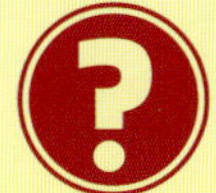

Did You Know

- Approximately one in 10 gastroesophageal reflux disease (GERD) sufferers will also develop Barrett's esophagus, which can be serious and may lead to esophageal cancer.
- Barrett's esophagus affects about one percent of US adults.

40 percent of patients who are diagnosed with esophageal adenocarcinoma deny having typical symptoms of heartburn, such as burning chest pain or regurgitation of acid.[6]

Barrett's esophagus is three times more prevalent in males than in females,[7] and predominantly affects white males[8] with a history of chronic heartburn or GERD. This fact puts white males at highest risk for development of esophageal adenocarcinoma; though the incidence of this cancer among white females has risen dramatically over the last three decades. Children rarely develop this condition. In fact, the average age at diagnosis of Barrett's esophagus is 50,[9] and one study found that Barrett's esophagus was twice as likely to be present in patients in their 70s as compared to patients 40 years of age or less.[10]

Risk factors for development of Barrett's esophagus include obesity, inflammation, age, and, to a lesser and less certain degree, family history.[11] Studies indicate that a high-fat diet may also be a risk factor.[12] Increased fat deposits in the abdominal area are thought to increase pressure on the stomach, especially when lying down. As to family history, findings are inconclusive and indicate that family members of patients with Barrett's esophagus or esophageal adenocarcinoma may be at greater risk for developing these diseases if they have a history of chronic heartburn as compared to others with GERD.[13] (See the sections on GERD and Heartburn for information on risk factors associated with these disorders.)

What Are the Signs and Symptoms?

Patients suffering from Barrett's esophagus typically suffer from GERD-like symptoms, which may include:[14]

- Heartburn
- Regurgitation
- Angina-like chest pain
- Asthma
- Laryngitis
- Chronic cough
- Sleep disturbance
- Loss of dental enamel
- Vomiting and weight loss

Some Barrett's patients may also suffer from other complications of GERD such as esophageal peptic ulcers, and stricture—a narrowing of the esophagus that comes from scarring.[15] This scarring may give rise to dysphasia (food getting stuck in the esophagus).

How Is It Diagnosed?

Barrett's esophagus cannot be diagnosed solely on the basis of symptoms, as these symptoms may have other causes. A definitive medical diagnosis can only be made through application of a special procedure called esophagogastroduodenoscopy (EGD) or upper endoscopy with biopsy. Esophageal capsule endoscopy is another procedure that has recently gained attention as a patient-friendly diagnosis and screening tool for Barrett's.[16]

If the esophagus, which is normally pinkish-white, is lined with red, Barrett's esophagus is suspected. With the aid of the endoscope, the doctor can then take a tissue sample (a biopsy) that will later be examined for the purpose of confirming the diagnosis. It's been recommended that patients who have a history of GERD for at least five years

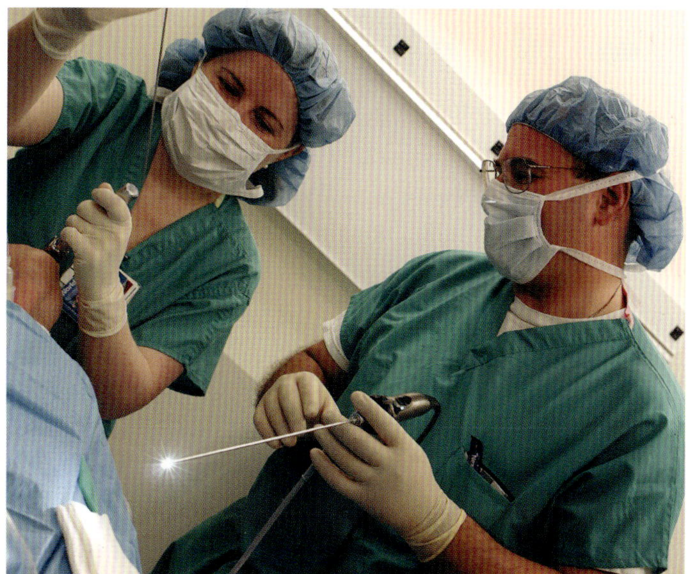

An esophagogastroduodenoscopy (EGD) procedure

and are age 50 or older should undergo upper endoscopy to look for Barrett's esophagus.[17]

A PET (positron emission tomography) may also be used for diagnosis.

What Is the Standard Medical Treatment?

There is no actual cure for Barrett's esophagus short of surgical removal of the esophagus (an esophagectomy) in part or in full. An esophagectomy is a high-risk surgery with a high mortality rate, so this radical procedure is generally reserved for cancer patients and those with high-grade dysplasia (pre-cancerous cell changes).

"While acid-suppressive drugs can protect the delicate tissues of the esophagus from harm, they have a vast array of undesirable side effects that may offset their therapeutic value."

Photodynamic Therapy (PDT) is a non surgical treatment for Barrett's esophagus that has been shown to be successful in a majority of cases.[18] This procedure involves the use of a photosensitizing drug called "PHOTOFRIN®" and an argon dye laser. First, endoscopic biopsies are done to confirm the diagnosis of Barrett's esophageal tissue. Then, a photosensitizing drug is injected into the body through a vein where it concentrates in the dysplastic (pre-cancerous) and cancerous tissue. Two to three days later, a specially designed balloon placed next to the endoscope delivers laser light. A chemical reaction occurs creating intracellular free radicals that kill the abnormal cells but minimally affect normal cells.[19]

PDT was developed by researchers at the Thompson Cancer Survival Center in collaboration with the College of Veterinary Medicine at the University of Tennessee. For more information on this treatment, contact the Thompson Cancer Survival Center's Laser Treatment Center at 865-541-1433.

Another non-surgical treatment available for Barrett's, which is similar to PDT, is radio frequency ablation therapy. Instead of using a laser, radiofrequency is used to treat the damaged esophageal tissue. This therapy has been found to have a high success rate.[20]

Apart from esophagectomy (removal of the esophagus) and experimental approaches, medical treatment of Barrett's esophagus is generally aimed at controlling underlying GERD symptoms.

There are five main approaches to doing this:

- Use of acid-suppressing medications
- Surgery to strengthen the lower esophageal sphincter (LES) and thereby prevent reflux
- NSAIDs or aspirin use
- Lifestyle and dietary changes
- Avoiding toxins in foods

See the subsequent section on GERD found in this chapter for details on these approaches.

The use of some of the most potent acid-suppressive drugs, such as the proton pump inhibitor, as well as anti-reflux surgery can cause some of the normal esophageal lining to partially grow back inside of the Barrett's esophagus lining.[21]

However, even where it appears that abnormal cells have been replaced with normal ones, it is unknown if these effects are lasting and if they result in reduced cancer risk. It is worth noting that, in some cases, normal cells may simply mask abnormal ones rather than replace them.[22]

While acid-suppressive drugs can protect the delicate tissues of the esophagus from harm, they have a vast array of undesirable side effects that may offset their therapeutic value. These are described in the GERD section.

Surgical repair is another approach to treating GERD. But while it may control reflux symptoms, it does not appear to cure Barrett's esophagus.[23]

The use of nonsteroidal anti-inflammatory drugs (NSAIDs) is sometimes recommended by mainstream doctors for Barrett's esophagus treatment, but the use of these drugs can actually damage the stomach and esophagus doing more harm than good.

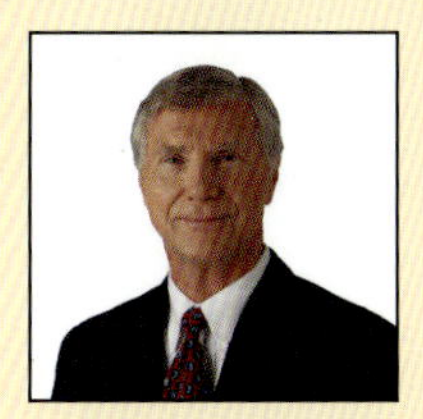

Dr. Smith's Comments

A daily diet that includes organic green and yellow fruits and vegetables, including plenty of cruciferous vegetables such as cabbage, broccoli, and cauliflower, may lower the risk of developing squamous cell cancer of the esophagus. The benefit of fruits and vegetables is generally thought to be due to the high antioxidant and phytonutrient content, which tends to decrease the intracellular free radical damage that seriously affects cell function. This intracellular free radical damage leads to damage of the DNA in the nucleus of esophageal cells that may then produce aberrant cells leading to Barrett's or cancer.

Paradoxically, there are studies that have shown that the use of nonsteroidal anti-inflammatory drugs or NSAIDs (such as aspirin, ibuprofen, naproxen, indomethacin, and Celebrex) is associated with a reduced risk of developing both squamous cell cancer and adenocarcinoma of the esophagus.

Use of NSAIDs, however, has many serious complications including gastrointestinal bleeding, kidney damage, strokes and heart attacks. The mechanism by which these drugs may prevent cancer center around decreasing inflammation. Inflammation leads to intracellular and intranuclear damage. It would seem that diet and lifestyle should be the primary way to protect from cancer, and the use of NSAIDs be reserved for times when appropriate food choices and an exercise program cannot be followed. Even then, the drugs should be used sparingly and for as little time as possible.

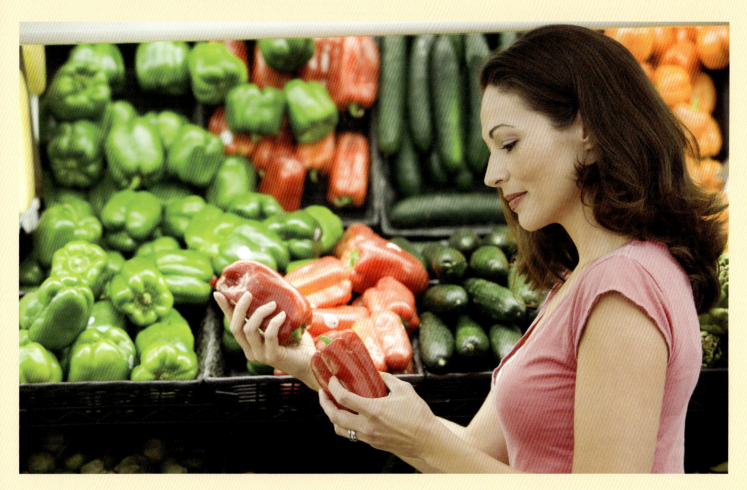

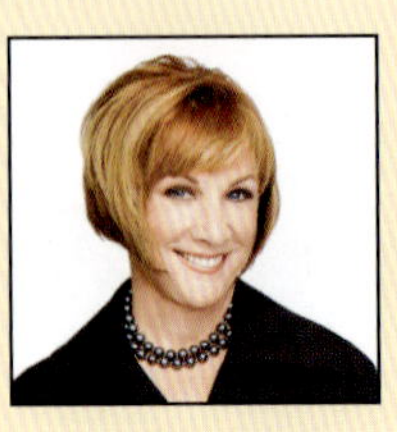

Brenda's Bottom Line

Even though Barrett's esophagus has no known cure, and quality of life can be greatly compromised, approaching this condition from the natural perspective of diet, lifestyle, complimentary therapies and supplementation should be considered.

In many cases, this disease state develops after a prolonged period of GERD or acid reflux. Unfortunately traditional medicine is not looking at the underlying causes of indigestion, heartburn and GERD, so these conditions may develop into more dangerous conditions like Barrett's esophagus.

It's never too late to start a program of natural healing no matter what disease the body has developed. There is an ever-growing scientific body of evidence to show that probiotics, L-glutamine, fiber, digestive enzymes and omega-3 oils are not only helpful, but critical for good gut health. In an effort to regain esophageal health, it would be prudent to follow the suggestions below in helping the body heal itself.

Recommended Testing

- The Heidelberg pH test (See the Appendix.)
- Because food sensitivities can be a source of inflammation in the body, food sensitivity tests are recommended. (See the Appendix.)
- In many cases, following up with a comprehensive stool analysis (CSA) is suggested.

Diet

If Candida is found, then follow the Candida Diet (see the Appendix) along with the following suggestions:

- If you are in pain, a juicing diet for 2 to 3 days may be helpful.
- Slowly move to the Fiber 35 Eating Plan when feeling better. (See the Appendix.)
- Eat small meals slowly.

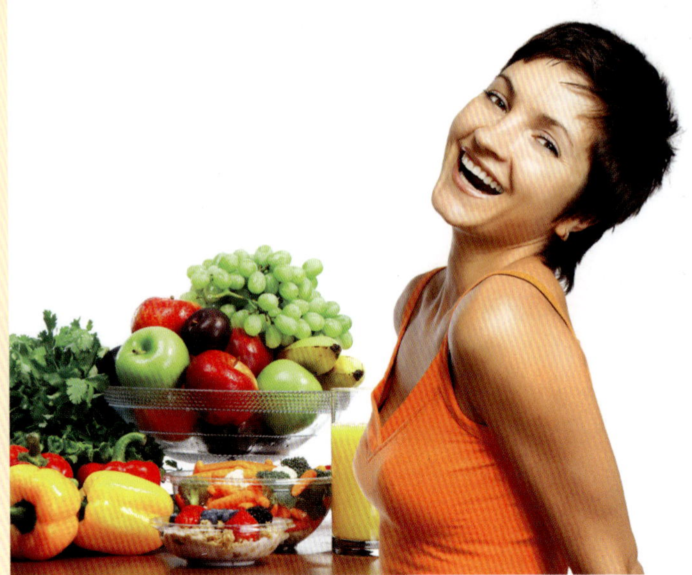

- Chew foods well, to mush or liquid, before swallowing.
- Do not drink cold liquids with meals. Have no more than half a glass of water at room temperature with meals.

Lifestyle

- Sleep on your left side to avoid heartburn and reflux.
- Do not lie down for at least three to four hours after eating.
- Elevate the head of the bed four to eight inches when sleeping.
- Make sure you have good bowel elimination daily.
- Exercise daily, at least walking.

Complementary Mind/Body Therapies

- Stress-reduction therapies such as yoga, biofeedback, massage and meditation can be helpful when stress is an issue.
- Acupuncture may be helpful because it targets the meridians associated with the digestive system, and is also a stress reducer.
- Chiropractic may be beneficial.
- Colon hydrotherapy will be helpful in removing toxins.

Recommended Nutraceuticals	Dosage	Benefit	Comments
Critical Phase Daily maintenance recommendations should also be taken during this phase unless otherwise indicated.			
L-Glutamine Powder with Gamma Oryzanol	10 grams (10,000 mg) daily in split doses on empty stomach with water for two weeks	Helps repair and keep digestive lining healthy.	Best if taken in loose powder form for contact with esophageal lining.
Probiotics	200 billion culture count daily for two weeks	Protects digestive lining, reduces inflammation and stimulates immune system.	Best if taken in loose powder form for contact with esophageal lining.
Helpful			
Candida Cleanse	As directed on label for at least 30 days. See Appendix	Helps to eradicate Candida overgrowth.	Look for ingredients such as uva ursi, caprylic acid, undecylenic acid, barberry, garlic, neem, grapefruit and olive leaf extracts.
Daily Maintenance			
Antioxidant Supplement	Use as directed	Protects against tissue damage.	Look for high-potentcy formula containing vitamins A, C, E, zinc and selenium along with other antioxidants.
L-Glutamine Powder with Gamma Oryzanol	5 grams (5000 mg) daily on empty stomach with water after critical phase	Helps repair and keep digestive lining healthy.	Best if taken in loose powder form for contact with esophageal lining.
Probiotics	50 billion culture count daily after critical phase	Protects digestive lining, reduces inflammation and stimulates immune system.	Best taken in powder form for Barrett's. Open capsule if necessary.
Digestive Enzymes	Take with meals	Helps digest food and reduce reflux.	Look for one with high potency protease, amylase, lipase and cellulase.
Omega-3 Fatty Acids	At least 2 grams daily of EPA/DHA combination	Reduces inflammation.	Look for a concentrated, enteric coated high dose EPA/DHA formulation.
Fiber	4-5 grams twice daily as part of a 35 gram daily fiber diet	Helps reduce reflux and promotes bowel regularity.	Look for a flax-based fiber with added ingredients such as glutamine, probiotics and healing herbs.

See further explanation of supplements in the Appendix

Esophagitis

What Is It?

An "itis" anywhere in the body involves inflammation. Esophagitis, as the name implies, is inflammation of the lining of the esophagus. More than 19 million Americans have chronic esophagitis.[1]

What Causes It?

Esophagitis is most frequently caused by reflux (an abnormal backward flow) of gastric contents into the esophagus resulting in chemical esophageal burns. (See the section on gastroesophageal reflux disease (GERD) for information on the cause of reflux.)

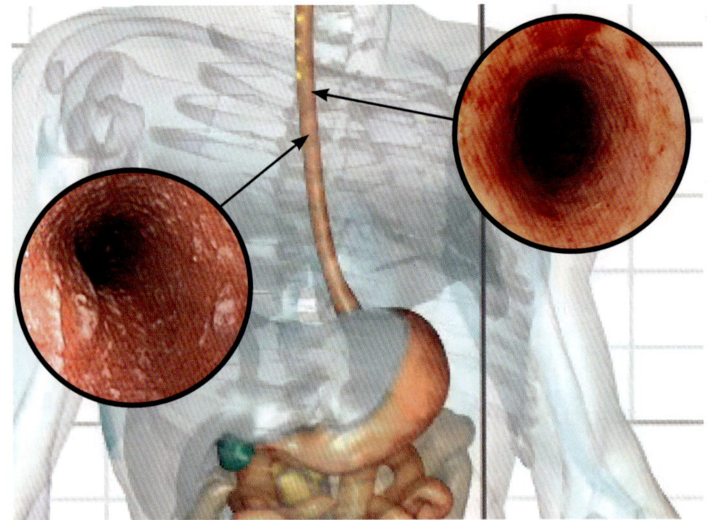

On the right is an internal scope of the esophagus that is inflamed and has esophagitis. On the left is a scope of Candidal esophagitis.

Esophagitis may also be brought on by infection, usually the result of a weakened immune system. Infections can be fungal, viral, bacterial or parasitic in origin. Candida (a yeast/fungus) and herpes (a virus) are the two most common forms of infectious esophagitis. Bacterial involvement is rarely a primary cause of esophagitis, though such infection may be secondary to a bacterial infection in the lungs.[2] Other fungi and viruses, such as human immunodeficiency virus (HIV) and cytomegalovirus (CMV), are possible rare causes of esophagitis. In these cases, immunosuppression is the underlying cause. Weakening of the immune system may itself be caused by certain medications such as corticosteroids.

"Certain medications, because of their caustic nature, may wear away the lining of the esophagus as they pass through it."

People with weakened immune systems may be at risk for developing infectious esophagitis. This would include patients with Candida, CMV, herpes simplex and HIV, as well as those taking immunosuppressive medications, undergoing chemotherapy or those who have had organ transplants. Heavy metal toxicity, often in the form of dental restorations, may be an unsuspected cause of immunosuppression. Patients with diabetes mellitus, adrenal dysfunction, alcoholism and those of advanced age can be predisposed to infectious esophagitis because of altered immune function.[3]

Erosive esophagitis is caused by irritation. Such irritation may be of a physical, chemical or energetic nature. The latter type of irritation is brought on by radiation. For example, 80 percent of patients receiving radiation therapy for cancer will develop esophagitis if the esophagus is exposed to radiation.[4] The risk level is increased if chemotherapy is administered in conjunction with radiation therapy.[5]

Strictures (narrowing anywhere along the esophageal tube) may also result as a consequence of an esophageal ulcer. These types of complications are most likely to occur in patients with esophageal motility problems, characterized by the inability to quickly move food through the esophagus. Certain medications, because of their caustic nature, may wear away the lining of the esophagus as they pass through it. The antibiotic doxycycline and the anticholinergic emepronium bromide are two of the most common culprits. Nonsteroidal anti-inflammatory drugs (NSAIDs) and slow-release forms of potassium chloride are also frequently implicated.[6] More than 20 percent of those who routinely take NSAIDs, such as aspirin or ibuprofen, will develop esophagitis.[7] Osteoporosis medications, such as alendronate (Fosomax), may also be caustic to the esophagus, contributing to esophagitis.[8]

Did You Know

- Probiotics produce important nutrients, eliminate toxins, destroy bad bacteria and enhance the body's immune system.
- Many modern-day farming practices include antibiotics in animal feed to protect them from disease and increased growth. When we eat the dietary products from these animals, we also consume the antibiotics they have ingested.
- The word antibiotic literally means "against life."
- The word probiotic literally means "for life."
- The over consumption of antibiotics is dangerous to our digestive health because we not only kill the problematic bad bacteria that make us ill, we also kill the beneficial good bacteria essential to good health.
- Some of the most beneficial probiotics are Lactobacillus and Bifidobacterium.
- Candidal esophagitis is a Candida infection in the esophagus. It most likely occurs when Candida in the mouth (thrush) moves into the esophagus, or Candida from the lower intestines moves into the stomach due to low stomach acid, and then into the esophagus.
- Proton pump inhibitor (PPI) use has been associated with the development of Candidal esophagitis.[9]

Repeated vomiting, sometimes self-induced, as with certain eating disorders, can cause an acid burn in the esophagus and may therefore be a cause of esophagitis. Esophagitis may also be the result of a hiatal hernia, where a portion of the stomach protrudes through the diaphragm muscle into the lower mediastinum (the lower portion of the chest). (See the Hiatal Hernia section for more information on this condition.)

What Are the Signs and Symptoms?

Signs and symptoms of esophagitis may include:

- A burning sensation behind the sternum (breastbone)
- Difficult and/or painful swallowing
- Mouth sores or ulcerations (herpes lesions)
- The sensation of having something stuck in the throat
- Gagging
- Nausea
- Vomiting
- Thrush (white patches) in the mouth (may be present with Candidal esophagitis)
- Rapid breathing/wheezing
- Mild to severe chest pain upon swallowing
- Loss of appetite
- Blood in stools
- Chronic reflux
- Anemia
- Increased salivation or drooling

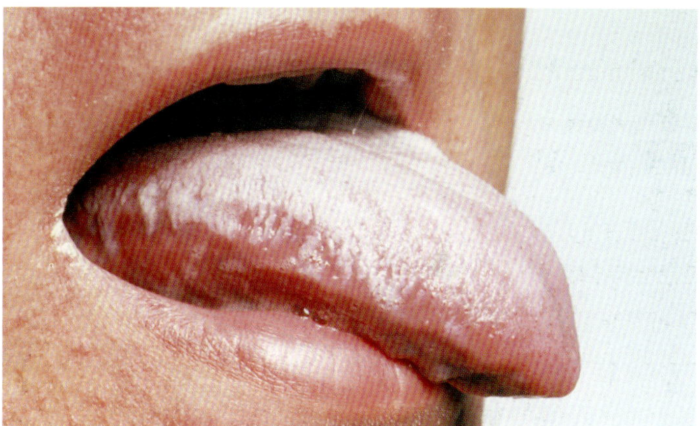

Oral thrush from Candida can lead to to Candidal esophagitis

Not all of these symptoms will be present with every patient who has esophagitis. Some symptoms, such as bleeding, are only present in advanced forms of the disease. The type of esophagitis will largely determine the nature of the symptoms experienced.

How Is It Diagnosed?

In addition to taking a medical history and doing a physical examination, if a doctor suspects esophagitis, he or she will order special tests. Some of the medical tests that may be used to diagnose esophagitis include: upper endoscopy with biopsy, upper GI series and throat swab culture to identify any infectious organisms. Blood tests, such as a complete blood count (CBC), may also be performed to check for infection. Additionally, the acidity/alkalinity of the esophagus may be measured. Esophageal motility tests may be done, as well, to evaluate the movement of food through the esophagus.

What Is the Standard Medical Treatment?

Treatment for esophagitis will depend on the type of esophagitis and the specific cause. To be fully effective, it must involve treatment of any underlying conditions such as GERD, Candida, diabetes, adrenal dysfunction, etc.

The traditional medical treatment for reflux esophagitis involves medications to suppress acid production. This is discussed more fully in the GERD section of this book. Also included in the GERD section is little-known information about the actual benefits of stomach acid and risks involved in suppressing it. Lifestyle changes and dietary restrictions are often also recommended when reflux is found to be the cause of esophagitis. These are discussed in the GERD section. For some difficult cases of reflux esophagitis where medications no longer control symptoms, or where complications such as stricture or ulceration are present, surgery may be performed to repair the esophagus.

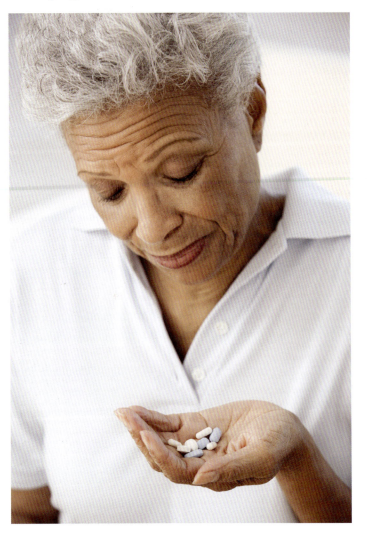

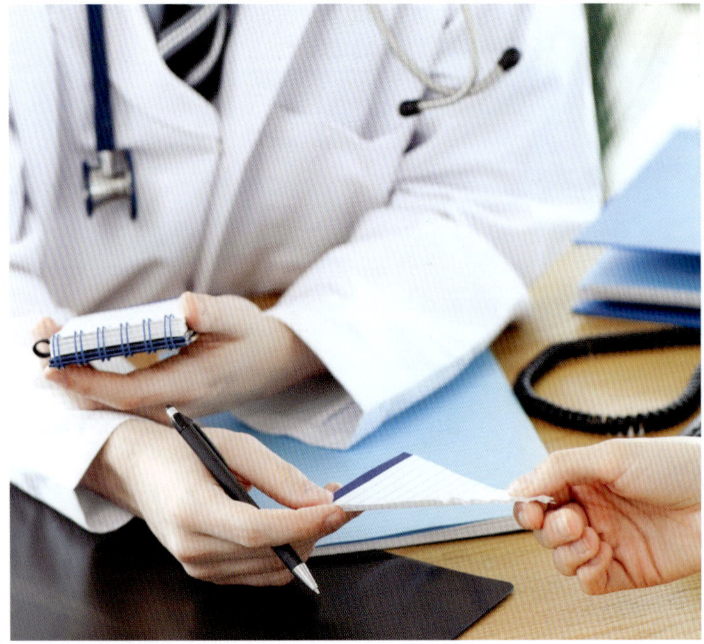

When infection is present, antibiotics are typically prescribed. Bearing in mind that antibiotics are only effective against bacterial infections, and most infectious esophagitis is not of a bacterial nature, the efficacy of such treatment is questionable. Even if the antibiotic is appropriately prescribed, adverse effects of such treatments—namely the killing off of all bacteria in the gut, both the good and the bad, may occur. This opens the door to a condition of bacterial imbalance (dysbiosis) and the subsequent onset of more gastrointestinal distress, unless beneficial bacteria are replaced. If the cause of infectious esophagitis is a viral infection, anti-viral medications will be prescribed. If the esophageal infection is found to be Candida, an antifungal medication will be prescribed.

Where esophagitis is caused by medications, it may be necessary to discontinue the offending drug (always under the guidance of a physician) and find an alternative treatment. Whatever the case, it's very important to always swallow pills with large amounts of water, especially if medication is taken just before bedtime. This helps prevent esophageal irritation.

Where esophagitis is due to injury from a caustic chemical, emergency medical treatment is required. Typically, the patient is given intravenous fluids and not permitted anything by mouth. Most often antibiotics and corticosteroids are used, although there is no good evidence documenting the efficacy of this approach.[10]

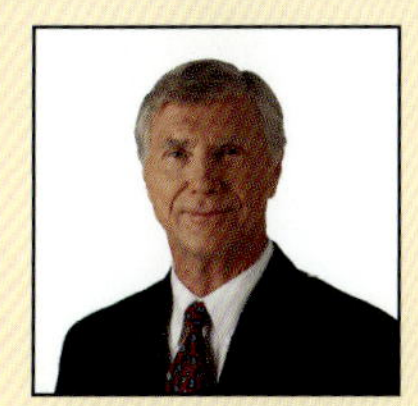

Dr. Smith's Comments

I have seen many patients who, after occasional episodes of heartburn, have been put on acid-blocking medications for indefinite periods of time. Often, I have found that if they will lose a little weight, improve their bowel function, eliminate foods that lower their esophageal sphincter pressure, remove sensitive foods and change their eating habits, they can get off of their medications. Since these medications can have significant and potentially serious side effects, it is wise to minimize their use. Implementation of more natural and safer nutritional options should be undertaken whenever possible.

I would like to point out that all esophageal conditions mentioned in this chapter, namely Barrett's esophagus, esophagitis, GERD, heartburn and hiatal hernia, have features in common that could be addressed from a nutritional standpoint:

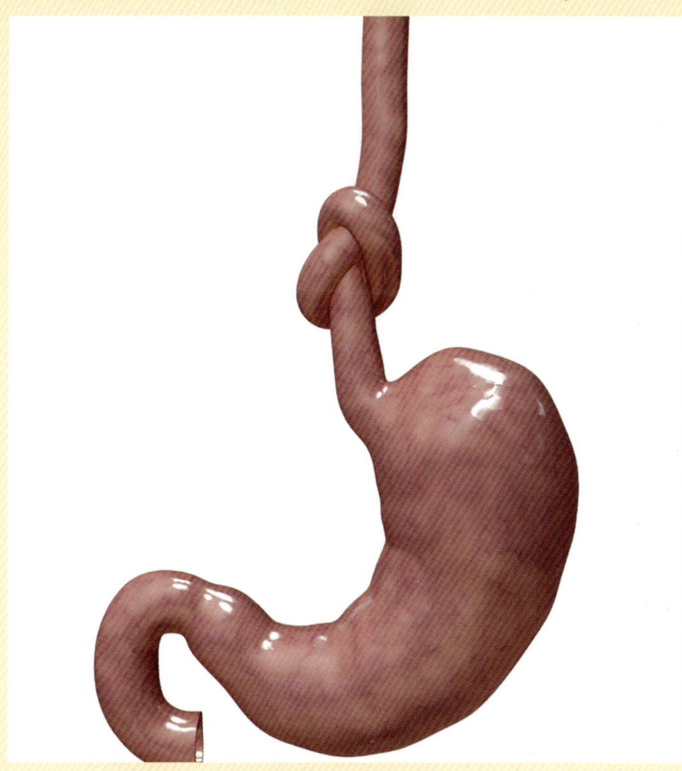

Do you sometimes feel like this?

- Material from the stomach periodically enters into the esophogus. This often causes an inflammatory reaction and can damage the esophageal lining. Researchers have recently observed that the damage to the lining may be due more to esophageal intracellular oxidative stress than to the direct contact of the acid and gastric contents. There are articles in the literature that support the fact that adequate antioxidant levels are protective against damage from reflux (Gut 2001;49;364-371). In this article, it was shown that pretreatment with antioxidants minimized damage and decreased inflammatory markers (malondialdehyde and NF kappa B). In addition, the antioxidants slowed down the loss of glutathione (a naturally produced beneficial antioxidant). It would be wise to supplement with vitamins A, C, E, and the minerals zinc and selenium.

- Mucus production has been shown to be variable, and people with lower levels tend to have more inflammatory problems in the esophagus and stomach. Normalizing cellular function with glutamine, glycine, and omega-3 essential fatty acids can be helpful. Mucus-producing nutrients (N-acetyl glucosamine, N-acetyl-galactosamine, fucose, galactose and sialic acid) and increased water intake are needed to make high quality and quantity of mucus. There is a good review article about probiotics and mucus and their role in intestinal health in the American Journal of Clinical Nutrition, 2003;78: 675-683.

Minimizing the possibility of inflammation is important. Checking for any type of infection, especially H. pylori or Candida, can be helpful. If found, short courses of appropriate anti-microbials should be implemented. After removal of pathogens, restoration of the beneficial bacteria (Lactobacilli and Bifidobacteria) is very important and may help prevent future infections. Liquid aloe vera has potent anti-inflammatory benefits as well.

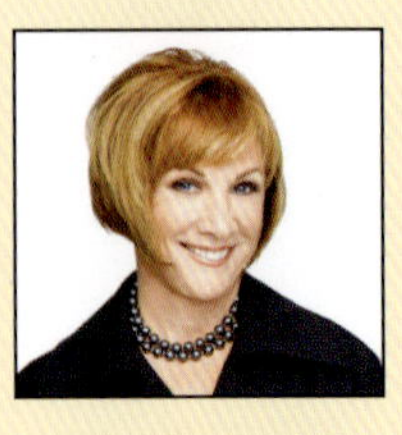

Brenda's Bottom Line

Esophagitis is another condition that results from a lack of knowledge, by both the patient and traditional doctors, of the underlying digestive causes which lead to esophageal inflammation. The one-pill-fixes-everything mentality associated with taking acid-blocking medication creates problems that lead to esophagitis in some people. Since esophagitis may be fungal in nature, this means that the fungal yeast has moved up the digestive tract from the intestines into the esophagus. When stomach acid is suppressed for long periods of time (as with acid-blocking medication) and the ratio of friendly to unfriendly microflora in the gut becomes imbalanced, the environment is set up for many of the inflammatory conditions of the upper GI tract to develop, including esophagitis.

In order to begin to heal esophagitis, it's best to take the approach of seeing the digestive tract as a whole, bringing the entire system back into balance. This is achieved through a combination of addressing the inflammation of the esophagus, finding the source of stomach involvement (often acid-blocking medications), and bringing the intestinal bacteria into balance. If individuals continue to use acid-blocking medication, and do not find the reason behind indigestion, the ability to help this condition will be compromised.

It's of utmost importance to rule out any underlying Candida or herpes conditions. (See the Candidiasis section.) If herpes is present, one should seek natural solutions for this condition when possible.

Recommended Testing

- A comprehensive stool analysis (CSA) will help to determine if the intestinal microflora is out of balance, as well as determine if Candida overgrowth is present. (See the Appendix for more information on this test.)
- A Heidelberg pH test can be used to find out what level of acid is present in the stomach. (See the Appendix for more information about this test.)

Diet

- If Candida overgrowth is an underlying problem, follow the Candida Diet found in the Appendix of this book.
- In an acute phase, a juicing diet for 2 to 3 days may be helpful.
- Slowly move to the Fiber 35 Eating Plan when feeling better. (See the Appendix.)
- Eat small meals, and eat them slowly.
- Chew foods to mush before swallowing.
- Do not drink cold liquids with meals. Have no more than 1/2 glass of water at room temperature with meals.

" In order to begin to heal the esophagus, it's best to see the digestive tract as a whole, bringing the entire system into balance."

Lifestyle

- Sleep on your left side to avoid heartburn and reflux.
- Do not lie down for at least three hours after eating.
- Elevate the head of bed four to eight inches when sleeping.
- Make sure you have good bowel elimination daily.
- Exercise daily—even if it's just taking a walk.

Complementary Mind/Body Therapies

- Stress-reduction therapies such as yoga, biofeedback, massage, and meditation may be helpful.
- Acupuncture may be helpful because it targets the meridians associated with the digestive system, and is also a stress reducer.
- Chiropractic may be beneficial.
- Colon hydrotherapy will be helpful in removing toxins.

Recommended Nutraceuticals	Dosage	Benefit	Comments
Critical Phase Daily maintenance recommendations should also be taken during this phase unless otherwise indicated.			
L-Glutamine Powder with Gamma Oryzanol	10 grams (10,000 mg) daily in split doses on empty stomach with water for two weeks	Helps repair and keep digestive lining healthy.	Best if taken in loose powder form for contact with esophageal lining.
Probiotics	200 billion culture count daily for two weeks	Protects digestive lining, reduces inflammation and stimulates immune system.	Best if taken in loose powder form for contact with esophageal lining.
Helpful			
Candida Cleanse	As directed on label for at least 30 days. See Appendix	Helps to eradicate Candida overgrowth.	Look for ingredients such as uva ursi, caprylic acid, undecylenic acid, barberry, garlic, neem, grapefruit and olive leaf extracts.
Daily Maintenance			
Antioxidant Supplement	Use as directed	Protects against tissue damage.	Look for high-potency formula containing vitamins A, C, E, zinc and selenium along with other antioxidants.
L-Glutamine Powder with Gamma Oryzanol	5 grams (5000 mg) daily on empty stomach with water after critical phase.	Helps repair the esophageal lining.	Best if taken in loose powder form for contact with esophageal lining.
Probiotics	50 billion culture count daily after critical phase	Protects digestive lining, reduces inflammation and stimulates immune system.	Best taken in powder form for esophagitis. Open capsule if necessary.
Digestive Enzymes	Take with meals	Helps digest food and reduce reflux.	Look for one with high potency protease, amylase, lipase and cellulase.
Fiber	4-5 grams twice daily as part of a 35 gram daily fiber diet	Helps reduce reflux and promotes bowel regularity.	Look for a flax based fiber with added ingredients such as glutamine, probiotics and healing herbs.
Omega-3 Fatty Acids	At least 2 grams daily of EPA/DHA combination	Reduces inflammation.	Look for a concentrated, enteric coated high dose EPA/DHA formulation.

See further explanation of supplements in the Appendix

Gastroesophageal Reflux Disease (GERD)

What Is It?

Gastroesophageal reflux disease (GERD) is a condition known by a variety of names, often referred to as acid reflux, chronic heartburn or acid indigestion. These terms are frequently used in advertisements to get you to buy the latest pill or tablet guaranteed to ease your pain. But if you are experiencing discomfort on a regular basis, the recurring sensation of heartburn is likely the symptom of a larger problem.

GERD is a digestive disorder in which partially digested food from the stomach, along with hydrochloric acid (HCl) and enzymes, backs up into the esophagus. This process is known as reflux.

HCl has a low pH, meaning that it is very acidic. Even if present in low amounts, HCl can cause damage when it comes into contact with the delicate lining of the esophagus. This mucous lining, or mucosa, of the esophagus, unlike the lining of the stomach, is not designed to withstand the caustic effects of acid and stomach contents.

Definitions of some conditions that involve reflux are listed below. Some of these terms are used interchangeably.

To clarify:

- **Heartburn** – painful burning sensation in the esophagus usually associated with regurgitation of stomach contents
- **Acid indigestion** – another name for heartburn
- **GERD** – chronic heartburn, usually defined as two or more times per week
- **Reflux esophagitis** – inflammation of the lining of the esophagus that has been caused by the backflow of stomach acid or contents into the esophagus

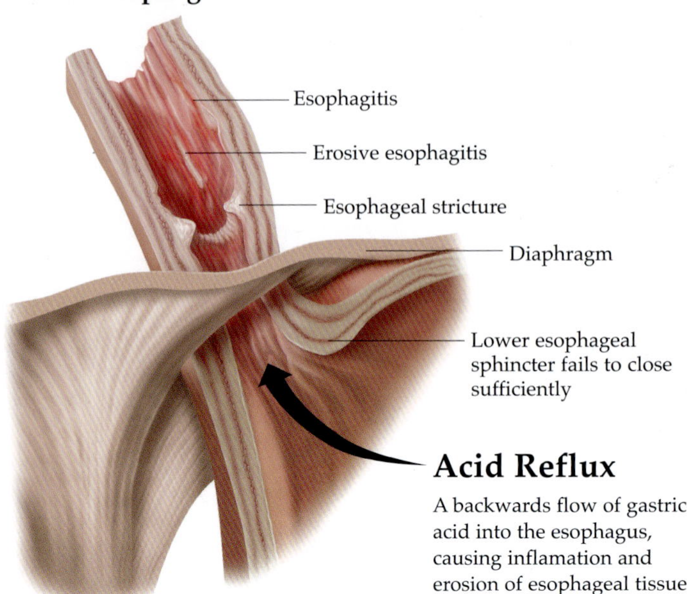

What Causes It?

Normally the lower esophageal sphincter (LES), the muscle that connects the esophagus to the upper portion of the stomach, opens to allow food from the esophagus into the stomach; then it closes immediately to prevent food and digestive stomach secretions from reentering the esophagus.

Reflux occurs when the LES weakens and malfunctions, staying open after food has entered the stomach, and allowing the contents of the stomach to flow backwards into the esophagus. This LES weakness causes GERD. But what causes the LES to weaken?

Hiatal hernia is one condition that weakens the LES and causes reflux. A hiatal hernia occurs when a portion of the stomach protrudes into the chest cavity through a small opening in the diaphragm, the muscle separating the abdomen from the chest wall. (See the Hiatal Hernia section for more information on this condition.)

There are also a number of dietary and lifestyle factors that may contribute to esophageal irritation and a weakened LES. These include:

- Overeating
- Eating too rapidly
- Inadequate chewing
- Swallowing large amounts of air when eating
- Overweight/obesity

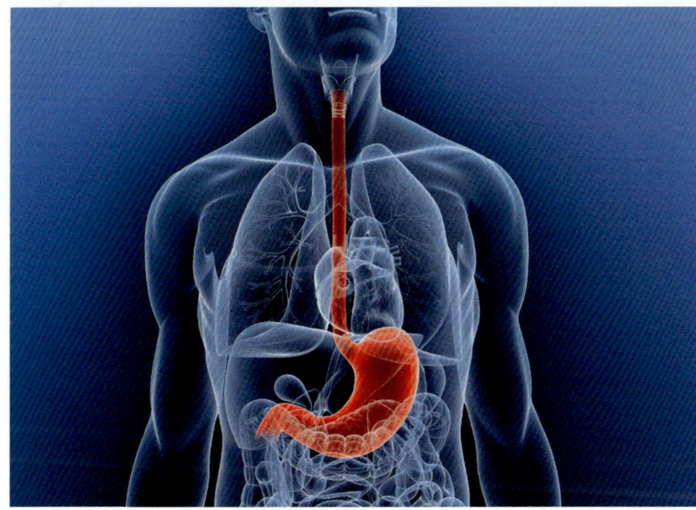

- Lying down after eating
- Intra-abdominal pressure
- Tight-fitting clothing that constricts the abdomen
- Stress (and eating when upset)
- Alcoholic beverages
- Smoking
- Chocolate, peppermint
- Spicy foods, including yellow onions and garlic
- Tomato-based foods and citrus, black pepper and vinegar
- Fatty foods and fried foods
- Sugar
- Insufficient water intake causing dehydration
- Coffee, tea and other caffeine-containing beverages
- Carbonated beverages
- Drugs that irritate the GI lining – non-steroidal anti-inflammatory drugs (NSAIDs), the antibiotic tetracycline, the antiarrhythmic drug quinidine, potassium chloride tablets and iron salts
- Pregnancy/birth control pills/estrogen replacement therapy

When food is eaten too quickly, the stomach becomes distended, and the food is pushed against the top of the stomach. This can force open the LES, and wash the food into the esophagus causing heartburn. This discomfort occurs from the partially digested food, gastric acid, enzymes and bacteria on the food, which can, at times, reach as high as the throat and windpipe, and occasionally cause aspiration pneumonia.

Swallowing air while eating—common when eating quickly or in an anxious state—warms the air to body temperature, which then expands, and is belched forcefully enough to push stomach acid into the esophagus causing heartburn.

Intra-abdominal pressure weakens the LES, and may be caused by bending from the waist, heavy lifting, straining at stool, pregnancy, and obesity—especially abdominal obesity or belly fat.[1]

Smoking inhibits production of saliva, salivary IgA (a protective antibody) and salivary epithelial growth factor (SEGF), which helps repair the intestinal lining. Both IgA and SEGF serve as protective barriers against damage to the esophagus. Smoking also weakens the LES.

NSAIDs (like aspirin, ibuprofen and naproxen), bronchodilating drugs used to treat asthma (like theophylline, albuterol, ephedrine), some blood pressure medications (calcium channel blockers, beta blockers), diazepam and nitroglycerine relax all muscles in the body, including the LES in the esophagus.[2]

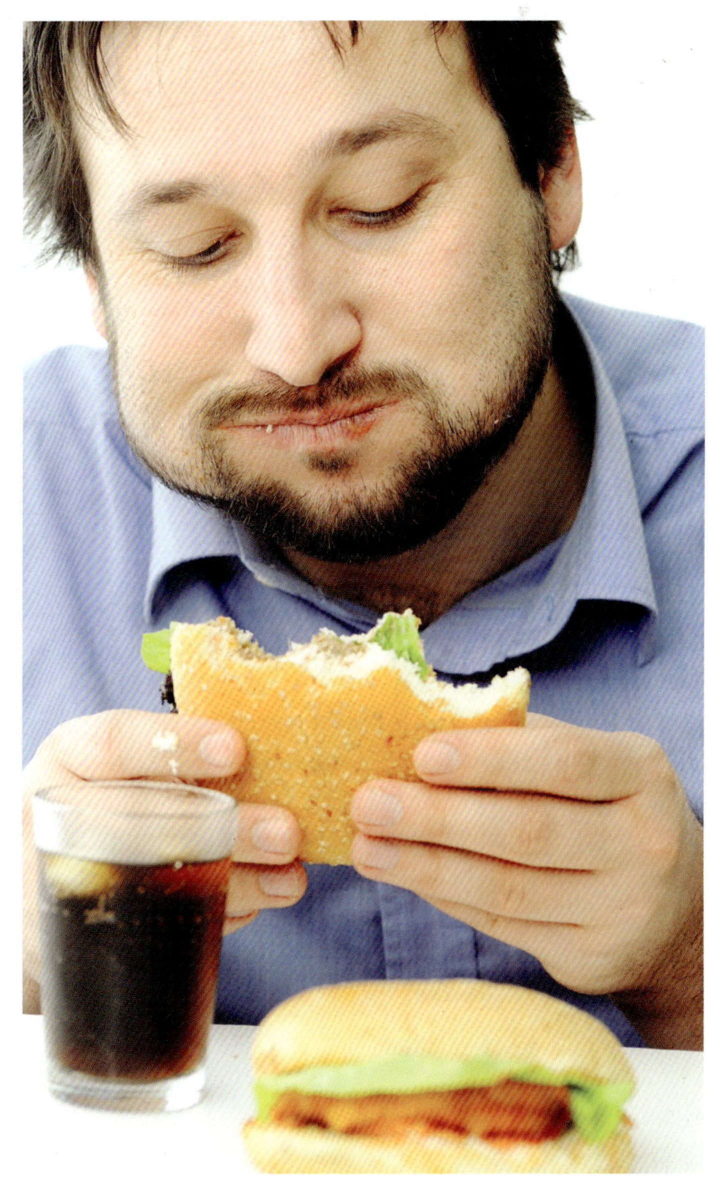

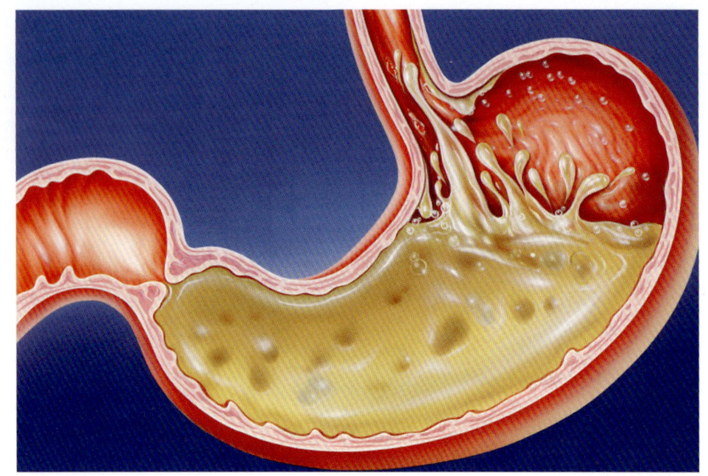

Because estrogens can weaken the LES, women who are pregnant, taking birth control pills or estrogen replacement therapy are more likely to suffer from heartburn than those who are not. More than 25 percent of pregnant women experience daily heartburn, and more than 50 percent have occasional distress.[3]

Other factors that can contribute to GERD are:

- Ulcers
- Food allergies and sensitivities, especially to wheat and dairy
- Gallbladder problems
- Enzyme deficiencies

It has been commonly accepted by the medical profession that heartburn and GERD are caused, solely, by excess stomach acid (hyperchlorhydria). Virtually all drugs used to treat GERD neutralize, reduce, suppress or inhibit HCl production.

This is very interesting in view of the fact that the 11th edition of the "Merck Manual," published in 1966, states quite clearly that "[heartburn] is not due, as formerly believed, to excessive gastric acidity per se, as the same symptom often occurs in achlorhydria [absence of stomach acid]."[4] The bottom line is that heartburn and GERD are more often caused by deficiency or lack of HCl than by too much of it.[5] Interestingly, both hypochlorhydria and hyperchlorhydria produce the same symptoms—a heartburn-like sensation that is sometimes accompanied by bloating and stomach pain.

Hypochlorhydria, or low HCl production, is more common than most people realize. With age, the production of stomach acid decreases.[6] It has been estimated that between 30 and 50 percent of people over 60 do not produce enough stomach acid.[7,8] To support healthy digestion, the stomach needs enough HCl to begin the breakdown of protein and activate pepsin, a protein-digesting enzyme found in the stomach.

Although it is difficult to comprehend taking acid to relieve heartburn, additional HCl helps the stomach to properly digest food, which ultimately helps to prevent putrefaction (the decomposition of animal proteins), a cause of gas production, reflux and heartburn.

So what causes low HCl production? Low HCl production can result from a deficiency of vitamin A and B complex, as well as from a low intake of protein.[9] Chronic stress and zinc deficiency are other factors that may result in suppression of stomach acid.[10] Low-salt diets may also contribute to HCl deficiency, as sodium and chloride are needed for HCl production.

HCl deficiency has some far-reaching consequences as far as overall health is concerned. HCl deficiency causes electrolyte deficiency, which in turn inhibits enzyme production.[11] The net result is poor metabolism of nutrients, disruption of homeostasis and development of degenerative disease conditions.

The most important step for people with GERD is to determine whether they have hypochlorhydria, or hyperchlorhydria. From there, the treatments are very

Did You Know

Because some calcium-based acid neutralizers are advertised as beneficial sources of supplemental calcium, some consumers, especially elderly women, overuse them in an effort to stave off osteoporosis. Ironically, the calcium contained in these products is calcium carbonate, an inorganic form of the mineral that is very poorly absorbed because it neutralizes HCl needed for its utilization. Because calcium requires an acid environment in order to be properly absorbed by the body, the carbonates, because they have an alkalizing effect, are a very poor dietary source of the mineral.

Did You Know

GERD is also common in infants. GERD may result in the frequent vomiting or spitting up that some infants experience. Usually reflux in babies is due to a poorly coordinated GI tract, although it can also be caused by a food allergy (usually to cow's milk, soy or wheat protein), or even poor feeding position. By the age of 1, most infants grow out of it when their digestive tracts mature.

Unfortunately, even infants are prescribed proton pump inhibitors (PPIs). A recent study that investigated the effects of PPIs on infants found that they were no more beneficial than placebo.[14] What's more, the rate of lower respiratory tract infections was higher in the infants taking PPIs.

In older children, GERD occurs for the same reason as in adults: the LES does not close properly. Factors such as obesity (a growing problem with today's youth), overeating, certain foods, beverages and medications may contribute to the development of GERD.

In children, as in adults, it may be more prudent to look at diet and other factors surrounding eating habits before medications are used. Interestingly, symptoms of GERD in infants may be indistinguishable from food allergies.

different. In fact, more health problems are created if treated improperly.

While chronic heartburn can strike anyone at any age, it is more common in older people than in younger people.[12] It is interesting that low HCl production also occurs more often in older people, suggesting a connection between low HCl and chronic heartburn.

What Are the Signs and Symptoms?

With GERD the amount and frequency of reflux differs individuals as does the degree of the acidity of the stomach contents being regurgitated into the esophagus. Therefore, one person with GERD may have mild symptoms while another could have severe symptoms. Along with reflux usually comes heartburn (in 70 to 85 percent of cases). Other signs and symptoms of GERD may include:

- Regurgitation
- Angina-like chest pain
- Dysphagia (difficulty swallowing)
- Bronchial spasms with asthma
- Laryngitis (voice problems or hoarseness)
- Shortness of breath
- Belching/bloating/gas
- A sense of fullness after eating (especially in conjunction with a chronic cough)
- Abdominal distention after eating
- Chronic sore throat
- Nausea
- Vomiting of blood (which may lead to anemia)

In addition, some people experience silent GERD, which does not produce the characteristic heartburn pain, but instead is associated with symptoms such as:

- Chronic cough, worse at night
- Inflammation of the gums
- Erosion of tooth enamel
- Bad breath
- Chronic throat irritation
- Hoarseness in the morning

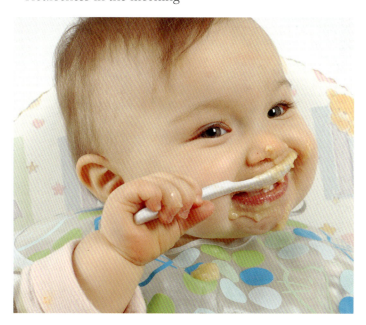

Not all people with GERD will experience all of these signs and symptoms. All GERD patients have reflux, but not all have burning, bloating and/or nausea.[13]

Bloating and gas, when present, can be the result of swallowing air, undigested food being acted upon by bacteria, overeating or by delayed gastric emptying. The stomach expands from gas, which travels up toward the esophagus, pushing HCl with it.

The resulting heartburn is caused, not by too much HCl, but by stomach contents, including undigested food, pathogens and even very low amounts of stomach acid that is in the wrong place—in the esophagus instead of in the stomach.

It is important to note that many of the symptoms of GERD may be indicators of other problems. For this reason, and because GERD can lead to the more serious Barrett's esophagus (covered extensively at the beginning of this chapter), or, for a small percentage of people, even cancer, physicians will often perform tests to establish a definitive diagnosis.

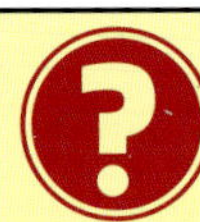

Did You Know

The use of proton pump inhibitors (PPIs) has been associated with:

- Increased risk of Clostridium difficile (C. diff) associated disease [15,16]
- Development of esophageal candidiasis[17]
- Osteoporosis-related bone fractures[18,19]
- Community- and hospital-acquired pneumonia[20]
- Vitamin B12 deficiency[21]
- Spontaneous bacterial peritonitis[22]
- Increased upper GI tract permeability ("leaky esophagus")[23]

Because PPI use leads to hypochlorhydria, bacterial overgrowth and acetaldehyde production, long-term use is potentially a risk factor for gastric and cardiac cancers.[24]

It has been determined that acid-reducing medicines lead to dependency.[25] This happens because, when the medication is discontinued, the GERD symptoms return.

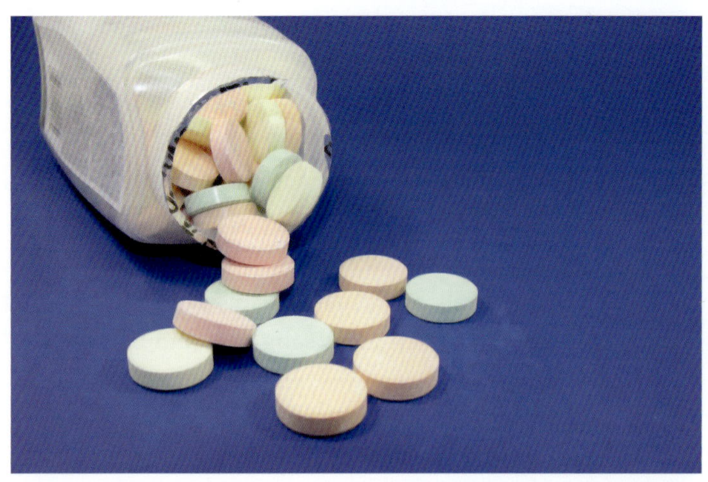

How Is It Diagnosed?

Unfortunately GERD is not usually diagnosed. Upon the presence of recurrent heartburn symptoms reported by the patient, the doctor may treat the symptoms with medication without performing any tests. Standard tests are available, however, and can help to determine the presence of reflux in the esophagus:

- Double-contrast endoscopy showing evidence of burning
- Biopsy confirmation

While these tests are used for diagnosing GERD, actual measurements of stomach acid production are not routinely done.

Recognizing that low stomach acid may play an important role in GERD, the progressive physician may do a gastric analysis to measure the stomach's acid-secreting capacity by testing the level of gastrin. The Heidelberg pH Diagnostic System, which does provide the actual measurements of stomach acid production, is very helpful in determining how to approach the treatment of GERD. (See the Appendix.) This test involves swallowing a "Heidelberg capsule," which contains a tiny pH sensor and radio transmitter. Then a series of bicarbonate challenges is introduced to see how quickly the pH changes from alkaline to acid.

Another test that may be ordered by a holistic physician is a comprehensive stool analysis (CSA). (See the Appendix.)

Conditions Associated with Low Gastric Acidity

- **Acne**
- **Allergies**
- **Anal Itching**
- **Asthma**
- **Cancer**
- **Celiac disease**
- **Chronic autoimmune disorders**
- **Chronic hives**
- **Diabetes mellitus**
- **Dilated nasal blood vessels**
- **Eczema (dermatitis)**
- **Food sensitivities**
- **Gallbladder disease**
- **Gastritis**
- **Grave's disease**
- **Hepatitis**
- **Hyper- and hypothyroidism**
- **Iron and calcium deficiencies**
- **Lupus erythematosis**
- **Osteoporosis**
- **Pernicious anemia**
- **Psoriasis**
- **Rheumatoid arthritis**
- **Rosacea**
- **Vitiligo**

Elevated levels of vegetable and meat fibers (especially meat) present in this stool analysis may be yet another indicator of insufficient HCl production.

The CSA also gives information about the levels of digestive enzymes, the degree of fat digestion and the microbial balance of the gut. This test can potentially identify problems not detected by standard GI tests, which are designed solely to identify structural, not functional problems.

What Is the Standard Medical Treatment?

For GERD, the hallmark of standard medical treatment is the routine use of acid-supressing drugs to neutralize or suppress stomach acid production. The thinking, with regard to use of such drugs, is that by reducing or neutralizing acid production, irritation to the esophagus will be minimized. Such thinking has given rise to widespread use of acid-supressing drugs to treat GERD.

These acid-supressing drugs may be divided into two categories:[26]

- Acid neutralizers
- Acid blockers

Acid Neutralizers

Acid-neutralizing drugs are alkalis, meaning they have an extremely alkaline (high) pH. Their active ingredients are mineral salts such as calcium, sodium, aluminum or magnesium. These minerals form a neutral salt upon contact with stomach acid, increasing the pH and reducing acidity.

Their effects are temporary. They do not halt the stomach's production of HCl. Acid neutralizing products are available over-the-counter without prescription. While their occasional use for isolated bouts of heartburn might not do much harm, habitual use can pose some serious problems.

Most serious of the potential problems is a syndrome called milk-alkali syndrome, characterized by excess calcium in the blood. This syndrome gives rise to a condition known as alkalosis (elevated blood pH), and to kidney failure. Milk-alkali syndrome may result from over-consumption of milk (which is high in the alkaline mineral calcium) along with the use of antacids over a long period of time. But it can also occur when no milk is consumed if calcium-based acid neutralizers are used habitually or excessively.

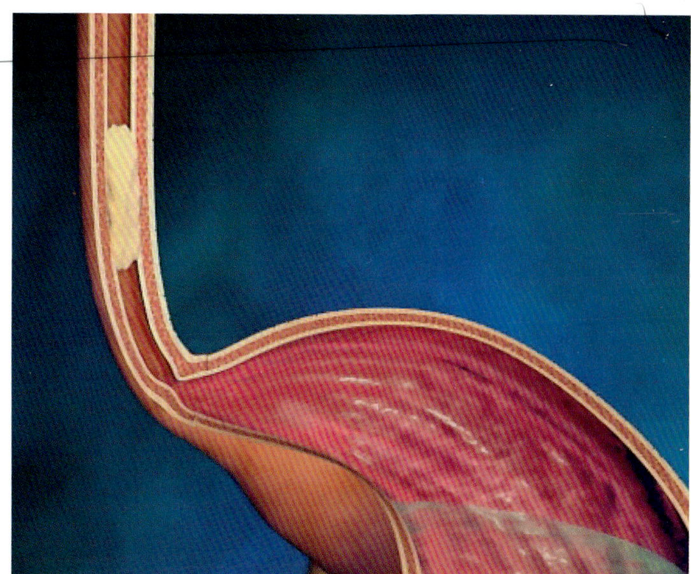

Illustration showing the location of the lower esophageal sphinctor (LES)

Some acid-neutralizing drugs contain aluminum, which poses an additional problem. This metal has been shown to be a possible cause of such brain dementias as Alzheimer's disease. It would therefore be advisable to avoid long-term use of aluminum-containing antacids.

Did You Know

The medical term used for chronic heartburn is "GERD" (gastroesophageal reflux disease). GERD is defined as a digestive disorder in which partially digested food from the stomach, along with hydrochloric acid (HCl) and enzymes, backs up (or regurgitates) into the esophagus.

Acid Blockers

There are two groups of acid-blocking drugs: histamine H2-receptor blockers (H2 blockers) and proton pump inhibitors (PPIs). H2 blockers prevent acid secretion by blocking the action of histamine. Histamine signals acid-producing cells to secrete HCl upon command of the hormone gastrin.

These drugs were originally developed to treat peptic ulcers, but came to be widely used to treat GERD instead when it was found that the bacteria H. pylori, and not excess HCl, causes ulcers. H2 blockers can shut off acid flow for hours at a time but, like many other drugs, they have serious side effects including GI disturbances such as:

- Constipation
- Diarrhea
- Nausea
- Vomiting
- Heartburn (the very condition they're prescribed to treat)

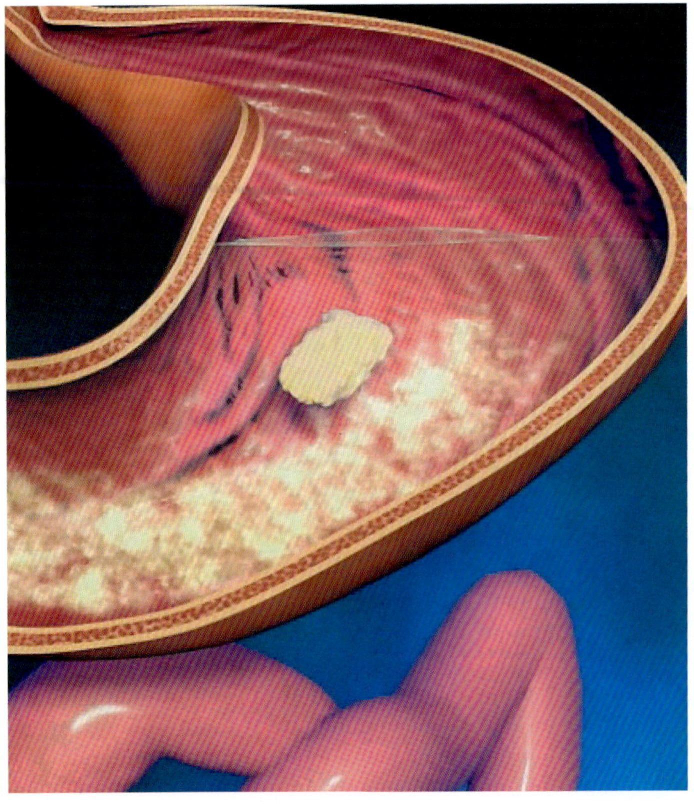

An illustration showing the digestion of protein by HCl in the stomach

Proton pump inhibitors (PPIs) are the strongest of the acid-blocking drugs. They block the action of the proton pump, the HCl producing and secreting mechanism inside cells in the stomach lining. **Long-term use of PPIs is associated with health consequences such as increased risk of pneumonia and Clostridium difficile infections, osteoporosis-related bone fracture, nutrient malabsorption and more. These medications lead to dependency and, once their use is stopped, a rebound effect can result in a problem that is worse than when it began.**

When a person with low stomach acid is treated with acid-blocking medications for heartburn, obviously the hypochlorhydria is exacerbated. And since inadequate HCl production is more often the cause of GERD than is excessive acid production, the problem is often made worse with the treatment.

Even if the lack of stomach acid was not a problem before treatment with acid-blocking medication, it can become one afterward. While they may provide short-term relief of heartburn, strong acid blockers, when used habitually, continually block the natural production of HCl. This knocks out one of the functions of stomach acid: to sterilize food before it enters the intestinal tract. Uncontrolled growth of every kind of microbe in the stomach, including yeast and Helicobacter pylori (H. pylori), the bacteria associated with gastric ulcers,[27] can result.

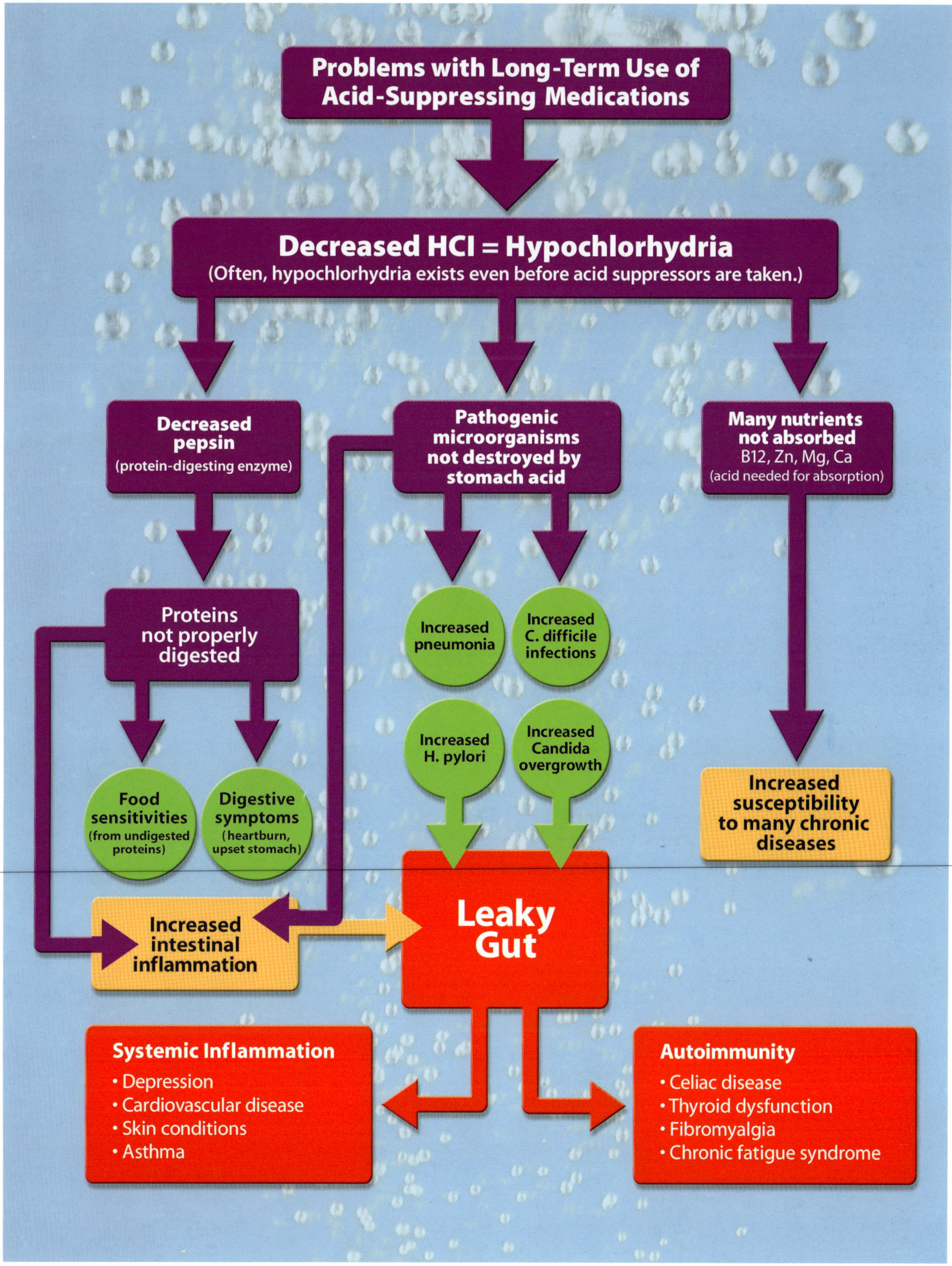

Problems with Long-Term Use of Acid-Suppressing Medications

Decreased HCl = Hypochlorhydria
(Often, hypochlorhydria exists even before acid suppressors are taken.)

Decreased pepsin
(protein-digesting enzyme)

Proteins not properly digested

Food sensitivities (from undigested proteins)

Digestive symptoms (heartburn, upset stomach)

Pathogenic microorganisms not destroyed by stomach acid

Increased pneumonia

Increased C. difficile infections

Increased H. pylori

Increased Candida overgrowth

Many nutrients not absorbed
B12, Zn, Mg, Ca
(acid needed for absorption)

Increased susceptibility to many chronic diseases

Increased intestinal inflammation

Leaky Gut

Systemic Inflammation
- Depression
- Cardiovascular disease
- Skin conditions
- Asthma

Autoimmunity
- Celiac disease
- Thyroid dysfunction
- Fibromyalgia
- Chronic fatigue syndrome

Healing HOPE Testimonial

"I began taking a digestive enzyme with HCl because I have problems with heartburn and acid reflux. The pills my doctor gave me were making me sick and I was taking over-the-counter antacids everyday. I knew that all this was just making things worse. Since taking the enzymes, I have noticed a big improvement in my symptoms, and have even found relief from constipation."
– Donna

Hydrochloric acid is one of nature's most essential antibiotics. Imagine a scenario where a patient with virtually no stomach acid production eats a salad and is incapable of destroying the bacteria present on all the raw vegetables.[28]

While acid-suppressing drugs may offer temporary relief of the symptoms of heartburn, they create many major problems. By alkalizing the lower stomach (the antrum), the hormone gastrin is released causing a huge rebound output of acid. This rebound requires more acid-supressors to neutralize the increased acid output in response to the gastrin.

Also important to note, acid-supressors create conditions conducive to yeast and fungus growth.[29] They can also mask symptoms of an ulcer, or even cancer of the stomach or esophagus.

Eventually the parietal cell mass that manufactures stomach acid ceases to function normally, resulting in low stomach acid (hypochlorhydria), or worse, no stomach acid (achlorhydria), which elevates the risk of stomach cancer.[30] While there is no outright proof that use of acid-suppressing drugs causes cancer, it is predicted that at least some of these drugs will be found to increase cancer risk, particularly when taken for a long time.

Motility-Enhancing Drugs

Because GERD is also considered to be a motility problem, motility-enhancing drugs may also be prescribed. They help strengthen the LES and move food through the stomach more rapidly. This certainly makes more physiological sense than suppressing acid production.

However, profound adverse side effects have limited the use of these drugs. For example, after a few years of clinical use, the FDA took one of the most potent motility enhancers off the market when it was found to cause heart failure.

Other Treatments

Should drugs and lifestyle/dietary adjustments fail to control symptoms of GERD, a physician may suggest surgery. A procedure known as fundoplication involves wrapping part of the stomach around the lower esophagus to strengthen the LES. This can be done laparoscopically with good results.[31]

Non-surgical alternatives are also available. Endoluminal therapy involves the use of an endoscope to tighten the junction between the esophagus and stomach with sutures. Radiofrequency therapy delivers energy waves to the muscles of the stomach and esophagus, which may have the ability to improve the function of the lower esophageal sphincter.[32]

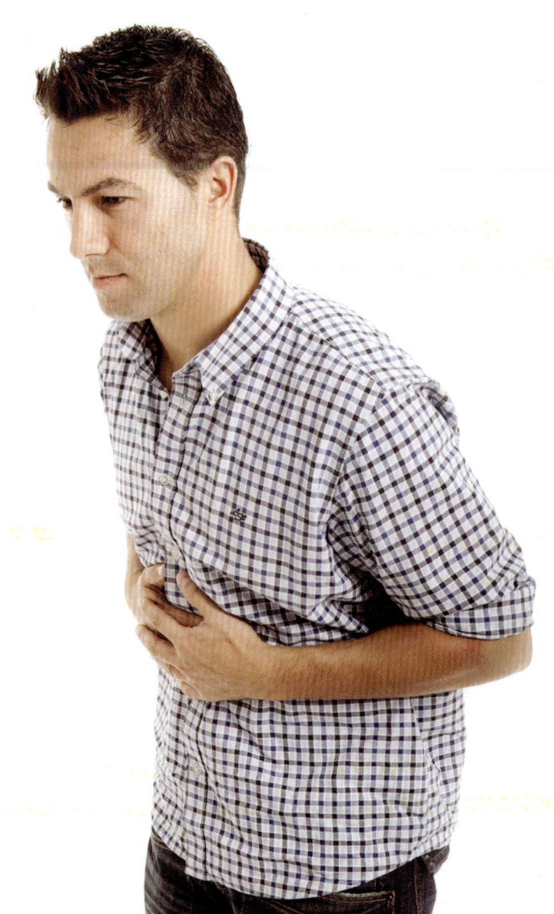

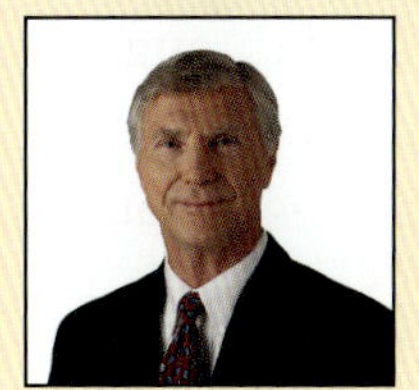

Dr. Smith's Comments

I have seen many patients who, after occasional episodes of heartburn, have been put on acid-blocking medications for indefinite periods of time. Often, I have found that if they will lose a little weight, improve their bowel function, eliminate foods that lower their esophageal sphincter pressure, remove sensitive foods and change their eating habits as mentioned in this chapter, they can get off of their medications. Since these medications can have significant and potentially serious side effects, it is wise to minimize their use. Implementation of more natural and safer nutritional options should be undertaken whenever possible.

I would like to point out that all esophageal conditions mentioned in this chapter, namely Barrett's esophagus, esophagitis, GERD, heartburn and hiatal hernia, have features in common that could be addressed from a nutritional standpoint:

- Material from the stomach periodically enters into the esophogus. This often causes an inflammatory reaction and can damage the esophageal lining. Researchers have recently observed that the damage to the lining may be due more to esophageal intracellular oxidative stress than to the direct contact of the acid and gastric contents. There are articles in the literature that support the fact that adequate antioxidant levels are protective against damage from reflux (Gut 2001;49;364-371). In this article, it was shown that pretreatment with antioxidants minimized damage and decreased inflammatory markers (malondialdehyde and NF kappa B). In addition, the antioxidants slowed down the loss of glutathione (a naturally produced beneficial antioxidant). It would be wise to supplement with vitamins A, C, E, and the minerals zinc and selenium.

- Mucus production has been shown to be variable, and people with lower levels tend to have more inflammatory problems in the esophagus and stomach. Normalizing cellular function with glutamine, glycine, and omega-3 essential fatty acids can be helpful. Mucus-producing nutrients (N-acetyl glucosamine, N-acetyl-galactosamine, fucose, galactose and sialic acid) and increased water intake are needed to make high quality and quantity of mucus. There is a good review article about probiotics and mucus and their role in intestinal health in the American Journal of Clinical Nutrition, 2003;78: 675-683.

Minimizing the possibility of inflammation is important. Checking for any type of infection, especially H. pylori or Candida, can be helpful. If found, short courses of appropriate anti-microbials should be implemented. After removal of pathogens, restoration of the beneficial bacteria (Lactobacilli and Bifidobacteria) is very important and may help prevent future infections. Liquid aloe vera has potent anti-inflammatory benefits as well.

Common Signs & Symtoms of Low Gastric Acidity

(often diagnosed as high gastric acid)

- **A sense of fullness after eating**
- **Acne**
- **Bloating, belching, burning and flatulence immediately after meals**
- **Chronic Candida infections**
- **Chronic intestinal parasites or abnormal flora**
- **Dilated blood vessels in the cheeks and nose**
- **Indigestion, diarrhea or constipation**
- **Iron deficiency**
- **Itching around the rectum**
- **Multiple food allergies**
- **Nausea after taking supplements**
- **Undigested food in the stool**
- **Upper digestive tract gassiness**
- **Weak, peeling and cracked fingernails**

From Encyclopedia of Natural Medicine, Revised 2nd edition by Michael Murray, ND & Joseph Pizzorno, ND

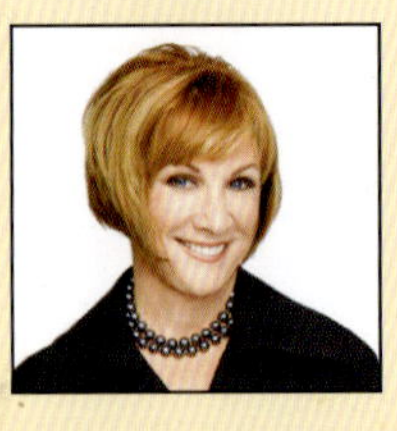

Brenda's Bottom Line

The condition of GERD causes distress to many people. Unfortunately, it can be a bit complicated because our traditional doctors do not take the necessary steps to find out why a person has GERD in the first place.

In cases where the patient is persistent about finding the underlying cause, the doctor will test for H. pylori infection. If found, antibiotics are given to treat the bacteria and acid-blocking medication to heal stomach irritation or ulcers. Other than recommending basic dietary and lifestyle changes, in traditional medicine the search for the underlying cause is over. The doctor does not heal the gut afterwards with nutrients like L-glutamine, NAG (N-Acetyl-D-glucosamine) and gamma oryzanol, nor does he know to replace the good bacteria that were destroyed by the powerful antibiotic.

Acid-blocking medication was originally developed for short-term treatment of gut irritation. If this were the only case in which people were given these drugs, it may not have escalated to the point it is today. If you go to a GI doctor with a symptom of heartburn, gas, bloating or even irritable bowel syndrome (IBS), they hand out these acid-blocking medications like they were candy with no testing to determine whether stomach acid is even the main problem!

People are kept on acid-blocking medication for years, which sets the stage for the development of serious health conditions down the road. Recent studies clearly show that these medications are over prescribed more than 53 percent of the time.

We have watched the pharmaceutical industry wreak havoc on our bodies with the over-prescription of antibiotics. And now we can see another travesty unfold long-term use of acid-blocking medications putting the health of millions of individuals in jeopardy. Instead of pulling out the prescription pad and writing another prescription, the doctor should be looking for the underlying causes. The Heidelberg pH test should be in every GI doctor's office, and this nonsense could stop. If you have GERD and are on acid-blocking medication long term, go to your doctor and tell him you are aware of the dangers and want to be taken off the medication. You can be carefully weaned off these drugs. (See the Appendix.) Then follow the protocol that follows.

In my experience, people who have these kinds of digestive problems have an underlying digestive issue in addition to stomach acid levels. If you have been on acid blockers long term, the chances that you have Candida overgrowth and other imbalances throughout the gut are highly probable.

Recommended Testing

- Stool test for Candida or parasites (See the Appendix.)
- HCl test (See the Heidelburg test in the Appendix.)
- Food sensitivity test if suspected (See the Appendix.)

Diet

- Follow the Fiber 35 Eating Plan found in the Appendix of this book. A high-fiber breakfast is important.
- If you suspect Candida overgrowth is an issue, follow the Candida Diet found in the Appendix.
- Some research suggests that a gluten-free diet can be useful in reducing GERD symptoms.
- Chew foods well, to mush or liquid, before swallowing.

Lifestyle

- Sleep on your left side to avoid heartburn and reflux.
- Do not lie down for at least three to four hours after eating.
- Elevate the head of the bed four to eight inches when sleeping.
- Make sure you have good bowel elimination daily.

Complementary Mind/Body Therapies

- Stress-reduction therapies such as yoga, biofeedback, massage, and meditation will be helpful.
- Acupuncture may be helpful as it targets the meridians associated with the digestive system.
- Chiropractic may be beneficial.
- Colon hydrotherapy should be considered.

Recommended Nutraceuticals	Dosage	Benefit	Comments
Critical Phase	Daily maintenance recommendations should also be taken during this phase unless otherwise indicated.		
L-Glutamine Powder with Gamma Oryzanol	5 grams (5000 mg) daily on empty stomach with water	Helps repair the esophageal lining and reduce inflammation.	Best if taken in powder form for contact with esophageal lining.
Probiotics	200 billion culture count daily for two weeks	Protects digestive lining, reduces inflammation and stimulates immune system.	Best if taken in powder form for contact with digestive lining.
Natural Heartburn Formula	Chew only in acute situation only when needed.	Temporarily neutralizes acid and soothes digestive tract.	Look for ingredients such as fava bean, ellagic acid, calcium, magnesium and aloe.
Helpful			
Antioxidant Supplement	Use as directed	Protects tissue from damage.	You can purchase a high-potency antioxidant formulation from most health food stores.
Melatonin	3-5 mg at bedtime	Study shows may be an effective treatment for GERD.	Start with lower dosage and build up to 5 mg.
Daily Maintenance			
Fiber	4-5 grams twice daily as part of a 35 gram daily fiber diet	Helps to reduce reflux and promotes digestive motility.	Look for a flax-based fiber with added ingredients such as glutamine, probiotics and healing herbs.
Probiotics	50 billion culture count daily after critical phase	Protects digestive lining, reduces inflammation and stimulates immune system.	Best taken in loose powder for contact with digestive lining. Open capsule if necessary.
Digestive Enzyme with HCl	1-2 capsules with every meal	Reduces fermentation, pressure, replaces low HCl, and helps tighten LES.	Do not use HCl if ulcer or stomach irritation is present. Switch to enzyme without HCl.
Omega-3 Fatty Acids	At least 2 grams daily of EPA/DHA combination	Reduces inflammation.	Look for a concentrated, enteric coated high dose EPA/DHA formulation.

See further explanation of supplements in the Appendix

See the Appendix for a protocol on weaning off of long-term acid blocking medication

HEARTBURN

What Is It?

Heartburn, also known as acid reflux, is a condition wherein gastric juices back up into the esophagus creating a burning sensation that then radiates upward. It is usually part of a larger symptom complex known as dyspepsia or indigestion. The term "heartburn" is used to describe an individual event. The medical term used for chronic (frequent) heartburn is gastroesophageal reflux disease (GERD). Heartburn is considered GERD when it occurs two or more times per week.

What Causes It?

See the GERD section for detailed information on the causes of heartburn.

What Are the Signs and Symptoms?

Twenty-five million adults experience heartburn daily.[1] Apart from the burning sensation in the chest, the heartburn sufferer may experience:

- Nausea
- Upper abdominal pain (usually comes after meals)
- Flatulence and belching (gas)
- Abdominal distention after eating
- A sense of fullness after eating

Frequent and persistent heartburn, particularly if it is accompanied by any of the symptoms listed below, may be an indicator of GERD:

- Hoarseness or wheezing
- Painful or difficult swallowing
- Vomiting
- Dramatic weight loss
- Increased severity of symptoms over time

Did You Know

Before taking acid blocking medication long term for this condition, make sure your stomach acid level is tested.

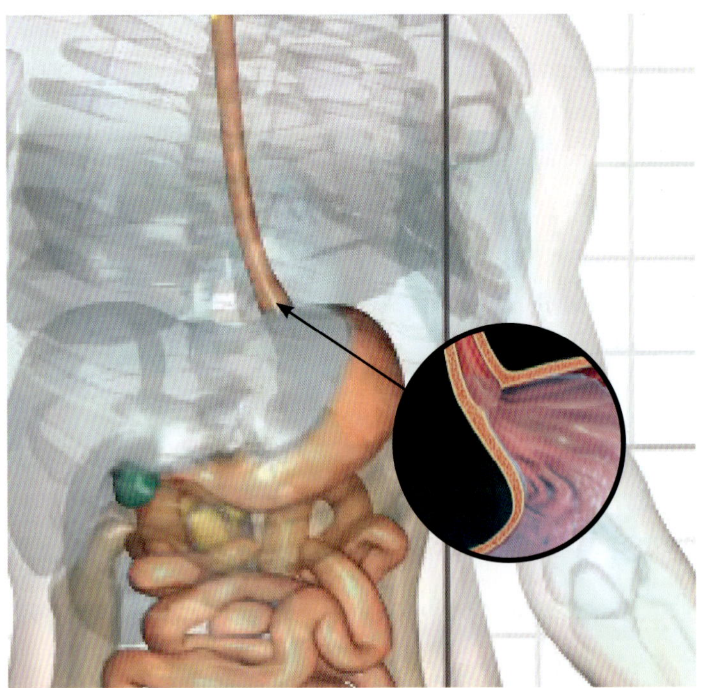

Illustration of stomach acid backing up into the esophagus because the lower esophageal muscle does not close properly

See the GERD section for more information if you have any of these symptoms.

How Is It Diagnosed?

Simple heartburn may be diagnosed on the basis of symptoms alone. However, your doctor may want to perform tests—upper GI series or endoscopy to be sure, and to rule out other conditions.

To distinguish heartburn from angina (heart pain), a Bernstein test (acid perfusion) may be performed.[2] This test involves introducing first a saline solution, then a weak hydrochloric acid (HCl) solution into the esophagus through a tube inserted into the nasal cavity. Theoretically, if pain is felt with the HCl but not with the salt, it is indicative of reflux. An EKG and stress test, as well as a 24-hour pH probe, may also be used to distinguish heartburn from angina. See the GERD section of this book for other tests that may be performed.

What Is the Standard Medical Treatment?

Standard medical treatment will involve the use of antacids or acid blockers. See the GERD section for a discussion of these medications, and the risks posed by using them on an ongoing basis.

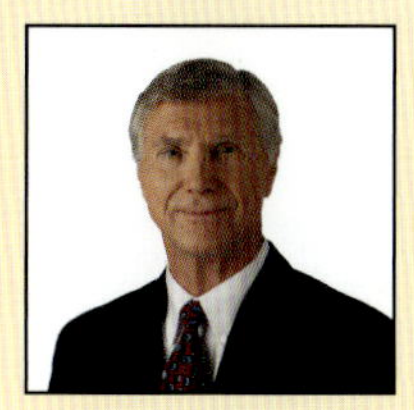

Dr. Smith's Comments

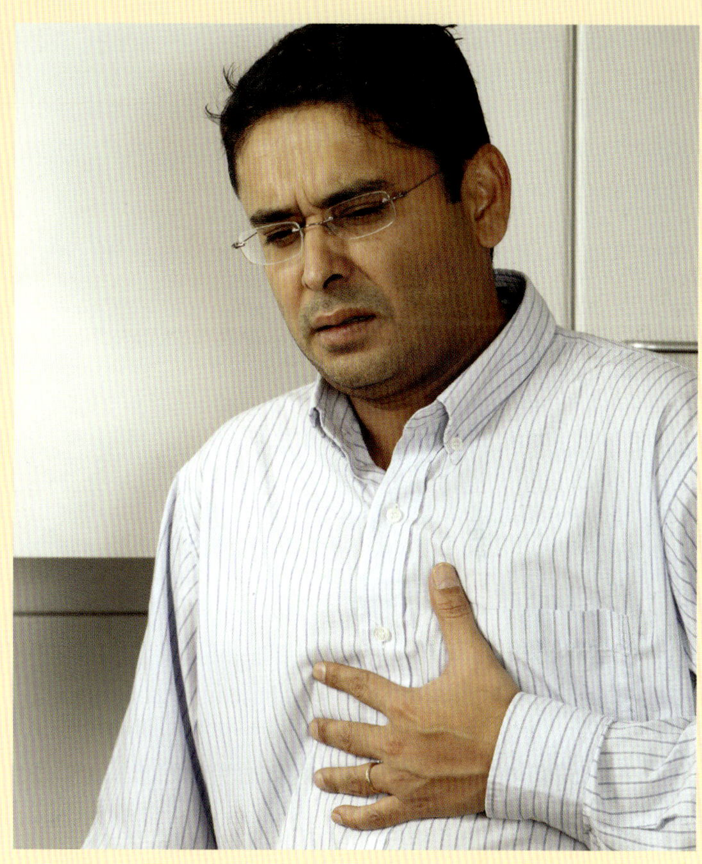

I have seen many patients who, after occasional episodes of heartburn, have been put on acid-blocking medications for indefinite periods of time. Often, I have found that if they will lose a little weight, improve their bowel function, eliminate foods that lower their esophageal sphincter pressure, remove sensitive foods and change their eating habits as mentioned in this chapter, they can get off of their medications. Since these medications can have significant and potentially serious side effects, it is wise to minimize their use. Implementation of more natural and safer nutritional options should be undertaken whenever possible.

I would like to point out that all esophageal conditions mentioned in this chapter, namely Barrett's esophagus, esophagitis, GERD, heartburn and hiatal hernia, have features in common that could be addressed from a nutritional standpoint:

- Material from the stomach periodically enters into the esophogus. This often causes an inflammatory reaction and can damage the esophageal lining. Researchers have recently observed that the damage to the lining may be due more to esophageal intracellular oxidative stress than to the direct contact of the acid and gastric contents. There are articles in the literature that support the fact that adequate antioxidant levels are protective against damage from reflux (Gut 2001;49;364-371). In this article, it was shown that pretreatment with antioxidants minimized damage and decreased inflammatory markers (malondialdehyde and NfkappaB). In addition, the antioxidants slowed down the loss of glutathione (a naturally produced beneficial antioxidant). It would be wise to supplement with vitamins A, C, E, and the minerals zinc and selenium.

- Mucus production has been shown to be variable, and people with lower levels tend to have more inflammatory problems in the esophagus and stomach. Normalizing cellular function with glutamine, glycine, and omega-3 essential fatty acids can be helpful. Mucus-producing nutrients (N-acetyl glucosamine, N-acetyl-galactosamine, fucose, galactose and sialic acid) and increased water intake are needed to make high quality and quantity of mucus. There is a good review article about probiotics and mucus and their role in intestinal health in the American Journal of Clinical Nutrition, 2003;78: 675-683.

Minimizing the possibility of inflammation is important. Checking for any type of infection, especially H. pylori or Candida, can be helpful. If found, short courses of appropriate anti-microbials should be implemented. After removal of pathogens, restoration of the beneficial bacteria (Lactobacilli and Bifidobacteria) is very important and may help prevent future infections. Liquid aloe vera has potent anti-inflammatory benefits as well.

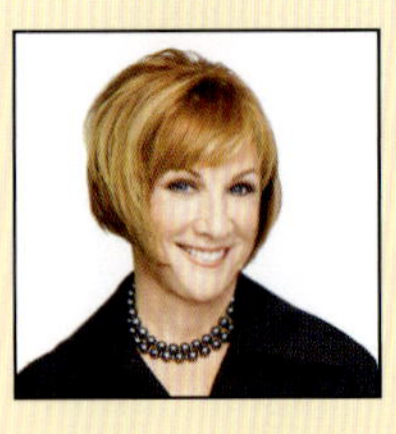

Brenda's Bottom Line

These suggestions are for the person who is just starting to suffer heartburn occasionally. It is important to recognize heartburn as a sign of imbalance in the body. Getting to the bottom of the problem at the beginning stages of heartburn is key.

Always start with your diet. This is the most important first step. Begin to carefully examine the timing of symptoms with food intake to determine which foods cause symptoms. Digestive enzymes can be used, not only for people who do not produce enough enzymes (from their pancreas or stomach) for digestion, but also when certain foods upset the stomach. Digestive enzymes help digest protein, starches, sugars, fibers and fat that are left undigested and can be responsible for the feeling of heartburn.

If the symptoms are not relieved with these suggestions, then you must determine if you have low stomach acid. You can do this with apple cider vinegar. If a tablespoon after eating relieves symptoms, this is a signal that you may not be making enough acid and may need to add a HCl acid supplement with meals. If you take the apple cider vinegar and you burn more, you may have too much acid. This should not be a reason to use acid-blocking medication long term, however.

The Heidelberg pH test is a more sophisticated test that can help to determine your level of stomach acid. (See the Appendix.) Most of the time when excess stomach acid is found, food sensitivities or a number of other factors listed in this chapter, are the underlying culprit. Please get to the bottom of the problem before resorting to prescriptions.

Suppressing stomach acid long term is a recipe for disaster, as we are now seeing with increased risk of C. difficile infections, pneumonia and osteoporosis in people taking acid blockers long term. These risks occur for two main reasons: key nutrients are not absorbed without acid, and potentially pathogenic organisms are not killed in the stomach if HCl levels are not normal.

Most people do not understand that malabsorption is going to create a host of complications because one of the major functions of food is to supply vitamins, minerals and antioxidants. Without these nutrients, we develop disease.

Another problem that is becoming more frequent in people with heartburn is the development of Candida overgrowth (see the Candidiasis section) in the intestines which can back up into the stomach if acid levels are too low to control it.

If you are just starting to suffer from heartburn, do something immediately to find out why! This could very well be the one thing that will keep you healthy for the rest of your life.

Recommended Testing

- Stool test for Candida or parasites (See the Appendix.)
- HCl test (See Heidelburg test in the Appendix.)

Diet

- Follow the Fiber 35 Eating Plan found in the Appendix of this book. Eating a high-fiber diet is essential.
- Eat smaller meals throughout the day. Eat meals slowly.
- Chew foods well to mush or liquid before swallowing.

Lifestyle

- Sleep on your left side to avoid heartburn and reflux.
- Do not lie down for at least three to four hours after eating.
- Elevate the head of the bed four to eight inches when sleeping.

Complementary Mind/Body Therapies

- Stress-reduction therapies such as yoga, biofeedback, massage and meditation can be helpful when stress is an issue.
- Acupuncture may be helpful because it targets the meridians associated with the digestive system, and is also a stress reducer.
- Colon hydrotherapy is helpful for heartburn.

Recommended Nutraceuticals	Dosage	Benefit	Comments
Critical Phase Daily maintenance recommendations should also be taken during this phase unless otherwise indicated.			
L-Glutamine Powder with Gamma Oryzanol	10 grams (10,000 mg) daily in split doses on empty stomach with water for two weeks	Helps repair the digestive lining and reduce inflammation.	Best if taken in loose powder form.
Natural Heartburn Formula	Chew only in acute situation only when needed.	Temporarily neutralizes acid and soothes digestive tract.	Look for ingredients such as fava bean, ellagic acid, calcium, magnesium and aloe.
Probiotics	200 billion culture count daily for two weeks	Protects digestive lining, reduces inflammation and stimulates immune system.	Best if taken in powder form for contact with digestive lining.
Helpful			
Antioxidant Supplement	Use as directed	Protects tissue from damage.	You can purchase a high-potency antioxidant formulation from most health food stores.
B-Complex with extra B-12	Use as directed	B vitamins needed for proper acid production.	Especially helpful as we age and decrease in vitamin B levels.
Daily Maintenance			
L-Glutamine Powder with Gamma Oryzanol	5 grams (5000 mg) daily on empty stomach with water after critical phase	Helps repair the digestive lining and reduce inflammation.	Best if taken in loose powder form for contact with esophageal lining.
Fiber	4-5 grams twice daily	Helps to reduce reflux.	Look for a flax-based fiber with added ingredients such as glutamine, probiotics and healing herbs.
Digestive Enzyme with HCl	1-2 capsules with every meal	Reduces fermentation, pressure, replaces low HCl, and helps tighten LES.	Do not use HCl if ulcer or stomach irritation is present. Switch to enzyme without HCl.
Probiotics	50 billion culture count daily after critical phase	Protects digestive lining, reduces inflammation and stimulates immune system.	Best if taken in powder form for contact with digestive lining. Open capsule if necessary.
Omega-3 Fatty Acids	At least 2 grams daily of EPA/DHA combination	Reduces inflammation.	Look for a concentrated, enteric coated high dose EPA/DHA formulation.

See further explanation of supplements in the Appendix

Hiatal Hernia

What Is It?

In order to understand what a hiatal hernia is, it is important to know that the esophagus passes through the diaphragm—the flat dome-shaped muscle that separates the chest cavity from the abdominal cavity—and into the stomach.

The opening in the diaphragm through which this passage is made is known as a "hiatus," which gives this syndrome its name.

When there is a weakness in the diaphragm muscles, a portion of the stomach rises up through the diaphragm causing a hiatal hernia.

The stomach is displaced to a position above the diaphragm, and the normal relation of the esophagus to the diaphragm is altered causing lower pressure at the junction of the stomach and the esophagus.

This area, known as the lower esophageal sphincter high pressure zone (LES-HPZ), is not really a valve or sphincter, but merely the site at which the diaphragm muscles attach to the junction of the esophagus and the stomach. The low pressure at this junction may cause gastroesophageal reflux (GERD), a backflow of stomach contents into the esophagus which causes a burning sensation. When this happens, the patient is said to have GERD. (See the GERD section for more information on this condition.)

What Causes It?

There are many contributing factors to hiatal hernia. Some include injury, trauma, obesity, thyroid dysfunction and age. By definition, the condition involves weakness in the diaphragm. It has also been theorized that, in some people, a congenital shortening of the GI tract[1] may be a causative variable. In this instance, the person would be born with a predisposition to hiatal hernia that could develop later in life as the result of some sort of stress, such as pregnancy or extreme physical exertion.[2]

Hernia Types

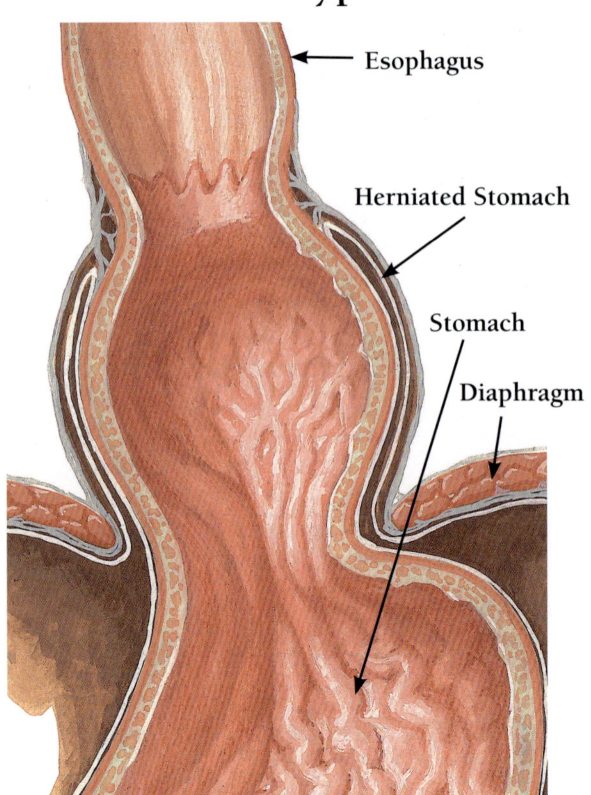

Sliding Hernia

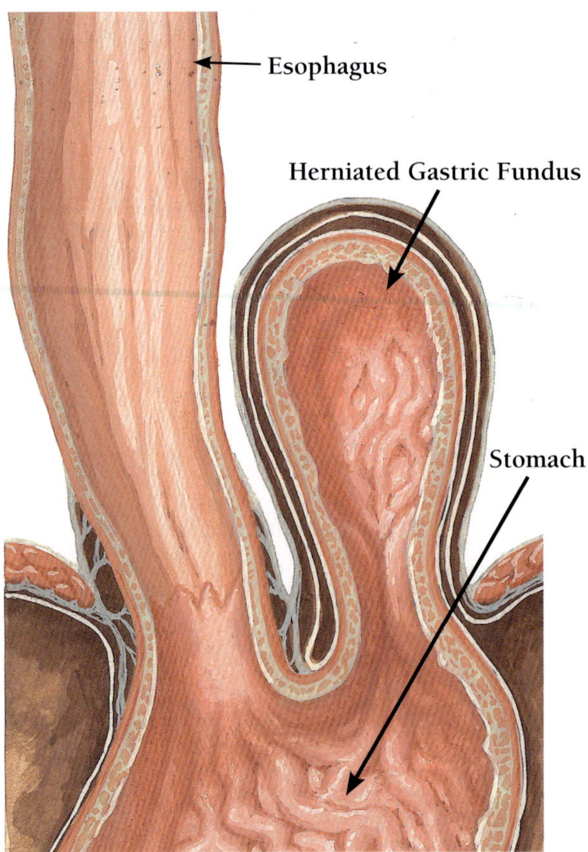

Para-esophageal Hernia

Other underlying factors that may play a role in hiatal hernia:

- Overweight and obesity
- Poor diet
- Constipation

Hiatal hernias affect women more frequently than men,[3] particularly pregnant women. They occur more often in people who are overweight than in people of normal weight[4] due to the increase in intra-abdominal pressure. These hernias also occur most often during middle age. In fact, the condition is so common that 25 percent of people aged 50 and over are estimated to have a hiatal hernia,[5] although, if there is no discomfort, they may not know it. Though not as common, it has been found that hiatal hernias can be hereditary.[6]

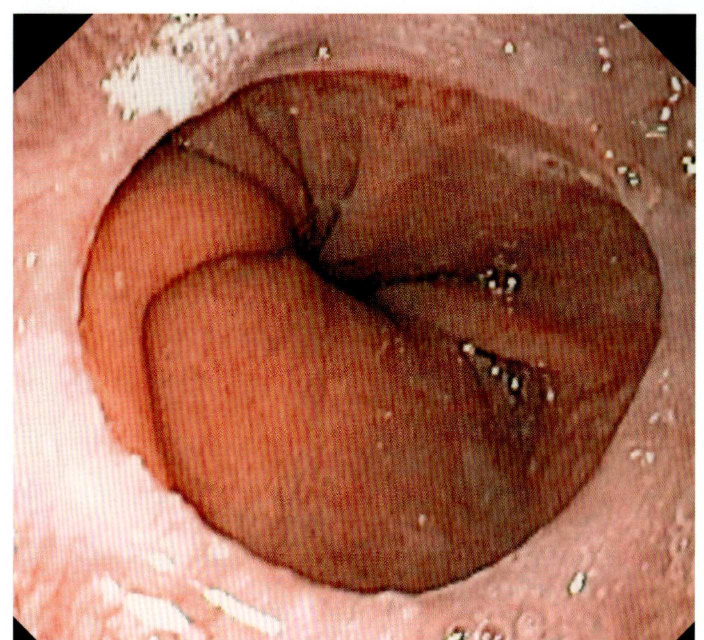

Endoscopic image of a hiatal hernia

What Are the Signs and Symptoms?

There are two types of hiatal hernias. The type and size of the hernia will largely determine the degree of distress experienced, if any. Most common is the sliding hiatal hernia. It occurs in 90 percent of all cases.[7] With this type of hernia, a portion of the stomach passes through the opening in the diaphragm. This condition may cause only mild, if any, symptoms. In fact, experts estimate that up to 40 percent of Americans have a sliding hiatal hernia and don't know it.[8]

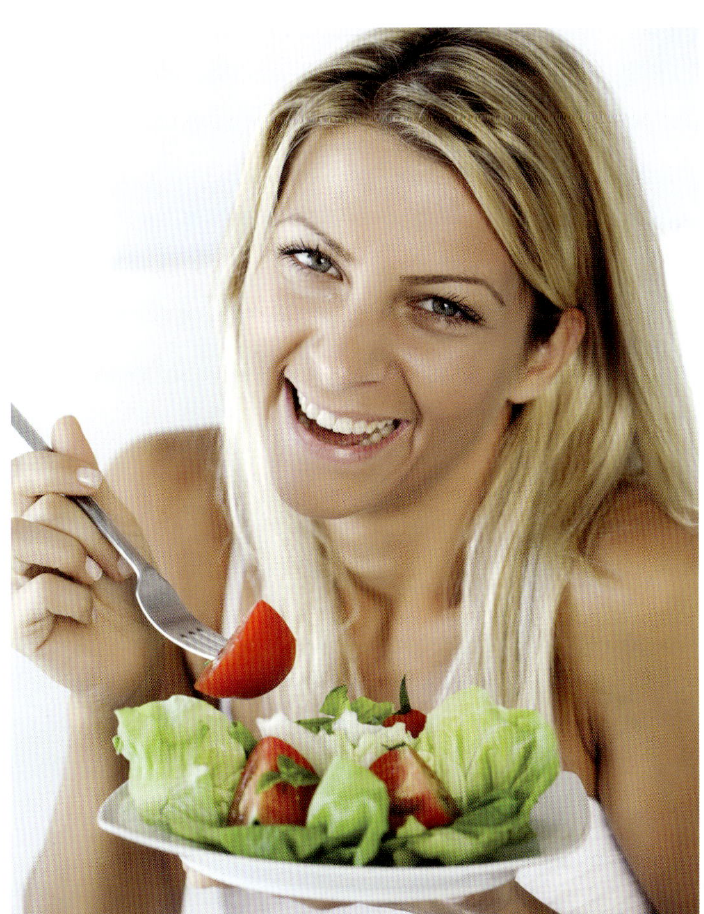

The second type of hiatal hernia is the para-esophageal hiatal hernia. Here, a portion of the stomach outpouches through the diaphragm and actually positions itself next to the esophagus. This type of hiatal hernia may produce no symptoms because the LES is not displaced. However, should the stomach get pulled higher into the chest and become pinched by the diaphragm, an emergency situation called "strangulation" may result requiring immediate surgical intervention.[9]

A sliding hiatal hernia may cause heartburn and other symptoms associated with GERD if the weakened LES permits reflux, the backflow of stomach contents into the esophagus. Both the sliding and the para-esophageal hiatal hernias may, on rare occasion, bleed (either a little or a lot) from their lining. A small amount of blood loss may lead to anemia, while massive blood loss can be life-threatening.[10]

How Is It Diagnosed?

The hiatal hernia is typically diagnosed by use of an upper GI series, also known as the barium swallow.

What Is the Standard Medical Treatment?

Many hiatal hernias, particularly if they're small, cause no symptoms and require no treatment. When GERD symptoms arise, they are likely treated with antacids. See the GERD section for information on the downside of habitual antacid use, as well as dietary and lifestyle modification recommendations. The section also offers nutritional approaches for managing GERD symptoms.

If it is confirmed that reflux is caused by a hiatal hernia and symptoms cannot be controlled through diet, medications and lifestyle modification, your physician may recommend surgical repair of the hernia.

Unfortunately there are no known ways to reverse hiatal hernia without surgery. However, the following nutritional options can enhance digestion, minimize reflux, and improve overall health and sense of well being.

General Recommendations For All Esophageal Problems

- Avoid foods and beverages that weaken the LES (such as chocolate, peppermint, fatty foods, caffeine-containing and alcoholic beverages).
- Decrease portion sizes at each meal.
- Don't lie down for at least three to four hours after eating.
- Don't wear clothing that constricts the abdomen.
- Reduce stress.
- Lose weight (if overweight).
- Quit smoking.
- Elevate the head of bed 4 to 8 inches when sleeping.
- Eat in a relaxed environment.
- Minimize activities (such as bending and heavy lifting) that might increase intra-abdominal pressure.
- Exercise regularly.
- Identify, reduce and/or eliminate any medications that may be contributing to the problem (under a doctor's supervision).
- Chew food thoroughly (until liquid).
- Drink more water (1/2 oz. for every pound of body weight—i.e., 50 oz. for a 100 lb. person).
- Keep a food diary to identify any food that may trigger an episode of GERD.
- Identify and avoid food allergens. (See the Resource section for testing information.)
- Combine foods properly (eat fruit alone; avoid eating starchy carbohydrates at the same time proteins are consumed.)
- Treat constipation if present.
- At the first sign of heartburn, drink a large glass of water.
- Take supplemental digestive enzymes at the end of each meal.
- Take a small amount of "bitters" (an aqueous blend of bitter herbs such as gentian root, artemisia, yellow dock, dandelion and barberry) about 15 minutes before eating. These will help stimulate the secretion of gastric acid, bile and pancreatic enzymes and assist in control of reflux by increasing the tone of the LES.[1]
- Drink raw potato juice (prepare with skin intact, drink immediately), diluted 50 percent with water, three times per day.[2]
- Drink a glass of fresh cabbage or celery juice daily.
- In lieu of HCl supplementation, if you wish, sip one tablespoon of apple cider vinegar [or lemon juice] diluted in a glass of water with meals.[3] Do not drink any other fluids with meals.
- Eat fresh pineapple and/or papaya. These fruits are rich in enzymes, which will aid digestion.
- Drink chamomile tea to relieve esophageal irritation.[4] This herb has anti-inflammatory properties.
- Consider a trial series of vitamin B12 injections. ("In cases of achlorhydria, it is an established fact that vitamin B12 is neither well digested nor well absorbed."[5])

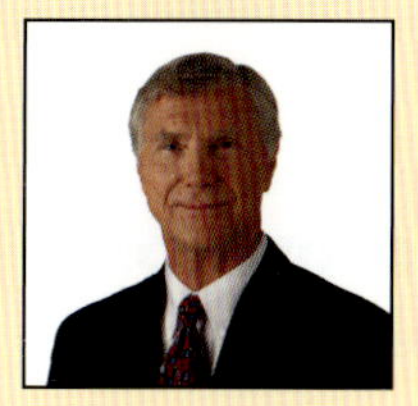

Dr. Smith's Comments

I have seen many patients who, after occasional episodes of heartburn, have been put on acid-blocking medications for indefinite periods of time. Often, I have found that if they will lose a little weight, improve their bowel function, eliminate foods that lower their esophageal sphincter pressure, remove sensitive foods and change their eating habits as mentioned in this chapter, they can get off of their medications. Since these medications can have significant and potentially serious side effects, it is wise to minimize their use. Implementation of more natural and safer nutritional options should be undertaken whenever possible.

I would like to point out that all esophageal conditions mentioned in this chapter, namely Barrett's esophagus, esophagitis, GERD, heartburn and hiatal hernia, have features in common that could be addressed from a nutritional standpoint:

- Material from the stomach periodically enters into the esophogus. This often causes an inflammatory reaction and can damage the esophageal lining. Researchers have recently observed that the damage to the lining may be due more to esophageal intracellular oxidative stress than to the direct contact of the acid and gastric contents. There are articles in the literature that support the fact that adequate antioxidant levels are protective against damage from reflux (Gut 2001;49;364-371). In this article, it was shown that pretreatment with

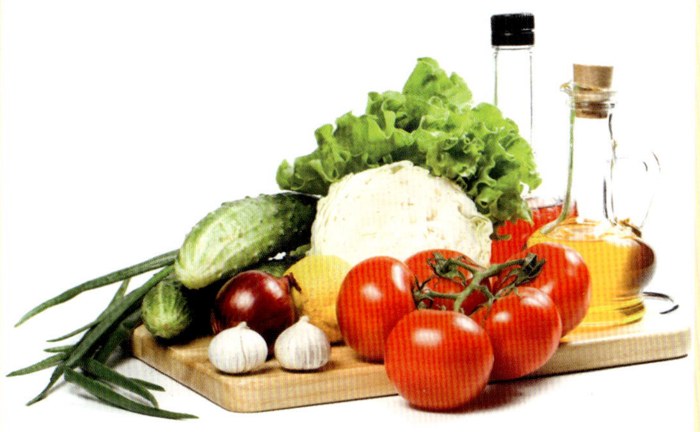

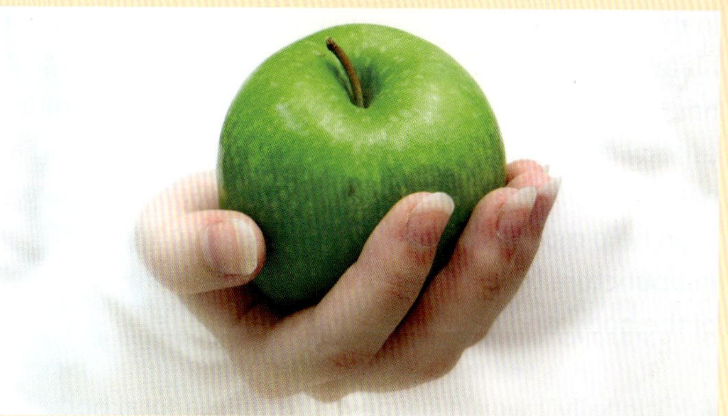

antioxidants minimized damage and decreased inflammatory markers (malondialdehyde and NF kappa B). In addition, the antioxidants slowed down the loss of glutathione (a naturally produced beneficial antioxidant). It would be wise to supplement with vitamins A, C, E, and the minerals zinc and selenium.

- Mucus production has been shown to be variable, and people with lower levels tend to have more inflammatory problems in the esophagus and stomach. Normalizing cellular function with glutamine, glycine, and omega-3 essential fatty acids can be helpful. Mucus-producing nutrients (N-acetyl glucosamine, N-acetyl-galactosamine, fucose, galactose and sialic acid) and increased water intake are needed to make high quality and quantity of mucus. There is a good review article about probiotics and mucus and their role in intestinal health in the American Journal of Clinical Nutrition, 2003;78: 675-683.

Minimizing the possibility of inflammation is important. Checking for any type of infection, especially H. pylori or Candida, can be helpful. If found, short courses of appropriate anti-microbials should be implemented. After removal of pathogens, restoration of the beneficial bacteria (Lactobacilli and Bifidobacteria) is very important and may help prevent future infections. Liquid aloe vera has potent anti-inflammatory benefits as well.

Gastritis

What Is It?

An "itis" anywhere in the body involves inflammation. Gastritis is inflammation of the lining of the stomach that involves erosion of the uppermost mucosal layer. Erosion of this protective layer leaves the underlying stomach tissue vulnerable to damage from enzymes and hydrochloric acid (HCl) that may seriously affect gastric function.

Various types of gastritis and who they affect are:

- Acute gastritis – those receiving high-dose radiation therapy
- Acute stress gastritis – those who have experienced sudden onset of an illness or injury, especially one involving massive blood loss, or extensive burns or trauma
- Atrophic gastritis – chronic low-grade infection of the stomach usually due to H. pylori infection, or due to an auto-immune attack or hypersensitivity of the stomach lining
- Chronic erosive gastritis – alcoholics, chronic users of non-steroid anti-inflammatory drugs (NSAIDs), those with Crohn's disease, those with bacterial or viral infections
- Viral or fungal gastritis – those with an immunodeficiency (during or following a long illness)

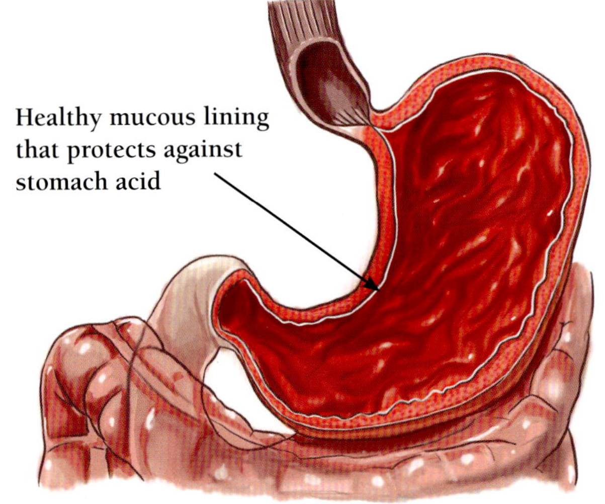

Normal stomach

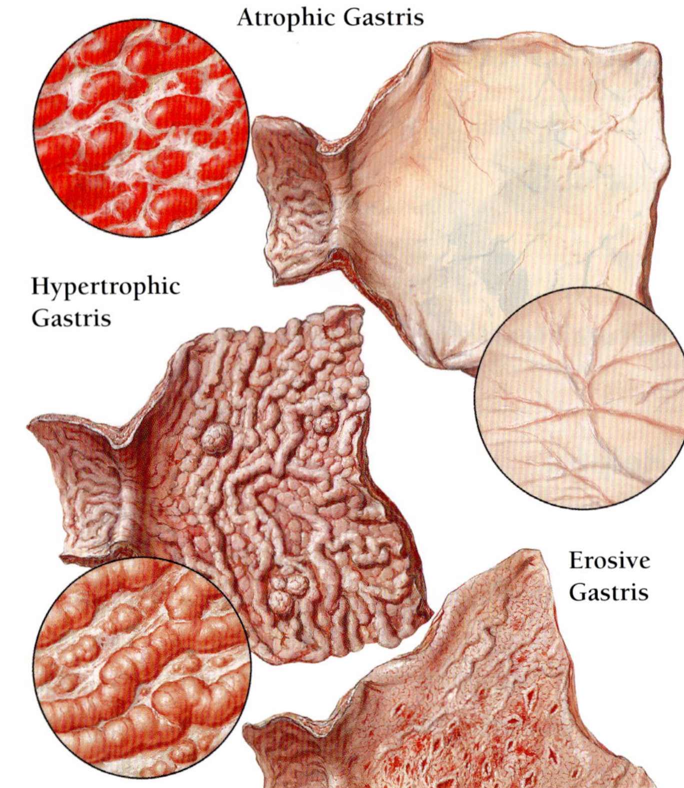

Different forms of gastritis

What Causes It?

Gastritis can have many causes, but recent research has shown that the bacterium Helicobacter pylori (H. pylori), which grows exclusively in the mucus-secreting cells of the stomach lining, is responsible for the majority of chronic gastritis cases.[1] It is interesting to note, however, that many people who are infected with H. pylori do not develop gastritis or any other GI disorder. While 25 percent of the U.S. population is infected with H. pylori, only 10 to 15 percent of this 25 percent will develop gastritis or ulcers.[2] It is not clearly understood why some people with the H. pylori infection develop problems and others do not.

However, the natural healing perspective holds the notion that it is not bacteria, but rather the context in which the bacteria are found that leads to disease. With that in mind, other factors such as diet and lifestyle can be viewed as important influences. One way in which H. pylori contributes to gut inflammation is that it increases stomach permeability ("leaky stomach") to undigested food particles. This stomach permeability may possibly lead to food allergies or sensitivities.[3]

H. pylori infection inhibits the secretion of gastric acid resulting in hypochlorhydria. When untreated, this infection can lead to the development of gastric cancer. Interestingly, people who have reflux esophagitis and H. pylori and are also taking proton pump inhibitors (PPIs) are at greater risk for developing gastritis.[4] These upper GI disorders often overlap, and the treatment for one can create problems for another.

Persons with H. pylori are at greater risk for developing chronic gastritis than people without this bacterial infection. The infection is transmitted from person to person through contaminated food and water; and through the use of diagnostic equipment, such as an endoscope, that has not been sterilized.[5] While the infection rate is only 25 percent in the U.S., it may be as high as 90 percent in underdeveloped countries where sanitation and hygiene are poor.[6] And while H. pylori is the bacterium most commonly associated with gastritis, E. coli can also play a role.[7]

Chronic erosive gastritis develops gradually as a result of the use of drugs that irritate the stomach lining (especially NSAIDs), and through alcohol abuse, smoking, Crohn's disease or from infections of a viral or bacterial nature. Acute gastritis, characterized by severe symptoms of short duration, is caused by ingestion of mucosal irritants or high doses of radiation.[8] Other irritants that may play a causative role in gastritis include heavy spices and tobacco.

Another type of acute gastritis is known as "acute stress gastritis." It is brought on by illness or injury, often an injury involving serious burns or profuse bleeding. Conditions such as high fever, heart attack and kidney failure may also give rise to acute stress gastritis.[9]

Indequate water intake is a major factor involved in gastritis. Water is needed to maintain a healthy mucosal layer in the stomach, which protects the stomach lining from stomach acid, pathogenic bacteria and other irritants.

What Are the Signs and Symptoms?

Many cases of gastritis will cause no symptoms at all.[10] Where symptoms do exist, the type of gastritis will determine their nature. The most commonly experienced gastritis symptoms include:

- Heartburn
- Pain in the upper abdomen
- Bloating
- Nausea/vomiting
- Belching
- Black, tarry stools (a sign of GI bleeding)
- Loss of appetite
- Weight loss

With its rapid onset, acute stress gastritis can lead to ulceration and bleeding, which can be fatal.[11]

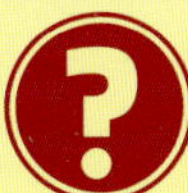

Did You Know

- Gastritis means inflammation of the stomach. It usually involves only the mucosal lining, not the entire stomach wall.
- Gastritis does not mean that there is an ulcer. It is simply inflammation — either acute or chronic.
- Helicobacter pylori is the name of a bacteria that has learned to live in the thick mucous lining of the stomach. It results in acute and chronic inflammation. It can occur early in childhood and remains throughout life. The infection can lead to ulcers and other gastric problems that are even more serious. Fortunately, there are now ways to treat this disorder.
- Currently in the United States, gastritis accounts for approximately 2 million visits to doctors' offices each year. Although gastritis can occur in people of all ages and backgrounds, it is especially common in:
  - Smokers
  - People over age 60
  - People who drink alcohol excessively
  - People who routinely use NSAIDs, especially at high doses
  - Viral infections – brief bouts of gastritis are common during short-term viral infections

How Is It Diagnosed?

As with all conditions, a thorough patient history is needed to assist in determining the cause of gastritis. A history of chronic NSAID use or alcohol abuse is particularly relevant.

Possible Gastric Irritants

- **Pepper**
- **Curry powder**
- **Cocoa**
- **Chili powder**
- **Chocolate**
- **Alcohol**
- **Caffeine-containing beverages**
- **Decaffeinated (and regular) coffee**

Gastritis is typically diagnosed through endoscopic examination. A small piece of stomach tissue can be snipped off (biopsied) using the endoscope, and later analyzed to help determine the type of inflammation. A biopsy can confirm the presence of H. pylori as can special blood and breath tests. With the aid of the endoscope, the doctor is also able to cauterize any damaged tissue, and thereby stop any bleeding that may be occurring.

In addition to gastroscopy, other tests may be performed. Physicians may order a stool analysis to detect blood or abnormalities. Holistic-minded physicians may order a specialized stool test called the comprehensive stool analysis (CSA), described in the Appendix. This test yields comprehensive information about the patient's digestive capabilities.

What Is the Standard Medical Treatment?

Unfortunately, Western-trained medical doctors in most cases do not ask enough questions of their patients' lifestyle, such as diet and NSAID use, to determine the root cause of gastritis. If an irritant, such as alcohol or a drug, is found to be the cause of gastritis, the condition can be expected to resolve following removal of that irritant. If the culprit is H. pylori, standard treatment will involve a course of antibiotics and the use of an acid-suppressing drug. Bismuth, an element that protects the stomach lining by protecting the mucous membranes from being dissolved by acid and pepsin,[12] may also be added to the regimen.

In acute gastritis or in painful flare-ups of chronic gastritis, the patient, if hospitalized, is given no solid food for 24 to 48 hours depending upon the severity of symptoms. Parenteral nutrition (placing nutrients directly into the bloodstream through an IV) may be administered if the patient is undernourished. As recovery occurs, the patient will progress to a soft or bland diet. The soft diet is a low-fiber one that helps in the transition from a liquid to a solid diet. The bland diet eliminates foods that are irritating to the GI tract.

Fried foods may be eliminated as well, as these have been found to reduce gastric emptying.[13] Some patients may find dairy products cause problems and will need to avoid these as well. The person with chronic gastritis would do well to eat small, frequent meals and avoid excessive fat intake.

The chronic form of gastritis may reduce the ability to secrete stomach acid and intrinsic factor,[14] both needed to absorb vitamin B12. For this reason, supplementation of B12 may be best accomplished through injection.

In addition, low stomach acid can cause malabsorption of most B vitamins, iron, zinc and amino acids. Iron is best supplemented through whole-food nutritional supplements or food sources.

Major iron-rich foods include:
- Eggs
- Fish
- Liver
- Meat
- Poultry
- Leafy green vegetables
- Whole grains

Nonsteroidal Anti-Inflammatory Drugs (NSAIDs)

- **Aleve**
- **Bayer**
- **Advil**
- **Excedrin**
- **Naproxen**
- **Acetaminophen**
- **Ibuprofen**
- **Aspirin**
- **Motrin**

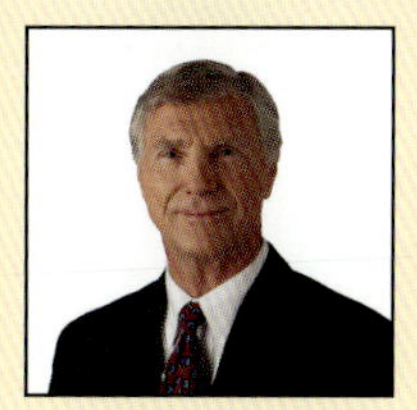

Dr. Smith's Comments

Chronic gastritis can have many causes, as mentioned in the text. However, at least 85 percent of them seem to be associated with H. pylori. In these cases, probiotics may be of considerable value. A literature review found seven out of nine human studies evaluating probiotics for improvement of H. pylori gastritis showed a decrease in the density of H. pylori in the stomach.[15] Adding probiotics to triple antibiotic therapy with PPIs (proton pump inhibitors) has been shown to be beneficial in treating H. pylori with less side effects. I would think it wise to continue the use of probiotics, in addition to vitamin C, as a good overall nutritional program indefinitely after the pharmaceutical therapy of gastritis.

Celiac disease or gluten sensitivity is at least one other cause of atrophic/autoimmune gastritis involving activation of T cells and B cells. Damage is done to the gastric lining parietal cells causing hypochlorhydria and B12 deficiency that leads to the same problems as are found with H. Pylori damage. In fact, a recent study from my alma mater, the University of Miami, documented a statistically significant 8- to 9-fold increase in gastric carcinoids since the introduction and widespread use of PPIs.[16]

In addition, diagnostic testing, such as the breath urease test, would be wise as annual follow-up, since there is a high recurrence rate of H. pylori infection.

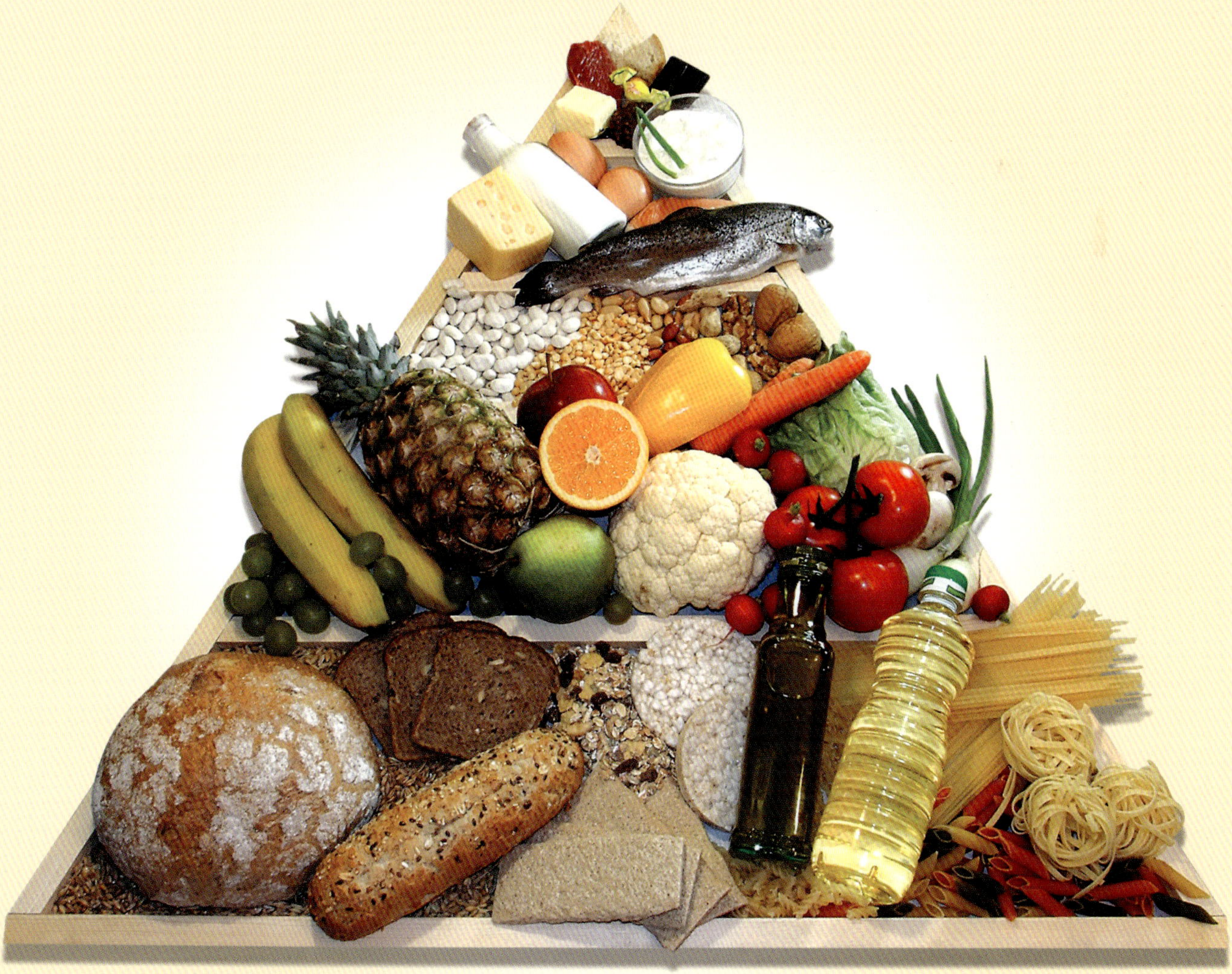

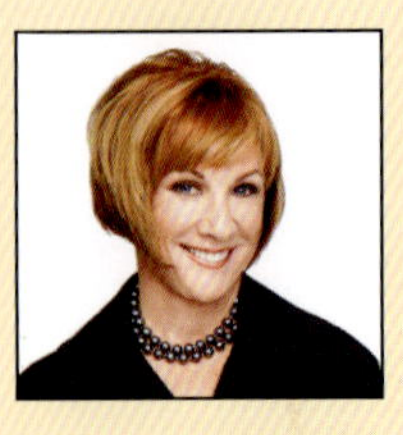

Brenda's Bottom Line

Gastritis can be a serious condition because it may lead to more serious stomach issues, most notably cancer. Usually gastritis starts as a mild condition, often as recurrent stomach upset that may or may not have an explainable cause.

The more this stomach irritation recurs, the more severe the gastritis. One major culprit in gastritis development is infection with the organism H. pylori. A test will be done to determine if this infection is present and, if found, antibiotic and acid-blocking medications will be prescribed. This is okay for a short-term period, but usually acid-blocking medications are unnecessarily prescribed long-term, which leads to serious health consequences including increased risk for developing C. difficile infections, pneumonia, osteoporosis-related bone fractures and nutrient deficiencies which lead to further problems yet.

I cannot emphasize enough the dangers of long-term blocking of acid production. The stomach produces acid for very good reasons: to kill off any potentially pathogenic organisms that pass through the stomach; to help with the absorption of key nutrients like vitamin B12, selenium and zinc; to help break down proteins from food; and to stimulate the production of pepsin, a protein-degrading enzyme. Decreasing stomach acid production treats symptoms, but does nothing for treating the underlying cause of the condition.

The other underlying issues that lead to stomach irritation and gastritis are multiple. One major factor is diet. A poor, low-fiber diet will lead to digestive imbalances that may be further worsened by overuse of non steroidal anti-inflammatory drugs (NSAIDs), Candida overgrowth, food sensitivities or dehydration. All of these factors may contribute to gastritis and should be ruled out. (See the Candidiasis section, Gluten Sensitivity section and the Allergies section for more information on these conditions.)

Recommended Testing

- Heidelberg pH test (see the Appendix) to determine stomach acid level
- Comprehensive stool analysis (CSA) (See the Appendix.)
- Food sensitivity test (See the Appendix.)

Diet

- Drink eight ounces of room temperature water 30 minutes before each meal
- Eliminate fatty, spicy and acidic foods that are known to irritate the stomach (such as cocoa, chili, high-sugar and processed foods) at least until healed.
- Slowly move to the Fiber 35 Eating Plan when feeling better. (See the Appendix.)
- Cabbage juice is excellent for the stomach.
- Slippery elm or ginger tea may be helpful to soothe stomach irritation.

Lifestyle

- Stop smoking and drinking alcohol, at least until healed.
- Avoid NSAIDs (nonsteroidal anti-inflammatory drugs) as these can worsen gastritis.

Complementary Mind/Body Therapies

- Stress-reduction therapies such as yoga, biofeedback, massage and meditation can be helpful when stress is an issue.
- Acupuncture may be helpful because it targets the meridians associated with the digestive system, and is also a stress reducer.
- Colon hydrotherapy will be helpful for gastritis.

Recommended Nutraceuticals	Dosage	Benefit	Comments
Critical Phase	Daily maintenance recommendations should also be taken during this phase unless otherwise indicated.		
L-Glutamine Powder with Gamma Oryzanol	10 grams (10,000 mg) daily in split doses on empty stomach with water for two weeks	Helps repair the stomach lining and reduce inflammation.	Best taken in loose powder for contact with stomach lining.
Natural Heartburn Formula	Chew in acute situation, and only when needed	Temporarily neutralizes acid and soothes digestive tract.	Look for ingredients such as fava bean, ellagic acid, calcium, magnesium and aloe.
Helpful			
B-Complex with extra B-12	Use as directed	B vitamins are needed for proper acid production.	Especially helpful as vitamin B levels decrease with age.
Daily Maintenance			
Probiotics	200 billion culture count per dose	Stimulates immune system and reduces inflammation.	Best taken in loose powder for contact with stomach lining.
L-Glutamine Powder with Gamma Oryzanol	5 grams (5000 mg) daily on empty stomach with water after critical phase	Helps repair the stomach lining and reduce inflammation.	Best taken in loose powder for contact with stomach lining.
Antioxidant Supplement	Use as directed	Protects tissue from damage.	You can purchase a high-potency antioxidant formulation from health food stores.
Digestive Enzymes	Take with meals	Helps digest food and reduce reflux.	Look for one with high-potency protease, amylase, lipase and cellulase.
Omega-3 Fatty Acids	At lease 2 grams daily of EPA/DHA combination	Reduces inflammation.	Look for a concentrated, enteric coated high dose EPA/DHA formulation.
Fiber	4-5 grams twice daily	Reduces stomach acidity.	Look for a flax-based fiber with added ingredients such as glutamine, probiotics and healing herbs.

See further explanation of supplements in the Appendix

Peptic Ulcers

What Is It?

"Peptic" means pertaining to pepsin (the protein-digesting enzyme produced in the stomach), or to digestion, or to the action of gastric juices.[1] An ulcer is a sore or lesion. A peptic ulcer is a sore that develops in the mucous lining of the stomach (gastric ulcer), duodenum (duodenal ulcer), or the esophagus (esophageal ulcer) and the underlying tissue as a result of exposure to stomach acid and pepsin. One in 10 Americans will develop a peptic ulcer at some time in their lives.[2] Gastric, duodenal and esophageal ulcers all fall under the category of peptic ulcer. The duodenal ulcer is the most frequent type, occurring four to five times more frequently than the gastric ulcer.[3] Esophageal ulcers are quite rare. They can develop as a consequence of gastroesophageal reflux disease (GERD), which involves regurgitation of stomach acid (and pepsin) into the esophagus where it burns delicate tissue. (See the GERD section.)

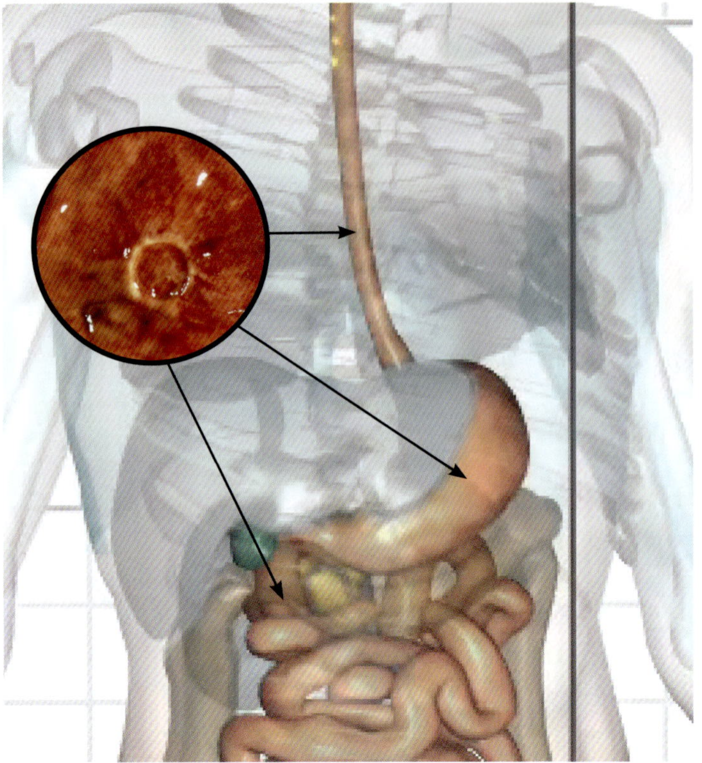

Illustration of the human body with an endoscopic image of a peptic ulcer

What Causes It?

Stress was once viewed as the major cause of peptic ulcers. The thinking was that stress caused an over-production of stomach acid which irritated the mucosal lining giving rise to an ulcer. While it is true that ulcers occur in the presence of stomach acid, it does not necessarily follow that excessive quantities of hydrochloric acid (HCl) are the cause of the condition.

In fact, given the fact that some people who have ulcers produce too little gastric acid, and others without ulcers have too much acid,[4] it seems safe to conclude that the amount of acid produced is not a critical variable in determining who will get ulcers and who will not.

More relevant seems to be the integrity of the protective mechanisms designed to shield tissues from the caustic effects of stomach acid. Ulcers occur due to an imbalance between the stomach acid and the mucosal lining of the stomach. The key player in this balance is the mucosal lining. If this lining is compromised, even a small amount of stomach acid can produce an ulcer.[5]

The stress-causes-ulcer model was largely abandoned in the earlier 1980s when Dr. Barry Marshall, an Australian researcher, discovered the presence of a bacterium, Helicobacter pylori (H. pylori), between the lining of the stomach and the protective mucous layer in ulcer patients. To prove the cause-effect relationship between H. pylori[6] and ulcers, researchers actually ingested the bacteria themselves and subsequently developed ulcers.[7]

It has been widely reported that the majority of patients with peptic ulcers have H. pylori, which is thought to weaken the mucosa over time leaving the stomach vulnerable to the caustic effects of its own acid.[8] H. pylori has been identified in many patients with peptic ulcers, but not all of them. Once H. pylori was estimated to be present in 65 to 100 percent of peptic ulcer sufferers. However, recent studies have suggested that the number is much lower, and could be below 50 percent.[9]

If H. pylori were the sole cause of ulcers, it would be found in all ulcer patients, and would be absent in those without ulcers. This is not the case, however. Many people

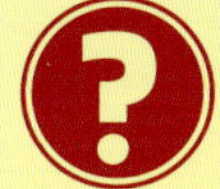

Did You Know

The prevalence of H.pylori in developing countries is higher than in developed countries, with most infections occurring during childhood.[13] Up to 70 percent of children under age 15 have been found to be infected with the bacterium.[14] In the US, 20-50 percent of people are infected with H.pylori.

in the U.S. have tested positive for H. pylori (about 20 percent for those under 40, and more than 50 percent of those over 60), but most people with H. pylori will never develop ulcers.[10] It is estimated that 40 million people in the U.S. have H. pylori, but only 10 to 20 percent of them will develop an ulcer.[11]

While H. pylori does not appear to be the sole cause of peptic ulcers, it seems to be an important contributing variable. When H. pylori is successfully eradicated, the rate of recurrence of these ulcers is greatly diminished.[12]

It would appear that the cause of peptic ulcers is multi-faceted—that is to say, there is more than one cause. However, most of the agents which lead to ulcer development reduce the integrity of the mucosal lining. Some important factors include:

- Regular use of nonsteroidal anti-inflammatory drugs (NSAIDs) such as aspirin (See the Gastritis section for the full list.)
- Use of steroid drugs like cortisone
- Alcohol consumption (moderate to excessive)
- Heavy smoking
- A family history of peptic ulcer disease
- Stress
- Nutrient deficiencies
- A low-fiber diet
- Food allergies
- Caffeine-containing beverages
- Dehydration
- Severe illness or trauma (causing a "stress ulcer")

It has been found that aspirin use at any level is a risk factor for developing peptic ulcers, although higher doses cause more gastrointestinal bleeding.[15] Those taking low-dose aspirin therapy in an effort to prevent heart disease, may therefore be putting themselves at risk for developing peptic ulcers.

Aspirin and other NSAIDs interfere with the stomach's ability to produce protective mucus and acid-neutralizing bicarbonate. They also affect blood flow to the stomach and interfere with cell repair.[16] Between two to four percent of patients who take NSAIDs for a year develop serious gastrointestinal complications, including ulcers and bleeding from the stomach and small intestine.[17]

Stress is certainly not the major culprit in ulcer formation as it was once thought to be. In fact, several studies have shown that the number of stressful life events is not significantly different in peptic ulcer patients than in carefully selected, ulcer-free controls.[18] However, stress hormones do affect stomach acid secretions, and ulcer patients do tend to have flare-ups during stressful times. Stress would therefore appear to be a factor contributing to peptic ulcers.

Dehydration as a cause of ulcers was recognized in the striking work of Dr. Batmanghelidj, an MD who found that the stomach needs plenty of water in order to produce adequate mucus. Amazingly, while imprisoned in Iran, he was able to successfully treat ulcers in fellow inmates using nothing but water.[19]

Food allergies, especially to dairy products, have been found to be a primary factor in many cases of peptic ulcer.[20] The truth is, population studies show that the higher the milk consumption, the greater the likelihood of ulcer.[21] This is because food allergies can initiate histamine release, which in turn stimulates HCl-producing cells, and produces more acid.

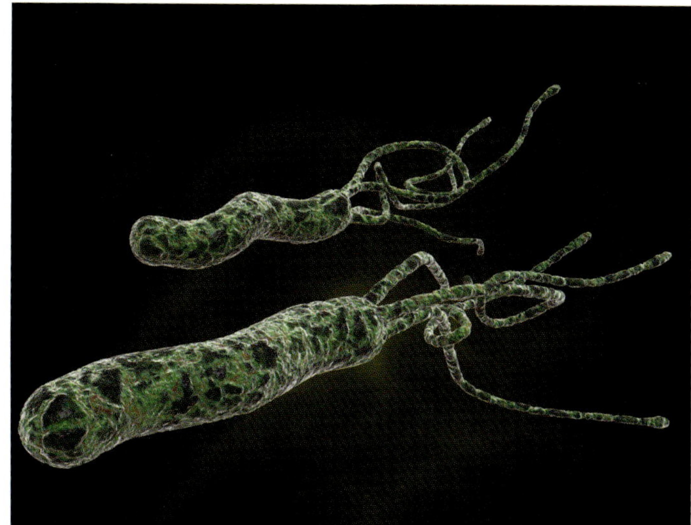

Helicobacter pylori organism

Antioxidant nutrients—vitamins A, C and E and the mineral zinc—protect the stomach lining from irritation by combating free radical damage. Free radicals are renegade chemical fragments that are injurious to cells. Inadequate levels of antioxidant nutrients, as well as a deficiency of vitamin B6 and the amino acid glutamine, may contribute to ulcers.[22] Where the antioxidant content of the GI tract lining is low, the likelihood of H. pylori infection is increased.

People who eat high-fiber diets have a lower rate of ulcers than those who consume low-fiber diets.[23] Fiber is found in whole grains, fruits and vegetables and is notoriously lacking in the processed Standard American Diet (SAD). Not only will a high-fiber diet help prevent ulcers, it has been shown to reduce the recurrence of recently healed duodenal ulcers by half.[24]

Lifestyle and dietary choices play a key role in ulcer formation. For instance, smoking appears is a major contributor to peptic ulcer disease. Those who smoke can expect to have a higher incidence of peptic ulcers, a higher rate of return of ulcers, and a decreased response to treatment.[25]

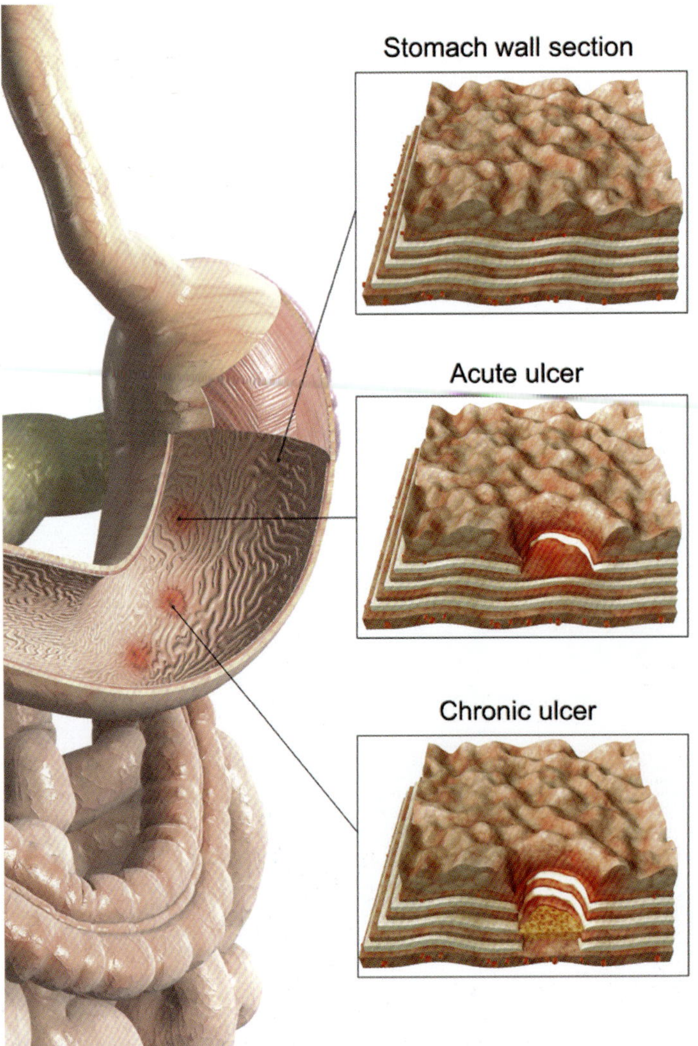

There are several reasons for this. The most significant is that smoking increases the reflux (backflow) of bile salts into the stomach causing irritation to the stomach and duodenum.[26] Smoking also contributes oxidants to the blood which can further hinder the healing process. Alcohol consumption is another problem for peptic ulcers. Alcohol irritates the stomach lining, and continued use of it interferes with ulcer healing.

The rationale for the avoidance of coffee and other caffeine-containing beverages and drugs is that caffeine seems to stimulate acid secretion in the stomach, which increases ulcer pain. Interestingly, decaffeinated coffee has the same effect as regular coffee, so clearly adverse effects are due to something more than just the caffeine.[27]

Although ulcers can affect people of all ages, it is rare for children to develop them. The risk of ulcer formation increases with age. Duodenal ulcers tend to occur more often in men than in women. Also, the age at onset of a duodenal ulcer is lower (30 to 50 years of age) than the more rare stomach ulcers (over age 60). Interestingly, these rarer forms of ulcer affect more women than men.[28]

What Are the Signs and Symptoms?

Many people with ulcers have no symptoms.[29] Those who do experience symptoms will feel pain in the upper abdomen underneath the breastbone. It may be a cramping, burning or gnawing sensation that feels like a hunger pang. The pain may be constant or intermittent.

Those with gastric ulcers will feel the pain just below the rib cage to the left, while the pain of duodenal ulcers is felt a little to the right of the mid-abdominal region. Often this pain is worse at night and between meals because gastric acid is more likely to cause irritation when the stomach is empty.

Food acts as a buffer to neutralize acid, and quickly relieves the pain of duodenal ulcers. Certain foods, though, may irritate and cause more pain. (See the chart in the Gastritis section.) Although this food may irritate gastric ulcers initially, the burning generally subsides as acid is neutralized.[30]

Other possible signs and symptoms of peptic ulcers include:

- Headache
- A choking sensation
- Nausea/vomiting
- Back pain
- Black tarry stools
- Paleness
- Weakness
- Loss of appetite
- Weight loss
- Dizziness

Incidents of black tarry stools and paleness are signs of internal bleeding. The symptoms are dizziness and weakness. Blood may also appear in vomit (looking like coffee grounds). These signs of hemorrhage should be treated as an emergency, and one should seek immediate medical attention.

How Is It Diagnosed?

Ulcers cannot be definitively diagnosed by symptoms alone for two reasons:

1. Only half of those with ulcers have symptoms, and the symptoms typical of peptic ulcers are the same as those of stomach cancer.[31] Gastric ulcers may be malignant (cancerous), while duodenal ulcers are almost never malignant.[32]

2. Symptoms of peptic ulcer may be similar to those of gastroesophageal reflux disease (GERD) and gastritis.

Endoscopy, which involves the use of a camera at the end of a tube inserted through the mouth into the digestive tract, is typically used to detect ulcers. H. pylori can be identified through a biopsy taken with the endoscope. The bacterium also shows up in special blood and breath tests. All of these tests are about 90 percent effective in detecting H. pylori.[33] Endoscopic biopsy can also rule out malignancy in gastric ulcers.

Another test for identifying gastric or duodenal ulcers is the upper GI series, also known as a barium swallow. Additionally, special stool and/or blood tests may be done to check for hidden (occult) blood.

A test that is often performed by progressive physicians is the comprehensive stool analysis (CSA). In this test, stool samples are taken at home and submitted to a laboratory. (See the Appendix.) The test helps identify problems with digestion and absorption, as well as microbial imbalances in the gut. This can be helpful in terms of getting to the cause of the problem, for H. pylori infection often results from an imbalance in the ecology of the gut.

A stool antigen test, used to measure antibodies for H. pylori in the stool, and the urea breath test, which measures urea (a metabolic by-product of H. pylori) in the breath, are effective tests for indicating the presence of H. pylori in the stomach.[34]

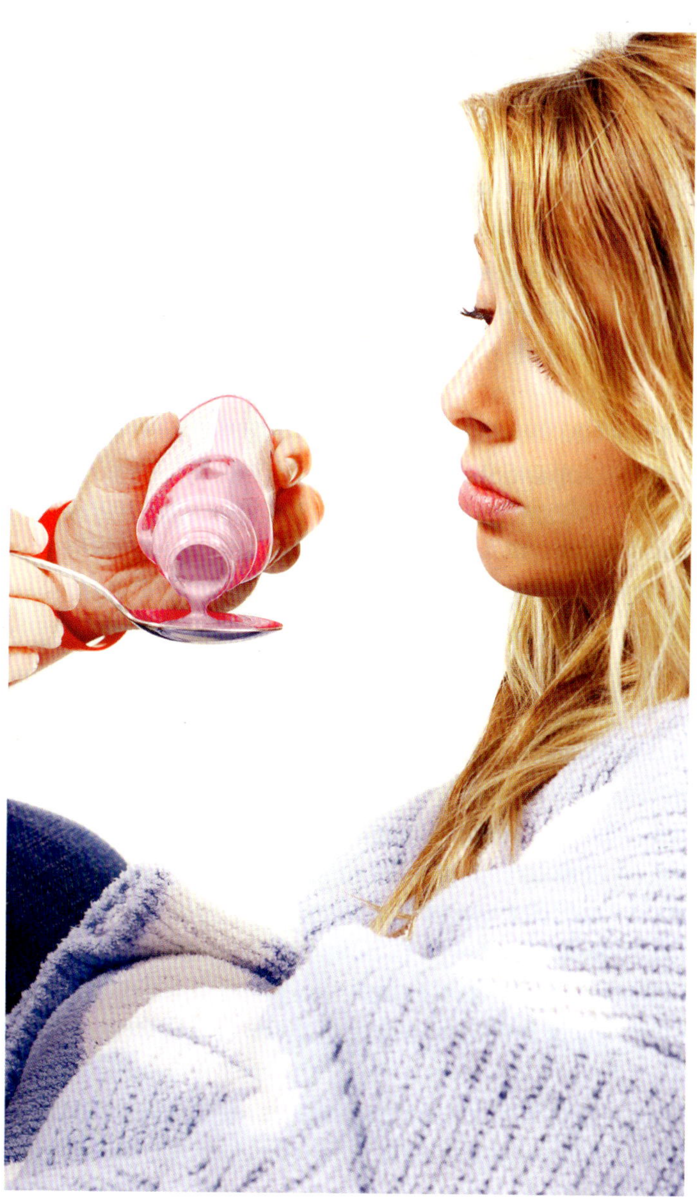

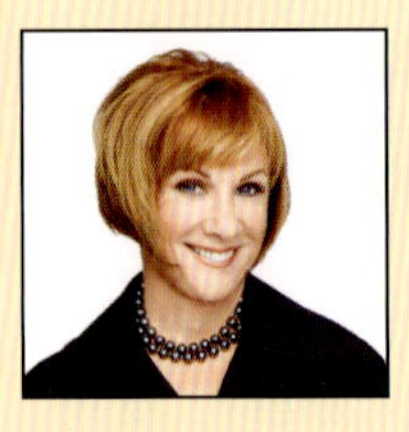

Brenda's Bottom Line

Though peptic ulcers can be considered serious in many cases, if you look at the reasons most people develop this problem, we are back to the same old song – a poor diet low in fiber. People do not eat a high-fiber breakfast, if they eat breakfast at all, and this sets the stage for imbalance in the digestive system. When you wake up, you begin to produce stomach acid that needs to be buffered with a high-fiber food. (See the Fiber 35 Eating Plan in the Appendix.) In addition, overuse of nonsteroidal anti-inflammatory drugs (NSAIDs) damages the gut lining leading to the development of ulcers and leaky gut.

Also notable, I encounter food sensitivities as a culprit in many people with these conditions. Food sensitivities should be ruled out as an underlying issue. (See the Gluten Sensitivity section or Allergies section.) In cases of suspected food sensitivity, I suggest stool tests from EnteroLab to rule out gluten, dairy or soy sensitivities.

Certainly a test for H. pylori should be administered as part of the traditional medical practice. If positive, antibiotics and acid-blocking medications will be prescribed. You can become reinfected with H. pylori again and again. You must start HCl production in the stomach to keep the bacteria from coming back. From that point on, it is essential to heal the gut with L-glutamine and gamma oryzanol and rebalance with probiotics. Additionally, Candida overgrowth needs to be ruled out. Follow a Candida Diet (see the Appendix) for at least a month.

Most importantly, do not, under any circumstances, take acid-blocking medication long term. I was speaking to an audience one night when a woman in her senior years stated that she had H. pylori, and that her doctor had put her on acid-blocking medication. I told her that it's okay short term, as long as they also give antibiotics to kill the bacteria.

I asked her how long ago she had the infection, to which she replied, "Fifteen years." She had been on acid-blocking medication for 15 years! I am shocked at the level of credibility we give doctors who would do such a thing. It never ceases to amaze me!
Taking acid-blocking medications increases risk for pneumonia and C. difficile infections, osteoporosis-related bone fractures and malabsorption of key nutrients like B12, zinc and selenium.

Rule out or treat H. pylori infection. The following recommendations are for healing and repair of the stomach lining.

Recommended Testing

- H. pylori test
- Heidelberg pH test (See the Appendix) to determine stomach acid level
- Comprehensive stool analysis (CSA) (See the Appendix.)
- Food sensitivity test (See the Appendix.)

Diet

- Eliminate fatty, spicy, and acidic foods known to irritate the stomach (such as cocoa, chili, high sugar and processed foods), at least until healed.
- Begin to incorporate the Fiber 35 Eating plan when feeling better. (See the Appendix.)

Lifestyle

- Drink plenty of water and decaffeinated herbal teas.
- Stop smoking and drinking alcohol, at least until healed.

Complementary Mind / Body Therapies

- Stress-reduction therapies such as yoga, biofeedback, massage and meditation can be helpful when stress is an issue.
- Acupuncture may be helpful because it targets the meridians associated with the digestive system, and is also a stress reducer.
- Chiropractic may be beneficial.
- Colon hydrotherapy may be helpful.

Recommended Nutraceuticals	Dosage	Benefit	Comments
Critical Phase Daily maintenance recommendations should also be taken during this phase unless otherwise indicated.			
L-Glutamine Powder with Gamma Oryzanol	10 grams (10,000 mg) daily in split doses on empty stomach with water for two weeks	Helps repair the stomach lining and reduce inflammation.	Best taken in loose powder for contact with stomach lining.
Natural Heartburn Formula	Chew in acute situation, and only when needed	Temporarily neutralizes acid and soothes digestive tract.	Look for ingredients such as fava bean, ellagic acid, calcium, magnesium and aloe.
Helpful			
Antioxidant Supplements	Use as directed	Protects tissue from damage.	You can purchase a high-potency antioxidant formulation from most health food stores.
Daily Maintenance			
Omega-3 Fatty Acids	At lease 2 grams daily of EPA/DHA combination	Reduces Inflammation.	Look for a concentrated, enteric coated high dose EPA/DHA formulation.
Fiber	4-5 grams twice daily	Reduces acidity, reduces rate of recurrence.	Look for a flax-based fiber with added ingredients such as glutamine, probiotics and healing herbs.
Digestive Enzyme with HCl	Take with meals	Replaces low HCl, creates environment inhospitable to H. pylori.	Do not use HCL with active ulcer. Wait until healed and use as part of maintenance.
L-Glutamine Powder with Gamma Oryzanol	5 grams (5000 mg) daily on empty stomach with water after critical phase	Helps repair the stomach lining and reduce inflammation.	Best if taken in loose powder form.
Probiotics	200 billion culture count per dose	Stimulates immune system and reduces inflammation.	Best taken in loose powder for contact with stomach lining.

See further explanation of supplements in the Appendix

Appendicitis

What Is It?

The appendix is a small tubular structure attached to the right side of the cecum, the lower right portion of the large intestine (colon). Appendicitis is either an acute or chronic inflammation of the appendix. Normally, the appendix resembles the little finger, being three to four inches long and one quarter of an inch in diameter. When inflamed, the appendix can swell, and the wall can fill with dead white blood cells (pus). This local infection can rapidly spread to the rest of the body. The pathological definition of appendicitis is the microscopic presence of white blood cells in the wall of the appendix.

In the past, medicine has not been able to assign a particular function to the appendix. Today, however, it is becoming more apparent that the appendix and surrounding lymphatic tissue probably serve an important role in immunity. Bowel movements in a liquid or semi-solid state pass in and out of the appendix. Research now supports the concept that microbes found in stool have a dynamic communication with the intestinal lining, including the lining of the appendix. Signals are sent from these microbes to the lymph tissue creating a memory bank of immune information. Future exposure will then cause the immune system to either accept or reject previously recognized microbial populations.

Additionally, it has been determined that the appendix functions as a "safe house" for the beneficial bacteria in the gut.[1] The beneficial bacteria inside the appendix form a biofilm that offers protection against pathogens. When a bout of diarrhea comes through the intestine, these bacteria are protected and reinoculate the gut once the diarrhea subsides.

What Causes It?

The cause of appendicitis is not officially known, though there are several possible causes of the condition. The appendix may become obstructed with solid pieces of stool (faecaliths or appendicoliths). Occasionally, impaction of

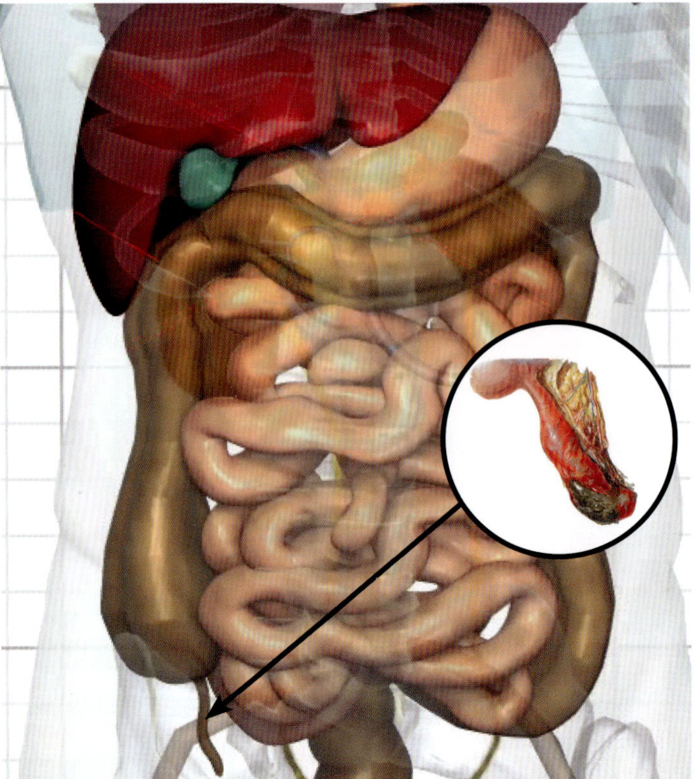

Illustration of the human body with a zoomed image showing an inflamed appendix

the appendix can occur secondary to parasites, especially pinworms.

Swollen lymph nodes at the base of the appendix can be another cause of appendicitis, secondary to a viral or bacterial infection. This swollen tissue can impede lymphatic or venous drainage, causing the appendix to swell. The pressure from the swelling may hamper arterial inflow resulting in decreased oxygen to the tissues followed by inflammation, more swelling and even gangrene and rupture of the appendix.

From the natural medicine perspective, chronic constipation, high concentrations of bad or pathogenic bacteria, absence of friendly bacteria, and decreased fiber could all play a role in appendicitis. In addition, tumors may be found in the appendix, both benign and malignant, usually found incidentally during surgery.

People of any age may develop appendicitis, but it most commonly occurs in pre-teens, teenagers and young

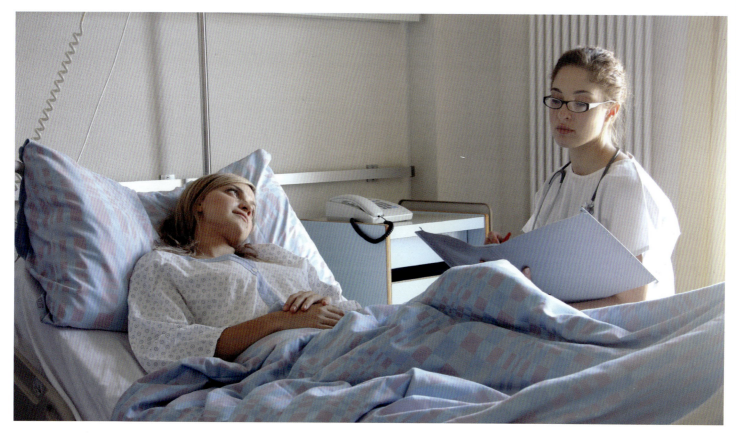

adults. It is most common between the ages of 10 and 30. Aside from trapped hernias, appendicitis is the most common cause of sudden abdominal surgery in the United States.[2] Younger children and elderly adults are at higher risk of developing a rupture—a perforation of the appendix that allows its contents to enter the abdominal cavity. This is a serious complication that requires immediate surgery.[3,4]

Interestingly, though men have appendicitis more than women, more appendectomies are performed on women.[6]

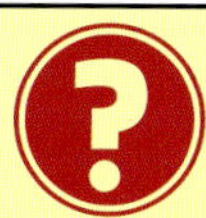

Did You Know

- The risk of appendicitis increases with age, and peaks between the ages of 15 and 30. However, appendicitis is also the main reason for abdominal surgery in children, with four of every 1,000 children requiring an appendectomy (surgical removal of the appendix) before age 14.[5]

- Although the duration of symptoms varies, most patients will seek medical attention within 12 to 48 hours because of the abdominal pain. In some cases, a low level of inflammation exists for several weeks before a diagnosis is made.

This is due to the fact that appendicitis can mimic other disorders, such as inflammation, and cysts of the ovaries and fallopian tubes. In these cases, a normal appendix may be removed to prevent further diagnostic dilemmas for the patient in the future.

The risk of developing appendicitis increases after a recent illness, especially a gastrointestinal infection or a roundworm infection.[7]

What Are the Signs and Symptoms?

The hallmark symptom of appendicitis is a pain running from the navel toward the lower right portion of the abdomen. This pain may come in waves initially, but becomes progressively more constant and pronounced. Pain typically worsens with movement, as with coughing or when the area is touched. Other signs and symptoms may include:

- Nausea/vomiting
- Change in bowel habits (constipation or diarrhea, inability to pass gas)
- Fever
- Abdominal swelling
- Tenderness in right abdomen

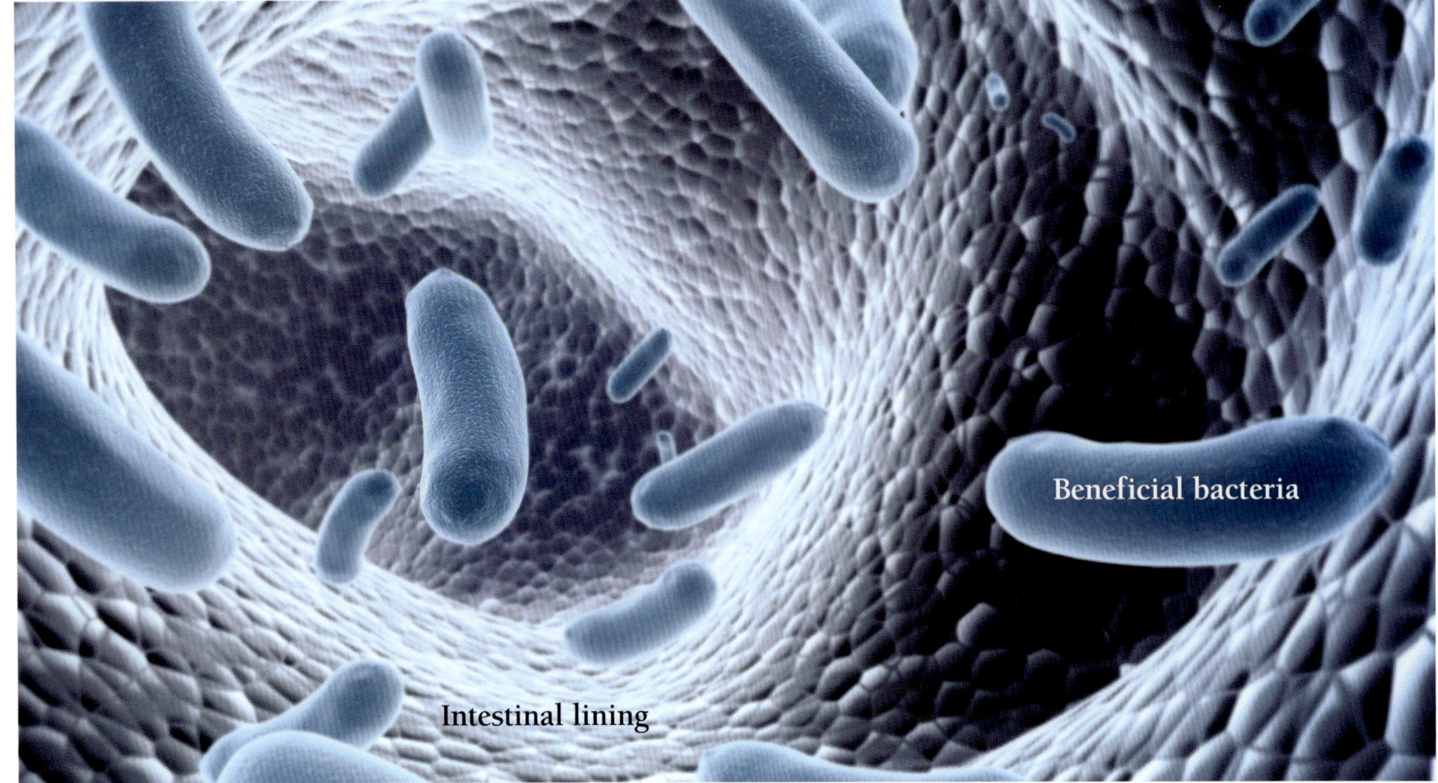

Beneficial bacteria reside in the appendix

- Loss of appetite
- Right-sided tenderness with walking, moving or coughing
- Elevated white blood count

Left untreated, an inflamed appendix can cause complications including tissue death (gangrene) of the appendix, a collection of pus (abscess) in, or in the vicinity of, the appendix, and blood poisoning (sepsis) caused by infectious bacteria or rupture of the appendix. When the appendix ruptures, fecal liquid and material plus pus spread throughout the abdominal cavity causing inflammation of the abdominal lining (peritonitis). This can be a life-threatening condition. The risk of these complications makes appendicitis an emergency condition. While the death rate for those whose appendix hasn't ruptured is quite low, it rises significantly if the appendix bursts.[8] These rates increase for the very young and the very old.

How Is It Diagnosed?

Appendicitis is generally diagnosed on the basis of medical history, physical exam and an ultrasound of the abdomen. Blood and urine tests may be done to check for infection. A recent study looked at 500 patients who underwent appendectomy. It was found that, for women, if a CT scan or ultrasound was done before the surgery, a healthy appendix was removed seven percent of the time compared to 28 percent of the time if a scan was not done. However, in some studies, this lowered rate did not hold up in men or children.[9] Ultrasound of the abdomen and pelvis is now a mainstay in the evaluation of the appendix.

What Is the Standard Medical Treatment?

Because of the risks of rupture, appendicitis is treated as a medical emergency with surgical removal of the appendix as the treatment of choice. An increasing number of surgeons are performing laparoscopic surgery in which a miniature camera and surgical instruments are inserted through tiny cuts in the abdomen. There are numerous claimed advantages to this procedure: less infection, fewer adhesions, less pain and scarring, and a more rapid recovery. There are instances, however, in which it is necessary to use traditional (open) surgical procedures to remove the appendix. Typically, antibiotics are administered as well as intravenous fluids, and if nausea occurs the patient will be given medication to control vomiting.

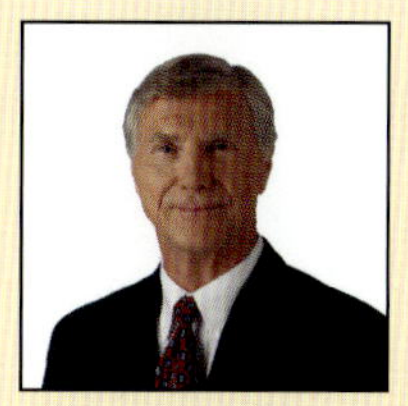

Dr. Smith's Comments

Appendicitis is a common surgical emergency requiring experience in making an accurate diagnosis. If the diagnosis is not clear, sometimes the judgment to proceed with the operation is best. Still, 10 to 20 percent of appendectomies are done when the diagnosis should have been for other conditions including diverticulitis, inflammation of the right fallopian tube or ovary, and lymphadenitis (swollen lymph nodes in the tissue surrounding the appendix).

CT scan has decreased the incidence of non-therapeutic appendectomy from about 14 percent to 7 percent. Ultrasound is less expensive, and sometimes is very good in confirming the diagnosis. Either of these studies can be done when the diagnosis is not clear. This is often be the case with young children and older patients whose history, signs and symptoms may not be classical. Delay in surgery can result in ruptured appendix, a very serious problem that can lead to recurrent intra-abdominal infection.

Nutrition may play a role in prevention. It has been shown that for societies with high-fiber intake there is a much lower incidence of appendicitis. High-fiber intake combined with probiotics produces short-chain fatty acids that fuel and maintain the health of colonic and appendiceal cells.

Many cases of appendicitis are due to either bacterial or viral infection. Dietary and supplemental antioxidants (especially vitamin C) as well as essential fatty acids may help avoid the inflammatory changes that accompany the infection (a Th1 cellular type of inflammatory immune response), and, thereby, prevent the swelling that leads to full-blown appendicitis. Probiotics might also help prevent appendicitis because they may decrease the incidence of pathogenic bacteria that can lead to appendicitis.

If surgery has already been performed, the following may be added to the above supplements:

- Take 5,000 mg. to 10,000 mg of glutamine powder with N-acetyl-glucosamine (NAG) and gamma oryzanol once to twice daily on an empty stomach. (See the Supplement section of the Appendix.)

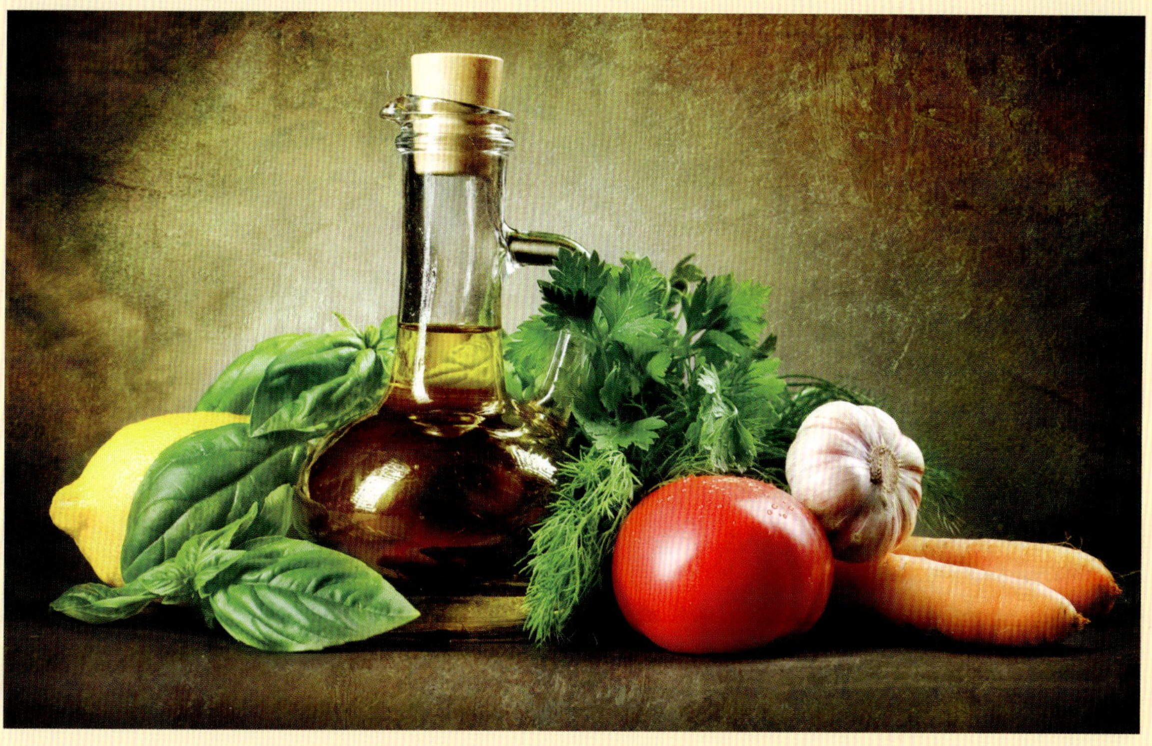

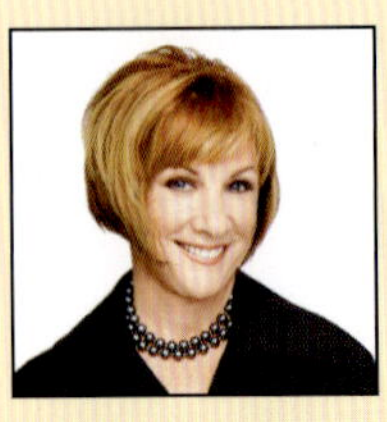

Brenda's Bottom Line

Because appendicitis is a medical emergency, a patient needs to tread lightly where alternatives are concerned. However, because of the potential for misdiagnosis, particularly for women, people should insist upon a complete diagnostic work up before electing surgery unless the appendix has ruptured, in which case immediate surgery must be performed.

Acute appendicitis is a condition that I have personal experience with. After years of being constipated, I developed appendicitis. When fecal matter is not moved out of the bowel regularly, it creates many problems in the intestines, one being irritation of the appendix. (See the Constipation section for more information on this condition.)

Getting to the root cause of constipation is an important part of preventing complications like appendicitis. Following the HOPE Program (High fiber, Omega oils, Probiotics and digestive Enzymes) helps to rebalance the digestive system and greatly reduces the chances of developing serious conditions like appendicitis.

Diet

- The Fiber 35 Eating Plan (see the Appendix) should be followed both as a preventive diet and after healing from an appendicitis episode.

Lifestyle

- Drink plenty of purified water daily. Ideally, drink half your body weight in ounces.
- For preventive measures, follow a Total Body Cleansing program twice a year.
- Exercise daily, even if just taking a walk. The mini trampoline can be beneficial to stimulate lymph flow.

Complimentary Mind/Body Therapies

- Colon hydrotherapy can be very helpful in prevention. Incorporate this into your cleansing program.
- Lymphatic massage is also beneficial for increasing movement of lymphatic fluid, thus stimulating the immune system.

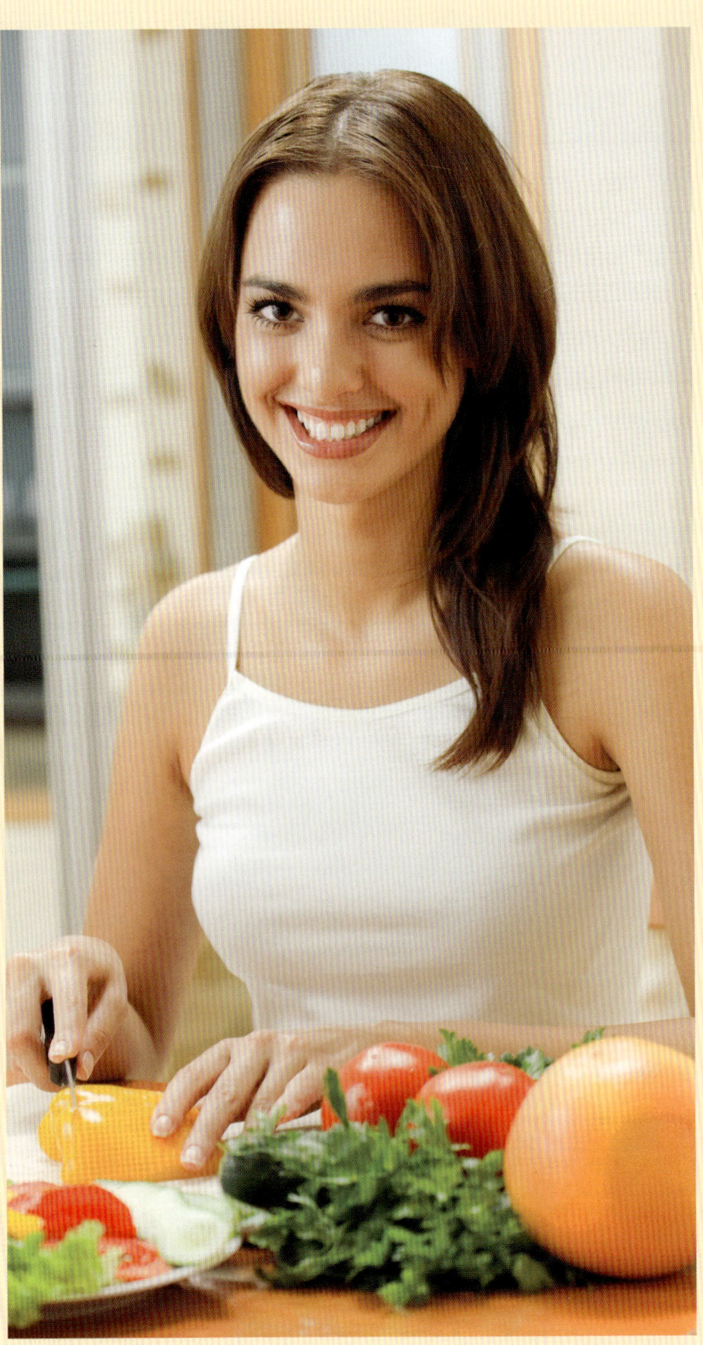

Recommended Nutraceuticals	Dosage	Benefit	Comments
Critical Phase	Daily maintenance recommendations should also be taken during this phase unless otherwise indicated.		
Follow daily maintenance protocol below.			
Helpful			
L-Glutamine Powder with Gamma Oryzanol	5 grams (5000 mg) daily on empty stomach with water	Helps repair and keep intestinal lining healthy.	Best if taken in loose powder form.
Daily Maintenance			
Probiotics	30 to 80 billion cultures daily	Helps reduce pathogenic bacteria from colonizing in the colon and appendix.	Look for a probiotic formulation with a high amount of bifidobacteria, the main bacteria for the colon.
Fiber	4-5 grams twice daily	Helps keep food moving through bowel, reduces toxic colon and accumulation of wastes.	Look for a flax-based fiber with added ingredients such as glutamine, probiotics and healing herbs.
Digestive Enzymes	Take with meals	Helps digest food matter into usable nutrients, reduces toxicity from undigested food.	Look for a supplement containing high amounts of protease, amalyase, lipase and cellulose along with others.
Omega-3 Fatty Acids	At least 2 grams daily of EPA/DHA combination	Reduces inflammation.	Look for a concentrated, enteric coated high dose EPA/DHA formulation

****See further explanation of supplements in the Appendix**

CANDIDIASIS

What Is It?

The presence of Candida albicans, a benign sugar-fermenting yeast, in various parts of the body—the skin, the genitals and especially the intestinal tract—is entirely normal. In small amounts, this yeast is an integral part of the intestinal ecology and, when kept in balance with other microorganisms, does no harm. Candidiasis, however, is a complex medical syndrome resulting from an overgrowth of Candida albicans. This yeast (or single-celled fungus) is one of 600 strains of Candida, and is among the minority that can become pathogenic (disease-causing).[1]

With candidiasis, normally harmless yeasts proliferate and change into a mycelial or hyphal form[2] where they take root in tissues and colonize. This upsets the ecological balance in the gastrointestinal tract. When the friendly gut bacteria that normally control Candida die off and Candida gains an upper hand, local problems can result—in the vagina (yeast infection), throat (thrush), nails (fungal infection), bladder (candidal cystitis), etc. When Candida colonizes in the gut, it can cause problems throughout the entire body due to the fact that potent, immune-suppressing toxins are absorbed into the bloodstream. Candida is actually a form of parasite, an organism that feeds off of the human body and can pollute the system with its toxic waste products if it is present in disproportionate quantities.

What Causes It?

There are multiple factors that may trigger the form change and proliferation of Candida that result in candidiasis. This condition develops when the balance between yeast and bacteria is upset as a result of:

- Immune dysfunction
- Disruption in ratio of good to bad bacteria in the gastrointestinal tract
- Upset in intestinal pH

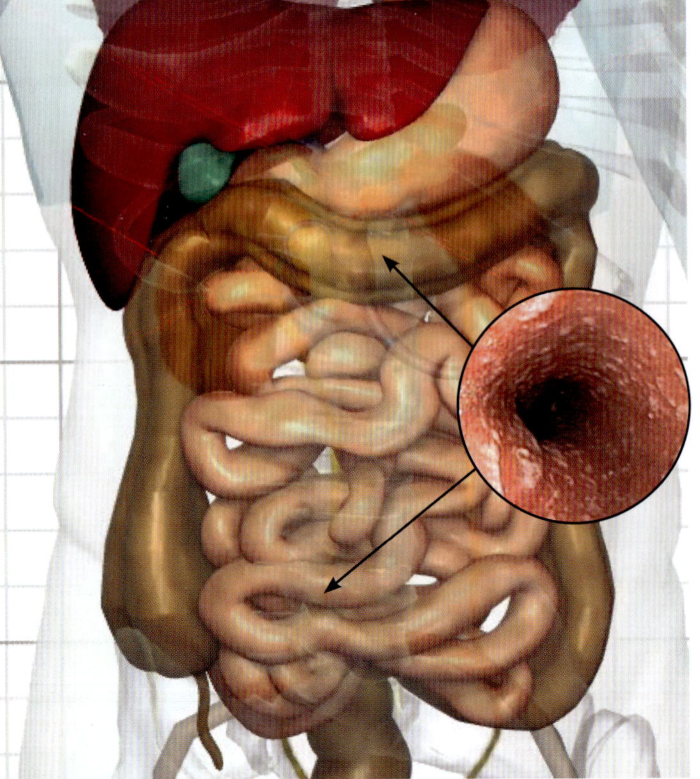

Illustration of the human body with an endoscopic image of Candida overgrowth

Immune dysfunction is caused by a number of factors:

- Ingestion of certain drugs (acid-blocking medication, antibiotics and corticosteroids)
- Exposure to toxic metals
- Internal toxins from poor digestion
- Consumption of refined carbohydrates
- Chemotherapy
- Stress

All of these factors create an imbalance of gut flora called dysbiosis, which can result in reduced or dysregulated immunity leading to candidiasis.

An alteration of the ratio of good to bad bacteria in the GI tract is a very common cause of candidiasis. In fact, the prolonged—and sometimes inappropriate—use (and overuse) of antibiotics is perhaps the most widespread cause of chronic candidiasis today. These drugs suppress not only pathogenic or bad bacteria, but also the friendly bacteria whose job it is to prevent yeast overgrowth. The net result is proliferation of Candida. As Candida proliferates, the fungus releases toxins (waste products called mycotoxins) that further weaken the immune system.

A by-product of Candida digestion of protein is beta-alanine. Beta-alanine is absorbed through the intestinal lining and secreted by the kidneys. It competes for reabsorption with the amino acid taurine in the kidneys and this lowers taurine levels. This is a significant problem because taurine enhances the intracellular uptake of magnesium and potassium. In addition, it helps to bind toxins and remove them from the liver. Thus, it has been clinically observed that patients with candidiasis of the intestinal tract may have problems absorbing magnesium and potassium, despite oral supplementation. (Personal communication with Dr. David Quigg, nutritional biochemist at Doctor's Data Laboratories.)

While the sources of heavy metals are many and varied, one of the most important with regard to candidiasis is the dental use of mercury. The silver amalgam dental filling routinely used by dentists is actually composed of from 50 to 53 percent mercury.[3] It will be extremely difficult for the person with amalgam fillings to rid the body of Candida because mercury has an antibiotic effect, killing off the friendly bacteria so they cannot control yeast overgrowth.[4]

Yeast-connected illness affects people of all ages and, although both sexes are affected, women are eight times more likely to experience the yeast syndrome.[5] Women may develop vaginal yeast infections following a course of antibiotics, during pregnancy, or while using oral contraceptives. Progestin from birth control pills changes the vaginal lining to make it more hospitable to yeasts, and also causes the release of yeast-feeding sugar into the bloodstream.[6] Candida may be transmitted sexually, and a mother may pass it on to her newborn.[7] Candidiasis in the form of oral thrush and/or diaper rash is common in babies.

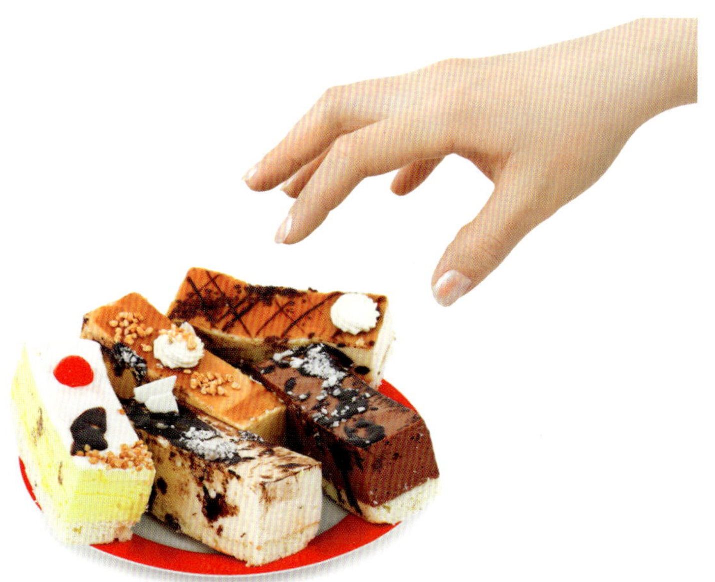

Factors that might predispose one to candidiasis include:[8,9]

- Use of antibiotics
- Use of corticosteroid drugs (which suppress the immune system and permit the overgrowth of yeast)

Healing HOPE Testimonial

"A few years ago I was suffering from severe fatigue. I was just tired all the time, and no matter what I did, it just kept getting worse. I went to several different doctors and had so many tests done—bloodwork, CT scans, X-rays—you name it, I had it done. Eventually I was referred to an infectious disease doctor, but after another round of testing, even he said there was nothing wrong with me and he just told me to go home and rest! It was so frustrating, and that's when I finally turned to Brenda who told me "Katie, it's all in your gut"—and it was...she changed my life!

One of the first things she did was a comprehensive stool analysis (CSA), and with her help I discovered that all my health problems were starting in my gut. Sure enough, I had dysbiosis, Candida overgrowth and a low immune response in my gut. Basically, I was a mess on the inside! So after balancing my system with the help of pharmaceuticals, natural supplements, and cutting things out of my diet like refined sugar, dairy, wheat and gluten, I now feel amazing."

–Katie

- A compromised immune system (evident in people with AIDS, cancer and autoimmune diseases, as well as those taking immunosuppressive drugs and those with a heavy body burden of toxins)
- A damp, moldy environment
- A diet high in refined carbohydrates and other yeast-promoting foods (See the Candida Diet in the Appendix.)
- Presence of mercury-containing silver amalgam fillings in the teeth
- Stress (which suppresses immune function)
- Decreased digestive secretions
- Nutrient deficiency
- Impaired liver function
- Dysbiosis

Also at increased risk for developing yeast infections are patients who have undergone surgical interventions, catheterizations or dialysis, as well as burn victims and those with diabetes mellitus and hypothyroidism.[10]

What Are the Signs and Symptoms?

Candidiasis can affect many parts of the body and may be characterized by a wide variety of local and systemic signs and symptoms, including:[11,12]

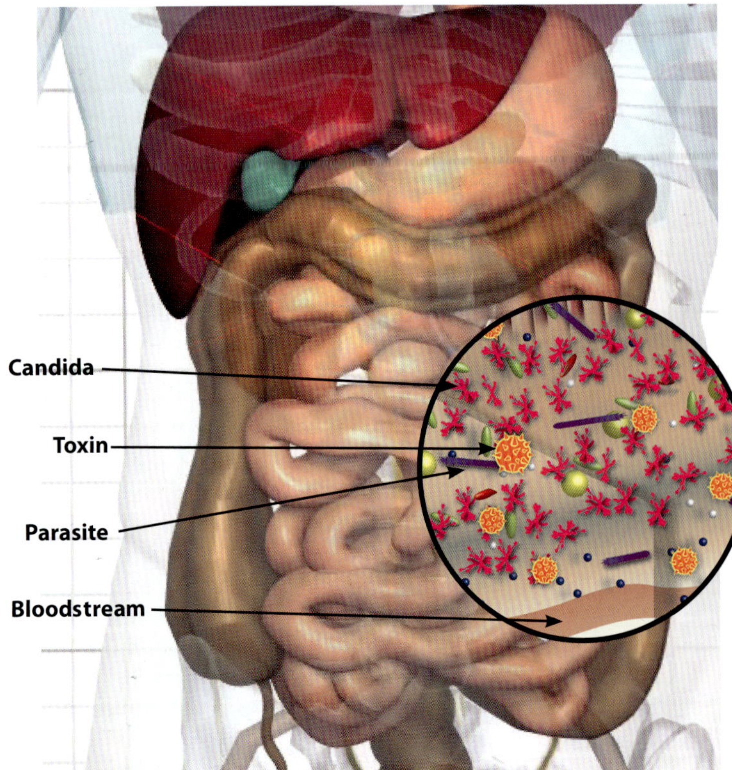

Illustration of the intestinal lining developing into leaky gut

Auto-Immune Diseases Resulting From Leaky Gut

- Lupus
- Rheumatoid arthrtis
- Polymyalgia rheumatica
- Multiple sclerosis
- Chronic fatigue syndrome
- Fibromyalgia
- Thyroiditis
- Crohn's disease
- Vitilego
- Vasculitis
- Ulcerative colitis
- Urticaria (hives)
- Diabetes

- Chronic fatigue
- Brain fog
- Anxiety
- Depression
- Food cravings (especially for sweets, fermented foods, alcoholic and carbonated beverages)
- Hyperactivity and learning disabilities in children
- Lack of libido
- Suppressed immune activity or autoimmune disorders
- Headaches
- Muscle aches
- Arthritis
- Bladder and kidney infections
- Gas and bloating
- Bad breath
- Rectal itching
- Clogged sinuses/sinusitis
- Acne
- Burning tongue
- White spots on tongue and in mouth
- Nail infections
- Diaper rash

As mentioned, Candida releases toxic waste products when it proliferates. One mycotoxin produced by Candida is acetaldehyde. Acetaldehyde is toxic to the central nervous system. It also interferes with normal hormone metabolism, affecting the pituitary, thyroid and adrenal glands.[13] Additionally, it has been shown that abnormal gut fermentation by yeast or bacteria can produce

Did You Know

It has been shown that abnormal gut fermentation by yeast or bacteria can produce increased blood-alcohol levels. This is known as auto-brewery syndrome.

increased blood-alcohol levels.[14] These processes explain how Candida can produce "brain fog" symptoms.

It is important to note that Candida is an underlying factor in many, if not most, diseases and conditions. Candida infection must be ruled out when addressing other health conditions.

The development of allergies and other autoimmune disorders is viewed by many progressive physicians and alternative practitioners as a consequence of mycotoxins entering the bloodstream. Normally, the semi-permeable lining of the intestinal tract will prevent contamination of blood with these and other toxins, microorganisms and undigested food particles. However, when the roots of Candida (known as rhizoids) burrow into the intestinal lining, they leave microscopic holes through which these contaminants may pass and enter into the bloodstream traveling throughout the body. The body sees undigested food particles as foreign substances and therefore launches an immune reaction that gives rise to autoantibodies that promote allergic responses, or even worse, autoimmune disease.

Candida toxins are carried through this leaky gut via the bloodstream to the liver. From there, they proceed to other organs of the body—the brain, nervous system, joints, skin, etc. If the liver's detoxification ability is impaired due to inadequate nutrition and toxic overload, these toxins will not be eliminated and can initiate states of chronic disease.

In addition to suppressing the immune system, Candida also disrupts the endocrine (glandular)[15] system, which has a regulating effect on the body. Leaky gut and dysbiosis, also contribute to the development of non-alcoholic fatty liver disease (NAFLD).[16] This condition is becoming more prevalent and can lead to the development of diabetes and even liver failure. These effects make it possible for Candida to cause, or contribute to, virtually any disorder anywhere in the body.

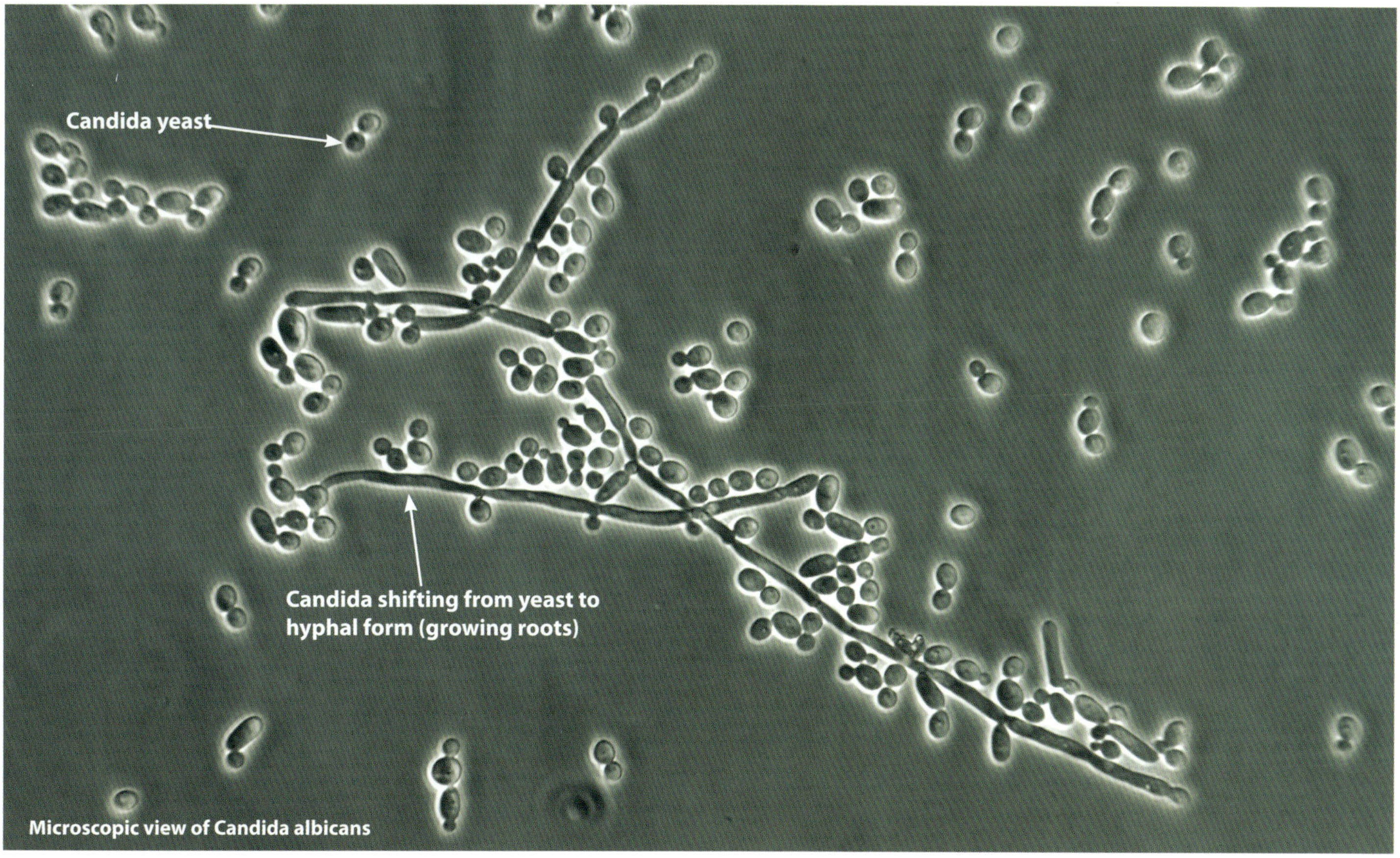

Candida yeast

Candida shifting from yeast to hyphal form (growing roots)

Microscopic view of Candida albicans

Constipation

What Is It?

Constipation may be defined as infrequent or incomplete bowel movements often characterized by stools that are hard, dry and difficult to pass due to slow transit time through the gastrointestinal tract. Gut transit time is the amount of time that elapses between ingestion of food and its excretion in the form of stool.

In conventional medical circles, it is considered normal to have a bowel movement as infrequently as three times a week.[1] In contrast, most holistic practitioners would consider the normal range of bowel movements to be one to three per day. The thinking is that three movements are ideal because we generally eat three meals daily. Ideally, when food enters the stomach, a nerve impulse is sent to the colon prompting it to contract and release its contents. This gastrocolic reflex, when functioning properly, would cause us to empty our colons after each meal.

Many people have just one bowel movement per day and think this is normal. A daily bowel movement may still be considered constipation especially when taking into consideration the amount of feces eliminated in the bowel movement. A daily bowel movement of approximately one and a half feet, which is about the size of the left side of the colon, would be considered normal by natural health practitioners. This may be broken up into two to three movements per day or, sometimes, in just one bowel movement.

What Causes It?

There are many possible causes of constipation, ranging from simple to complex. Among them are:[2-9]

- Insufficient fiber in the diet
- Too much fat in the diet and too many refined foods
- Side effects of some medications (antidepressants; tranquilizers; painkillers that contain codeine, morphine or opium; some blood pressure and heart medications)
- Lack of exercise
- Life changes

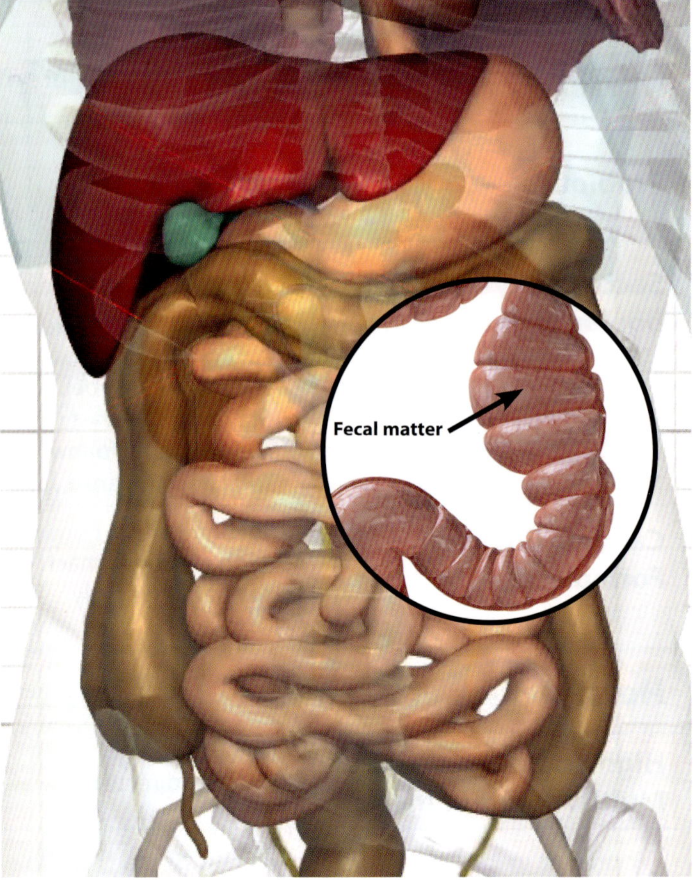

Illustration of the digestive system showing fecal matter built up in the colon causing constipation

- Travel (especially changing time zones)
- Pregnancy (hormonal and mechanical problems presented)
- Excessive use of laxatives or enemas (can damage nerve cells in the bowel interfering with its ability to contract)
- Ignoring the urge to defecate
- Surgery (such as hysterectomy or back surgery that may result in severance of nerves in the bowel)
- Dehydration
- Extreme stress/depression
- Magnesium deficiency
- Deficiency of peristalsis-inducing nutrients: vitamin B5, vitamin C, choline and arginine
- Prolonged bed rest
- Lack of sleep
- Advanced age
- Spinal cord injury
- Insufficient levels of digestive enzymes

Constipation is common in diseases such as:

- Parkinson's disease
- Autoimmune diseases such as lupus and diabetes
- Glucose intolerance
- Hypercalcemia (too much calcium in the blood)
- Hemorrhoids and anal fissures (produce spasms of the anal sphincter muscle, delaying bowel movements)
- Scleroderma and other neuromuscular disorders
- Multiple sclerosis
- Kidney failure
- Stroke
- Colon cancer
- Dysbiosis (imbalance in bowel bacteria, where bad bacteria outnumber the good)
- Food allergies
- Parasites
- Hypothyroidism
- Neurologic injuries such as spinal cord injuries
- Liver disease

Thyroid function is particularly important with regard to constipation. If the body were a car, then the thyroid would be considered the spark plug. If it is sluggish, eliminations will also be sluggish. Many people today have what has been called "subclinical hypothyroidism." This means that their depressed thyroid activity does not show up on standardized tests.

Subclinical hypothyroidism occurs in up to 20 percent of women. Alternative laboratory tests may be employed by progressive physicians to detect such thyroid problems. Some may test for and treat Wilson's thyroid syndrome, characterized by chronically low body temperature.[10] Identifying and treating a sluggish thyroid is important. (See Thyroid Dysfunction section for more information.)

A slow gut transit time (the time it takes for food to pass through the gastrointestinal tract—from mouth through rectum) is an underlying factor in many cases of constipation. The optimal transit time is 24 to 30 hours or less. However, in the U.S., the normal transit time can be 48 hours or more.[11]

Another possible cause of constipation has to do with the position we assume when having a bowel movement. In Western "civilized" cultures, we sit on a toilet, whereas in more primitive cultures the squatting posture is used. Actually, the squatting posture makes a good deal more physiological sense in terms of bowel stimulation and support achieved when the thighs come in contact with the abdominal wall.

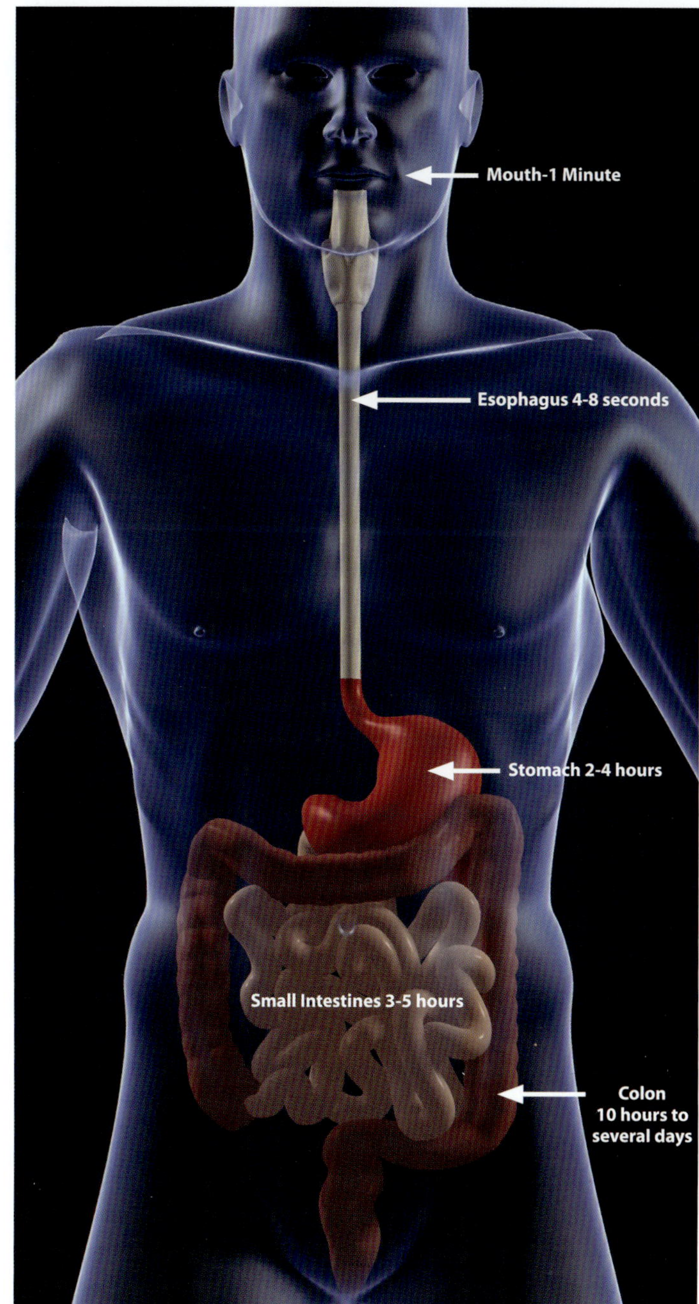

Average transit time through the digestive system

Constipation is much more common in Western cultures than elsewhere, also due to our sedentary lifestyles and consumption of processed foods. Fiber (indigestible complex plant carbohydrates found in fruits, vegetables and whole grains) is removed from most processed foods because it decreases shelf life.[12]

Chronic constipation is the top gastrointestinal complaint in the United States. According to the National Digestive Diseases Information Clearinghouse, more than four million Americans have frequent constipation. It affects people of all ages, but older adults are five times more likely than younger people to have the problem.[13]

Indigenous cultures that have a high intake of dietary fiber invariably enjoy superior intestinal health and are virtually free of the diseases of modern civilization.

High intake of dietary fiber has many benefits for constipated individuals including:

- Decrease of transit time of stools
- Decrease of absorption of toxins from stools
- Bulking and softening of stools
- Increasing frequency, quantity and quality of bowel movements

What Are the Signs and Symptoms?

With constipation, a wide range of symptoms may be experienced. These could include:

- Abdominal discomfort/fullness
- Rectal discomfort
- Bloating
- Nausea
- Loss of appetite
- Headache
- Lower back pain
- General feeling of malaise

When bowel transit time is slow, waste is not promptly eliminated from the body. It will consequently create prolonged bacterial fermentation of the retained fecal material which can produce harmful or poisonous chemicals. As toxins are reabsorbed into the body, the risk of developing colon diseases and other health problems increases.[14] Excessive bowel transit time means increased exposure to waste and toxins. These toxins stress the gallbladder, pancreas and liver giving rise to fatigue and headaches.

Toxins created in the constipated bowel damage digestive enzymes in the intestinal wall and cause digestive problems and nutrient deficiencies. The walls of the colon can weaken and herniate, giving rise to diverticulosis.[15] (See Diverticulosis section.) Besides diverticulosis, the excessive bowel transit time associated with constipation can contribute to such bowel disorders as irritable bowel syndrome and colitis.

In addition, studies suggest that constipation may indirectly cause estrogen to be reabsorbed.[19] With slow

Long-Term Non-Treated Constipation Can Lead To:[16,17,18]

- Appendicitis
- Bad breath
- Body odor
- Coated tongue
- Depression
- Diverticulitis
- Fatigue
- Gas
- Hemorrhoids
- Hernia
- Indigestion
- Insomnia
- Obesity
- Varicose veins
- Bowel cancer
- Malabsorption syndrome

The accumulation of toxins, antigens and undigested food particles may lead to:

- Diabetes mellitus
- Meningitis
- Thyroid disease
- Candidiasis
- Migraines
- Ulcerative colitis
- Skin conditions
- Allergies
- Anxiety
- Depression
- Female disorders

Types of Laxatives

Bulk-forming Laxatives – These increase the bulk and water content of the stools. Some commonly used bulk-formers are psyllium, methylcellulose, calcium polycarbophil and bran (used as a food and in supplement form). The only downside of the regular use of these products is that they can interfere with absorption of some drugs.

Osmotic Agents – These contain salts or carbohydrates that draw water into the colon to facilitate the passage of stools. While safe for occasional use, dependency can result if used habitually, and minerals can be washed out of the body. Examples of osmotic agents are lactulose, sorbitol, milk of magnesia and Epsom salts.

Stool Softeners – These wetting agents, acting as a lubricant, moisten and soften the stool so that it passes through the intestines more easily. An example of this type of laxative is mineral oil. These products should not be used on a regular basis. Mineral oil reduces absorption of fat-soluble vitamins, and docusate sodium, found in the mineral oil, may increase the toxicity of other drugs taken at the same time causing liver damage to occur.[21]

Stimulant Laxatives – These irritate the intestinal wall triggering muscular contractions (peristalsis). Prolonged use can lead to dependency, and can damage the bowel. Some examples of these are: bisacodyl, castor oil, casanthranol, senna, cascara sagrada, and phenolphthalein. It should be noted that phenolphthalein, which is actually the active ingredient in prune juice, was recently removed from the market. Overuse of this substance causes depletion of potassium in the blood and reduced absorption of vitamin D, calcium and other minerals.[22]

transit times, a low-fiber diet and low concentrations of beneficial Lactobacilli and Bifidobacteria, there will be reabsorption of estrogen. Elevated estrogen can give rise to many female problems including breast, ovarian and uterine cancer.

How Is It Diagnosed?

After taking a detailed medical history, physicians may perform a rectal exam and order a stool analysis to look for hidden (occult) blood. Blood and urine tests may also be performed.

Where constipation is long-standing (chronic), the physician may want to have special tests done to rule out bowel obstruction. Such tests may include sigmoidoscopy, colonoscopy, barium enema or virtual colonoscopy. Motility tests to measure movement within the colon, and a test to measure transit time may also be performed. Testing transit time involves X-rays of the colon on successive days after barium is swallowed.

There is a self-test which can determine bowel transit time.[20] In this test, 20 grains (5 to 12 tablets) of charcoal are swallowed all at once with water, and a note is made of the time. The time is again recorded when the black color of the charcoal is first seen in the stools. Ideally, this would be within 16 to 30 hours. Any longer indicates an excessive bowel transit time. If the black is not seen for 78 hours or never appears, this is indicative of significant constipation. A continuation of the black in stools for several more days is also a sign of a sluggish bowel.

Natural health practitioners may also suggest a comprehensive stool analysis (CSA). This test can give important information as to the cause of many cases of chronic constipation, such as bacterial imbalance, pH imbalance, pathogenic yeast or microorganism presence, parasitic infection, enzyme deficiencies and intestinal inflammation. (See the Appendix for more information.)

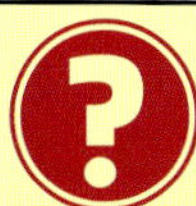

Did You Know

In the last ten years many people have been diagnosed with irritable bowel syndrome (IBS) instead of constipation. Constipation occurs in IBS, often alternating with diarrhea.

Healing HOPE Testimonial

"All my life I have been constipated, having a bowel movement every eighth day, only after using laxatives. I was not getting the help I needed through traditional medicine. I started on the HOPE program (High fiber, Omega oils, Probiotics and Enzymes) and got immediate results. I was able to enjoy food again. I used to always feel full and had a poor appetite. By following the diet suggestions and including plenty of fiber, I also managed to lose 17 pounds. I continue to take the supplements every day and look forward to a Total Body Cleanse every six months."
– Helen

Another test frequently suggested by natural health practitioners that may be helpful to determine causes of chronic constipation is a food sensitivity test. (See the Appendix.) Constipation is a common side effect of food sensitivities, such as sensitivity to wheat gluten.

What Is the Standard Medical Treatment?

Because lack of dietary fiber in the diet is thought to be the most common cause of constipation, many doctors recommend the use of fiber supplements as well as the addition of more high-fiber foods (fruits, vegetables, whole grains) to the diet. Bran, prunes, figs and apricots are particularly high in fiber. If this protocol is followed, bran should be added to the diet slowly because adding bran to the diet too rapidly can cause gas and bloating. (See the Fiber 35 Eating Plan in the Appendix for more information about adding fiber to the diet.) Additional fiber may also be obtained through the use of dietary supplements.

In addition to recommending the addition of more dietary fiber and, possibly, another form of laxative, many doctors will recommend lifestyle changes such as increasing water intake and exercise.

If medications are suspected as the cause of constipation, they may be discontinued or switched by the physician.

If a disease process, such as hypothyroidism, malignant tumor, polyps or an inflammatory bowel condition, is identified, appropriate treatment of that condition will be initiated.

Drugs and surgery are the major tools of the medical doctor, so some form of these will likely be employed regardless of the cause of the constipation. In fact, the cause may not even be established. If the constipation problem is due to parasites, candidiasis or food sensitivities, the traditional medical doctors are unlikely to discover this, as these conditions generally lie outside their area of knowledge.

One study showed that the majority of patients with slow transit times and defecation disorders did not benefit from fiber therapy.[23] For patients like this, the issue of insufficient peristalsis must be addressed. Medically, this is done with prescription drugs used to enhance bowel motility (movement). Unfortunately one recent drug, Zelnorm, was used for this purpose, but was taken off the market when it was found to cause serious cardiovascular adverse events.[24] Currently, Amitza is the drug of choice for increasing bowel motility.[25]

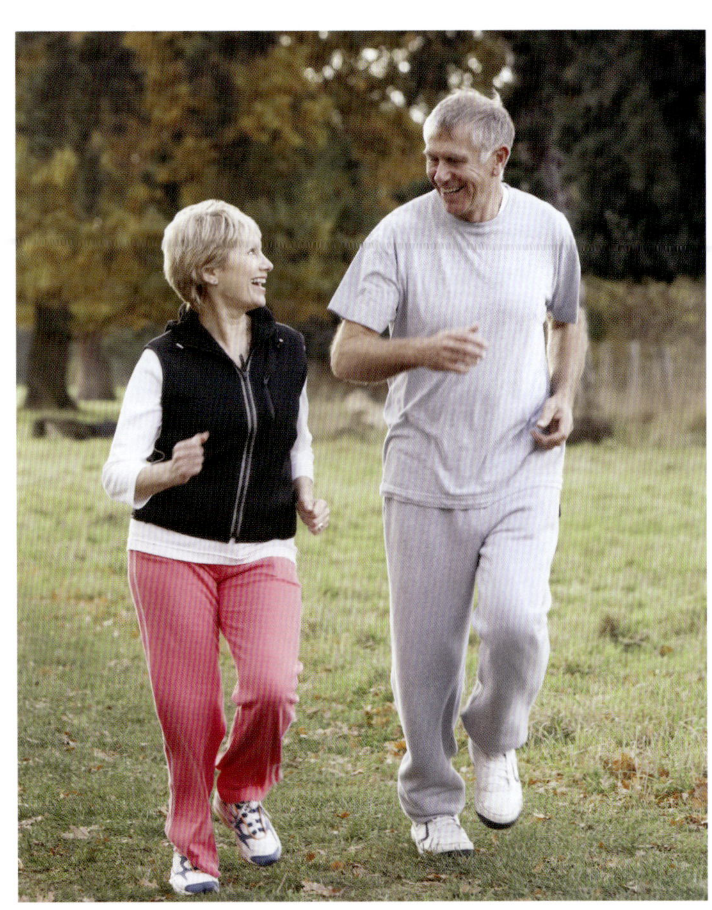

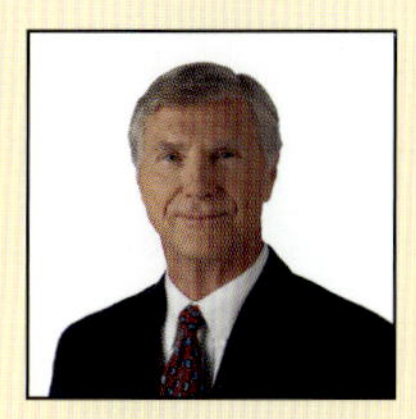

Dr. Smith's Comments

Constipation is one of the most common and expensive problems for Western society. A review article from the New England Journal of Medicine (349: 1360-1368, Oct. 2, 2003) describes this in detail. Constipation is a problem for up to 27 percent of the population of Western countries. There are 2.5 million visits to physicians and 92,000 hospitalizations per year involving constipation. Laxative sales exceed several hundred million dollars per year for constipation. The article goes on to divide constipation into three groups:

Normal transit time (most common) – responds well to hydration, fiber and osmotic laxatives to keep stool soft. Severe cases may require prescription drugs like Tegoserod (5-hydroxytryptamine receptor agonist).

Defectory disorders – often structural abnormalities like rectocoele, rectal intussusception or excessive perineal descent—are often due to lack of coordination of abdominal, rectoanal and pelvic floor muscles during defecation. The condition is often helped by biofeedback training. (See the Appendix.)

Slow transit time – usually occurs in young females who experience one or less bowel movements per week. It often starts at puberty with symptoms of bloating, abdominal pain and no urge to defecate. Fiber, water and osmotics help in mild cases, but severe cases are made worse with fiber. The worst of the slow-transit patients have histological changes with decreased Cajal cells (regulate motility) and in myenteric nerve plexus cells as well. Often these patients require total or subtotal colectomy (removal of a portion or all of the colon) to solve the problem. Thirty-two studies showed a patient satisfaction rate of 39 to 100 percent with this surgery.

In my own experience, constipation is certainly one of the most common complaints of hospital patients. I believe that it has, directly or indirectly, led to hospitalization and surgery, and kept patients in the hospital longer than necessary. I have had patients who

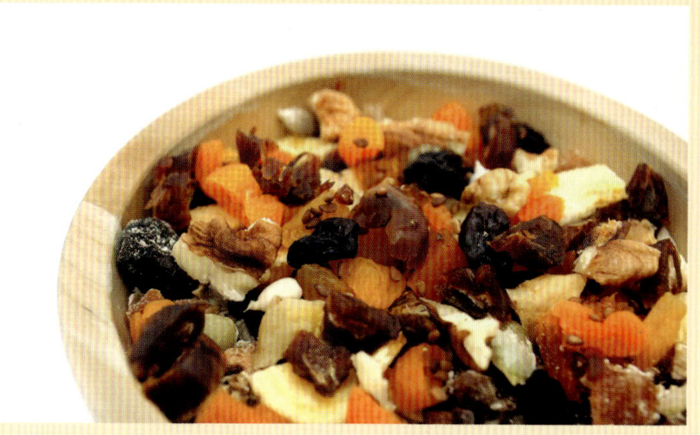

were slow to recover and, by treating their constipation, their problems rapidly resolved.

I have lectured for and worked with the International Association of Colon Hydrotherapists since 1999. In addition, I have personally experienced colon hydrotherapy. I believe it is an important therapy for anyone who cares about his or her health. It is interesting how often patients who try this therapy are amazed by the gentle and effective results they achieve. It is my opinion that all detoxification and chelation centers would be enhanced by adding colon hydrotherapy to their program.

I look forward to the day that colon hydrotherapy becomes a standard of care for the medical profession, both in the hospital and for outpatient settings. In fact, I believe that colon hydrotherapy should be the standard of care for prepping seniors and children for colonoscopy. In addition, it could become the mainstay treatment for constipation in childhood. Recent research has shown that childhood constipation is largely the result of fear of painful bowel movements that occur when children are forced to evacuate by giving them laxatives.

In summary, most everyone can enhance their colonic eliminative process with a balance of soluble and insoluble fiber, probiotics, oils, good hydration and exercise.

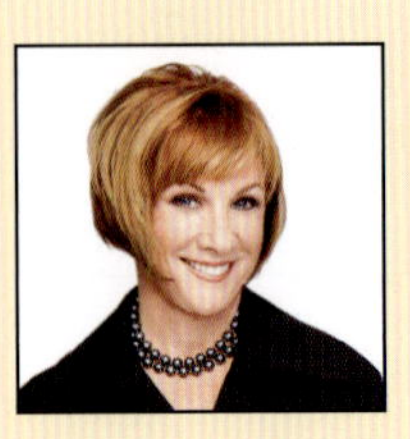

Brenda's Bottom Line

If you are not having at least one bowel movement every day, you are constipated. If you are having one bowel movement each day, and it is not one and a half feet long you are still constipated. If you are not eliminating one and a half feet of feces per day (the length of the descending colon), you are not getting enough dietary fiber in your diet. This comes as no surprise, as the average intake of dietary fiber in the US is 12 to 15 grams. I recommend at least 35 grams daily for optimal health.

"If you are not having at least one bowel movement every day, you are constipated."

Chronic constipation can lead to so many health problems. Take my own story, for example. As a result of chronic antibiotic usage in childhood, I became constipated. The first consequence of this constipation was migraine headaches in elementary school. In high school it had progressed to chronic fatigue. All of this stemmed from my chronic constipation. If I had only known then what I do now!

The underlying causes of constipation are numerous, and can be complex. The cause could be dehydration, lack of fiber, lack of beneficial bacteria, lack of B vitamins, certain medications, chronic stress or genetics, to name a few.

My hope is that you will get to the bottom of the problem without having to resort to long-term laxative use that can worsen the problem and lead to dependence. Think of it as an investigative journey with a destination of good health. The following recommendations will help you on your way.
Rule out and/or treat underlying issues and causes for chronic constipation mentioned earlier in this chapter.

Recommended Testing

- Comprehensive stool analysis (CSA) (See the Appendix.)
- Food sensitivity test (See the Appendix.)

Diet

- Follow the Fiber 35 Eating Plan found in the Appendix.
- If Candida is an underlying cause, follow the Candida Diet until bowel elimination is regular.
- Drink half your body weight in ounces of water daily. (Example: 140 pounds would be 70 ounces of water daily.)
- Limit beverages that have high tannin content, such as red wine and tea, as these can contribute to constipation.

Lifestyle

- Make time to go to the bathroom, even if it means getting up earlier in the morning.
- Use the LifeStep, a toilet step that will help raise your feet so that you are in natural squatting position for better elimination.
- Incorporate exercise into your lifestyle. Walking, swimming and using the mini trampoline are great exercises.

Complementary Mind/Body Therapies

- Colon hydrotherapy can be extremely beneficial alone, or in conjunction with the suggestions here.
- Yoga can help strengthen the abdominal muscles and colon.
- Chiropractic spinal adjustments can be helpful in resolving constipation.
- Acupunture could also be beneficial by stimulating the energy meridians of the colon and digestive tract.

Recommended Nutraceuticals	Dosage	Benefit	Comments
Critical Phase Daily maintenance recommendations should also be taken during this phase unless otherwise indicated.			
Natural Laxative Formula	Use as directed	Use initially to encourage elimination. Do not use long term.	Look for ingredients such as magnesium, aloe, rhubarb, and triphala.
Probiotics	200 billion culture count twice daily	Restores bacterial balance and pH of colon.	Look for high amount of bifidobacteria, the main bacteria in colon.
Helpful			
Total Body Cleanse	As directed for 30 days. See Appendix	Helps rid the body of waste and toxins from chronic constipation.	Herbal formula should support the seven channels of elimination.
Magnesium	400 mg daily	Magnesium deficiency is common cause of chronic constipation.	Make sure to take magnesium if you are taking a calcium supplement.
Daily Maintenance			
Probiotics	30 - 80 billion culture count twice daily after critical phase	Restores bacterial balance and pH of colon and promotes regularity.	Look for high amount of bifidobacteria, the main bacteria in colon.
Fiber*	4-5 grams two to three times daily.	Provides bulk needed for proper elimination.	*See note below. Start with once daily and work up to three times daily.
Omega-3 Fatty Acids	At least 2 grams daily of EPA/DHA combination	Helps restore moisture to the intestinal tract.	Look for a concentrated, enteric coated fish oil.
Digestive Enzymes	Take with meals	Helps to digest foods and absorb nutrients.	If low stomach acid is found find a formula that contains hydrochloric acid.

See further explanation of supplements in the Appendix

*** Note: If you have not had bowel elimination for three to seven days or more, delay the usage of fiber supplementation until elimination occurs.**

DIARRHEA

What Is It?

Diarrhea is the frequent passage of watery stools. It can occur for many reasons, a common reason being increased bowel motility that causes a rapid transit time (the time elapsed from ingestion to elimination of food). With an increase in gut motility there is insufficient time for water in the intestinal tract to be reabsorbed into the body. The result is that the stool retains water and remains liquefied.

Diarrhea may be either acute or chronic. Acute diarrhea takes the form of an isolated incident caused by a temporary problem—usually an infection that lasts three to seven days. Chronic diarrhea is much more complex with a multitude of causes, and can last for months.

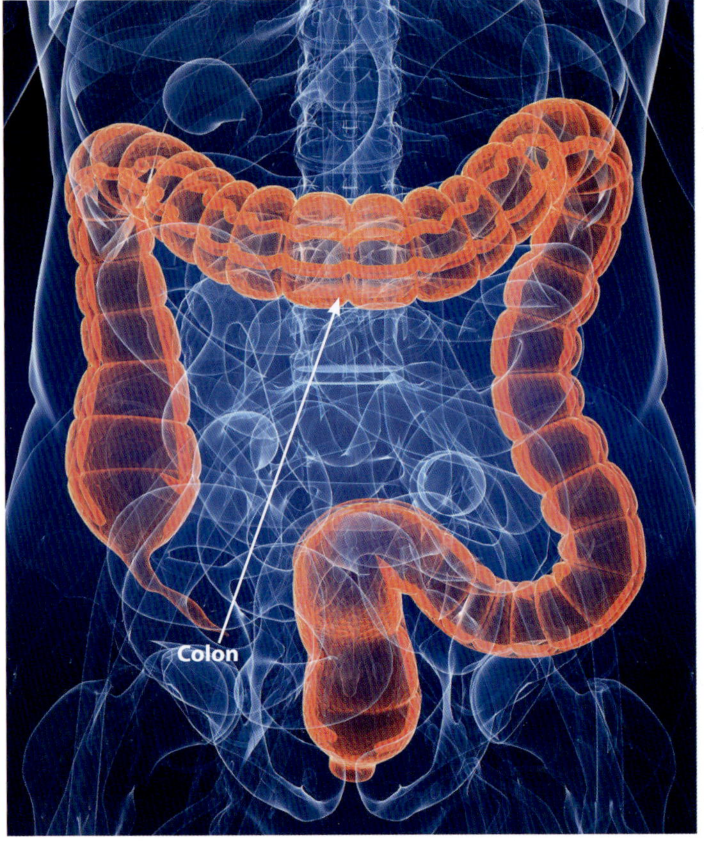

Illustration of the lower digestive system with the colon highlighted

What Causes It?

The causes of diarrhea are many and varied. Basically, the condition stems from intestinal irritation or increased motility (muscular action) in the intestinal tract that can be brought on by a variety of causes, including:

- Incomplete digestion of food
- Use of certain drugs (especially antibiotics like tetracycline, clindamycin and ampicillin and nonsteroidal anti-inflammatory drugs (NSAIDs), such as aspirin) that damage the gut lining
- Food poisoning
- Food allergies or sensitivities (especially to dairy, eggs, wheat)
- Excessive consumption of alcohol
- Regular or excessive use of caffeine-containing beverages (coffee, tea, sodas), foods (chocolate) and drugs (No-Doz, Excedrin)
- Laxative use/abuse
- Overuse of sugar and sweeteners such as sorbitol, xylitol, mannitol, fructose and lactose
- Infections: bacterial, viral, fungal (including Candida) and parasitic
- Pancreatic insufficiency or pancreatic tumor
- Emotional stress
- Bowel diseases: Crohn's disease, irritable bowel syndrome, diverticulitis, ulcerative colitis, cancer
- Consumption of contaminated water
- Radiation or chemotherapy
- Nutrient deficiencies (vitamin A and B complex, glutamine, zinc)[1]
- Deficiency of hydrochloric acid (HCl stomach acid)[2]
- Celiac disease or gluten sensitivity
- Surgical resection of the small intestine
- Short bowel syndrome
- Inadequate bile secretion (hepatitis or bile duct obstruction) causing malabsorption of fat
- Use of magnesium-containing antacids
- Bacterial toxins
- Malnutrition (deficiency of calories, protein)
- Heavy metal poisoning[3]
- Neurological disease (diabetic neuropathy)
- Metabolic disease (hyperthyroidism)
- Fecal impaction
- Long-distance running

Acute diarrhea can be of microbial origin which can be bacterial, viral or parasitic. One common way that people get diarrhea is food poisoning. Such food-borne illnesses include:

- Salmonella – from raw eggs, undercooked chicken or ham
- E. coli – from undercooked red meat
- Botulism – found in canned high-protein foods
- Staphylococcus – from infected food handlers

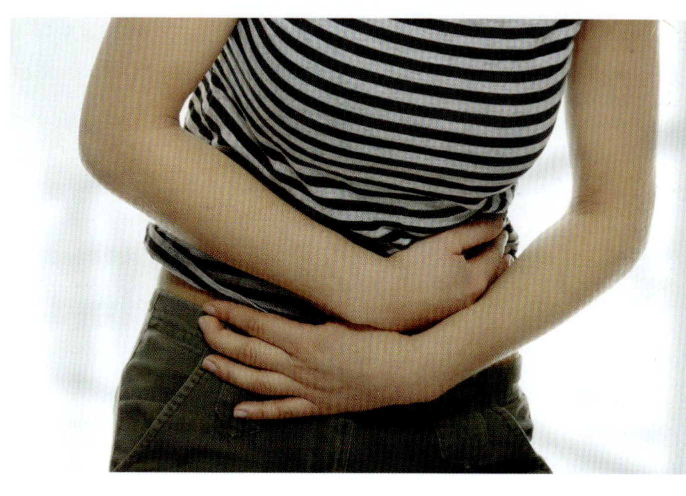

Bacteria like salmonella and E. coli both attack the intestinal lining giving off toxins that cause a profuse secretion of fluid, and gives rise to diarrhea. Parasites may be passed on from those who handle food and from the water supply. Parasites like Giardia lamblia, Entamoeba histolytica and Cryptosporidium interfere with digestion and/or damage the intestinal lining often causing diarrhea.

People who have insufficient stomach acid (HCl), often induced by acid-suppressing medications, will be more susceptible to parasitic and other infections. Food and water-borne diarrhea is frequently associated with travel to underdeveloped countries, but also occurs, to a lesser degree, in developed countries.

In fact, the parasite Cryptosporidium has been found in U.S. municipal waters. Current filtration and treatment methods are unable to ensure that Cryptosporidium is not present in U.S. tap water.[4] This is one good reason why water filtration systems in the home are so important.

Another important note, with regard to parasite diarrhea, is that parasites can still be present yet remain dormant. So fecal elimination may be normal or even constipated for a while, but parasites may be lying dormant.

Food allergens and sensitivities can be another cause of diarrhea. When a food allergen is ingested, histamine and other allergic compounds from white blood cells (known as mast cells) in the intestinal lining are released. These can have a strong laxative effect.

Chronic diarrhea, particularly as seen in irritable bowel syndrome (IBS), is often caused by chronic low-grade inflammation of the bowel lining that can be due to food sensitivities or microbial imbalances. With chronic diarrhea, the body is not absorbing all the nutrients from food, and the result is malnourishment. (See the IBS section for more information on this condition.)

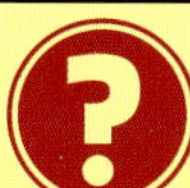

Did You Know

Antibiotic use can result in a type of diarrhea (pseudomembranous colitis) caused by overgrowth of the bacterium Clostridium difficile, sometimes called C. diff. This bacterium, common in hospitals, gives off toxins that damage the lining of the colon, causing severe diarrhea as well as lower abdominal cramps and fever.[5]

C. difficile is the most common cause of hospital-acquired diarrhea in developed countries. The incidence of C. difficile-associated diarrhea is increasing, and can include complications such as toxic megacolon, colonic perforation and even death. Antibiotic use is the most common risk factor for developing C. difficile diarrhea, but other factors include advanced age, severe illness, hospitalization and immunosuppressive therapy. As a matter of fact, it is estimated that 300 hospital deaths occur each day as a result of C. difficile infections.[6]

Recently, the use of proton pump inhibitors (PPIs) has been associated with C. difficile infections. A study in the American Journal of Gastroenterology showed an increased risk of developing C. difficile-associated diarrhea in hospitalized patients who used acid-suppressive therapy, especially proton pump inhibitors.[7] (See the GERD chapter.) They state that a possible cause for this increase results from the higher gastric pH in patients on acid-suppressing drugs. This facilitates the survival of C. difficile spores and their toxins throughout the stomach where, because of insufficient stomach acid, they are not destroyed.

People with gallbladder disease, or who have had their gallbladder removed, may experience diarrhea after eating a fatty meal. This usually improves in time, but may persist due to an imbalance in the ratio of bile produced to the amount of fat in the diet.

People of any age can develop diarrhea. It is a particularly serious condition when it occurs in the very old or very young. Diarrhea has long been the leading cause of death among infants and children worldwide. For most people in the U.S., it is an acute, self-limiting condition brought on by a pathogen. The average American will have a bout of diarrhea about four times a year.[8] Interestingly, younger adults seem to develop traveler's diarrhea slightly more often than older ones.[9]

What Are the Signs and Symptoms?

Diarrhea, which consists of the frequent passage of loose, watery stools, is often accompanied by:

- Abdominal cramps/pain
- Bloating/gas
- Malaise (generalized feeling of illness)
- Blood and mucus in the stools
- Rectal soreness
- Fever
- Weakness
- Loss of appetite/weight loss
- Intestinal rumbling sounds
- Increased thirst

The last symptom above, increased thirst, can be a sign of dehydration. Other signs may include a dry mouth, anxiety or restlessness, strong body odor, little or no urination, severe weakness, dizziness or lightheadedness. If any of these signs of dehydration occur, a doctor should be contacted immediately. Medical help should also be sought if diarrhea persists for more than a few days, if severe abdominal or rectal pain is experienced, if other family members are affected with the same symptoms, if fever exceeds 101 degrees F, or if there is blood in the stool (which will have a black, tarry appearance).

How Is It Diagnosed?

While diarrhea is obviously not difficult to recognize from symptoms, zeroing in on the cause can be more

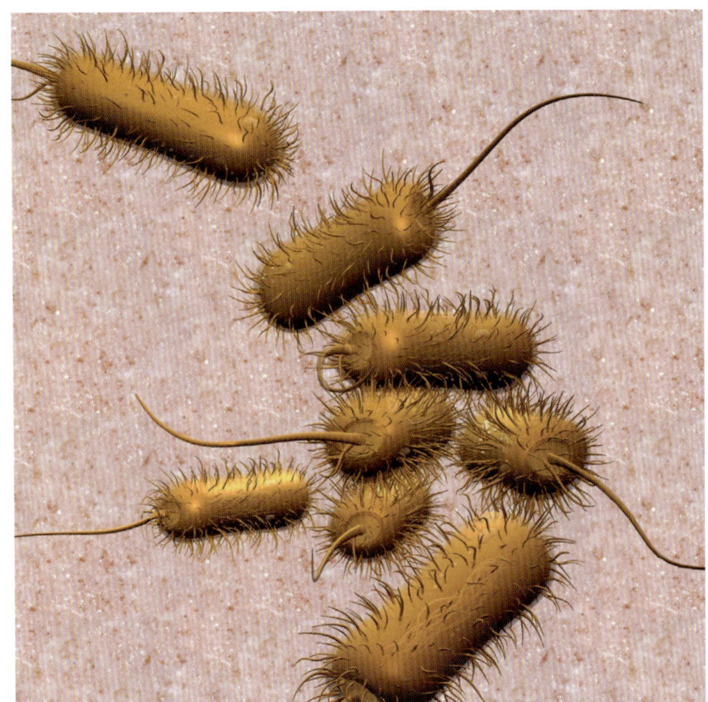

Illustration of pathogenic E. coli bacteria

problematic. As with other disorders, a thorough patient history can help point to possible causes. It is important to know what medications the patient is taking, if the patient has recently traveled outside the country, or is taking magnesium-containing supplements or products (like antacids or laxatives), or is taking large doses of vitamin C. In addition, tracking dietary habits for ruling out food allergy or sensitivities is helpful.

Because most cases of diarrhea in the U.S. are self-limiting and relatively mild, specific laboratory tests are not always done. With more severe cases, a stool test will help identify such pathogens as Shigella, Salmonella, Campylobacter or Yersinia.[10] If symptoms are severe, the stool will be cultured for abnormal bacteria to help determine the appropriate antibiotic to use.[11] In the case of traveler's diarrhea, a test for parasites will probably be ordered if diarrhea persists once the traveler has returned home. Unfortunately, many doctors will not order a parasite test unless the patient has traveled outside of the country.

Holistic physicians are more likely than traditional ones to test for parasites and digestive disorders in people with no history of travel. (See the Parasitic Disease section for more detailed information on parasites and testing for them.)

A stool test for the presence of fat will help detect malabsorption problems that may be due to a disease of the small intestine. **A hydrogen breath test may be performed to detect small intestinal bacterial overgrowth. In addition, a small bowel biopsy may be ordered.** If the biopsy is negative, then a sigmoidoscopy or colonoscopy may be performed. Another option is the upper GI series. These tests will help rule out inflammatory bowel disorders like Crohn's disease and ulcerative colitis.

Natural health practitioners may also suggest a comprehensive stool analysis (CSA). This test can give important information as to the cause of many cases of chronic diarrhea such as: bacterial imbalance, pH imbalance, pathogenic yeast or microorganism presence, parasitic infection, enzyme deficiencies and intestinal inflammation. (See the Appendix for more information.)

Another test frequently suggested by progressive health practitioners that may be helpful to determine causes of chronic diarrhea is a food sensitivity test. (See the Appendix.)

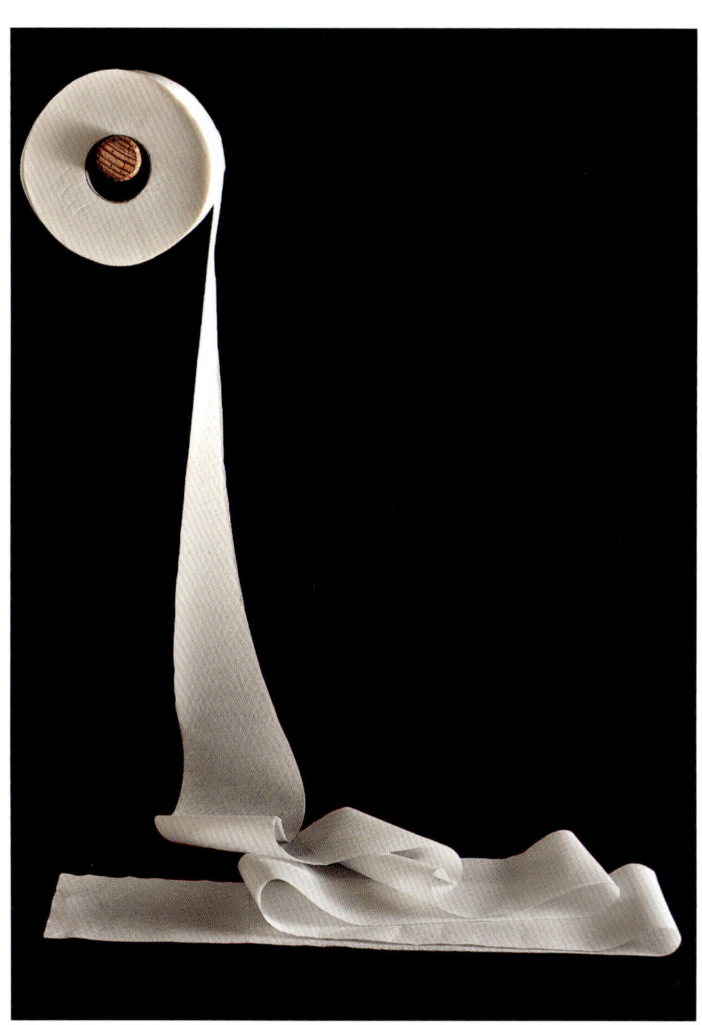

Healing HOPE Testimonial

"I decided to try probiotics after years of chronic diarrhea for which a cause had never been clearly determined by my doctors. Literally, within 30 minutes, the symptoms completely disappeared and have not returned since I started a daily dose of probiotics. I have to say it is like a miracle that I've had very normal bowel movements since I started this daily dose. I've researched EVERY ingredient and could find mounds of evidence supporting the benefits from universities all over the world. But my experience tells me everything I need to know.

As well, my partner, who has suffered from life-long acid reflux, then decided to give probiotics a try...and AGAIN, the next day, he was amazed that he didn't need his antacid which he's been taking for 20 years! He was completely surprised and so very happy to finally find something that helped his constant and severe acid reflux."

– Jim

What Is the Standard Medical Treatment?

There is some disagreement in medical circles with regard to the treatment of acute diarrhea. Some doctors will prefer to let a mild case run its course, while others will offer symptomatic relief through the use of drugs. Bismuth subsalicylate reduces the secretions of the intestines and has antimicrobial and anti-inflammatory effects.

Loperamide and diphenoxylale medications slow down the movement of the intestines and their secretions. However, they may actually worsen the diarrhea by retarding the elimination of organisms and toxins responsible for it.[12] While diphenoxylale and loperamide may offer temporary symptomatic relief, they should not be used if symptoms last more than a few days.[13]

Most cases of diarrhea are just the body's way of eliminating an irritant. Judicious use of antimotility drugs

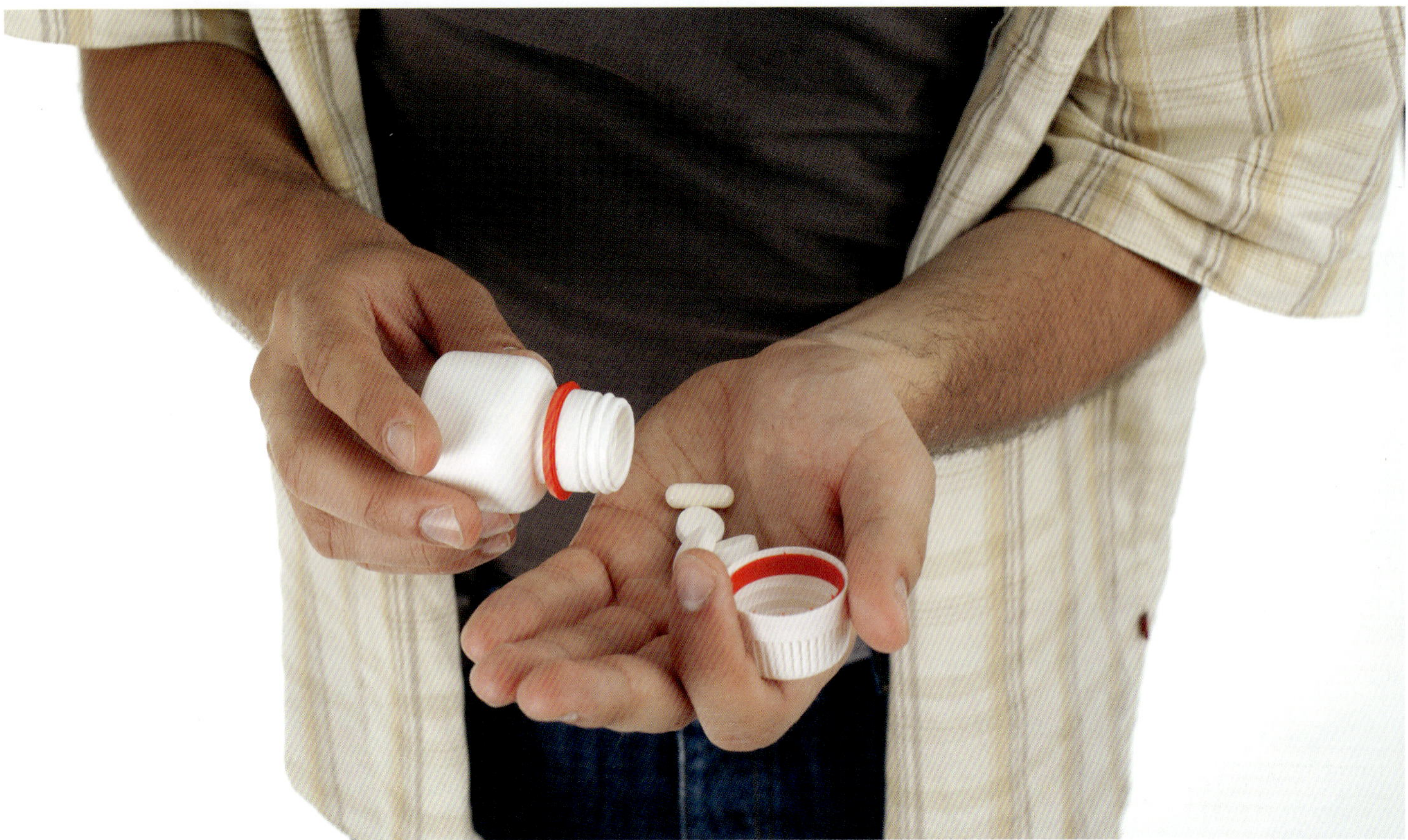

by a person in close communication with a doctor is acceptable. But a short-lived case of diarrhea can actually be therapeutic, as it will facilitate the removal of an undesirable substance from the body. In such a case, it's easy to see how a patient can make the situation worse through the use of symptom-suppressing medications.

Treatment of diarrhea depends upon the cause:

- If it is **lactose intolerance**, dairy foods will need to be eliminated from the diet
- If it is **Celiac disease**, gluten-containing grains must be avoided
- If it is **medication-related**, it will be necessary to adjust, switch or discontinue medications
- If it is a **food allergy or sensitivity**, the food allergen must be avoided or eaten infrequently on a rotating basis
- If the diarrhea is caused by **over-consumption** of alcohol, sweeteners, vitamin C, mgnesium (in supplement or other form), or caffeine, it will be necessary to reduce, or in some cases, discontinue intake of these items.
- Where **nutrient deficiency**—of HCl, digestive enzymes, zinc, glutamine, vitamins A, and B complex—is established to be a factor, supplementation of the deficient nutrients becomes part of the treatment plan. This is not apt to be the case in traditional medical circles where nutritional awareness is limited.
- Where **infection** is present, treatment involves the appropriate drug—usually an antibiotic, anti-fungal or anti-parasitic agent. Natural healthcare practitioners will gravitate more toward the use of herbal remedies, as described below, for this purpose. Some may combine antibiotic and herbal treatments.

When traveling to another country, especially a developing country, a good preventative measure for traveler's diarrhea would be to **avoid**:

- Drinking the local water
- Using ice cubes made from local water
- Eating raw vegetables
- Eating dairy products
- Eating unpeeled fruit

This will help to avoid ingesting any pathogenic bacteria that may be present in the food and drink overseas.

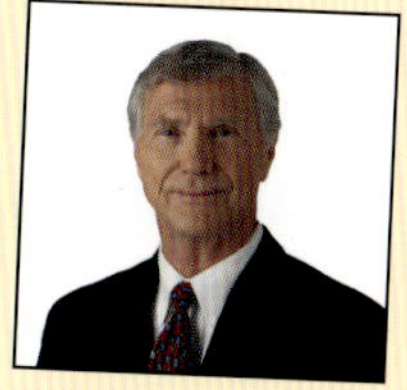

Dr. Smith's Comments

Diarrhea can cause inflammation and damage the intestinal lining. In viral diarrhea, there are changes in the cells of the small intestine, such as flattening and shortening of the villi, an increase in crypt cells and generally an increase in cellularity in the intestinal wall. The protective mucous barrier and brush border enzymes are damaged or destroyed, and there is a likelihood of increased intestinal permeability.

It follows that partially digested food particles could pass through, and, in the presence of an already activated immune system, cause an autoimmune type of reaction. This sets up the potential development of food sensitivities if foods with a higher allergic potential are eaten during, or even a few days after, an episode of diarrhea. Unfortunately, this would include many so called "comfort" foods, such as wheat, dairy, tomatoes, eggs, sugary foods, etc. I suspect that many childhood allergies, especially to wheat and dairy, could develop as the result of introducing these foods back into the diet while the child is in a hyper-immune and hyper-permeable state, which could last three to seven days after the diarrhea has subsided. I recommend starting with water, then rice water and progressing to vegetable juices, vegetable soup and then cooked vegetables. For convenience, a hypoallergenic, nutritionally balanced powdered drink could be very helpful.

Did You Know

Intestinal Toxins

Digestive Toxins Developed From

• Undigested Protein • Undigested Starches • Undigested Fat

Which can result in gas, bloating, heartburn and diarrhea

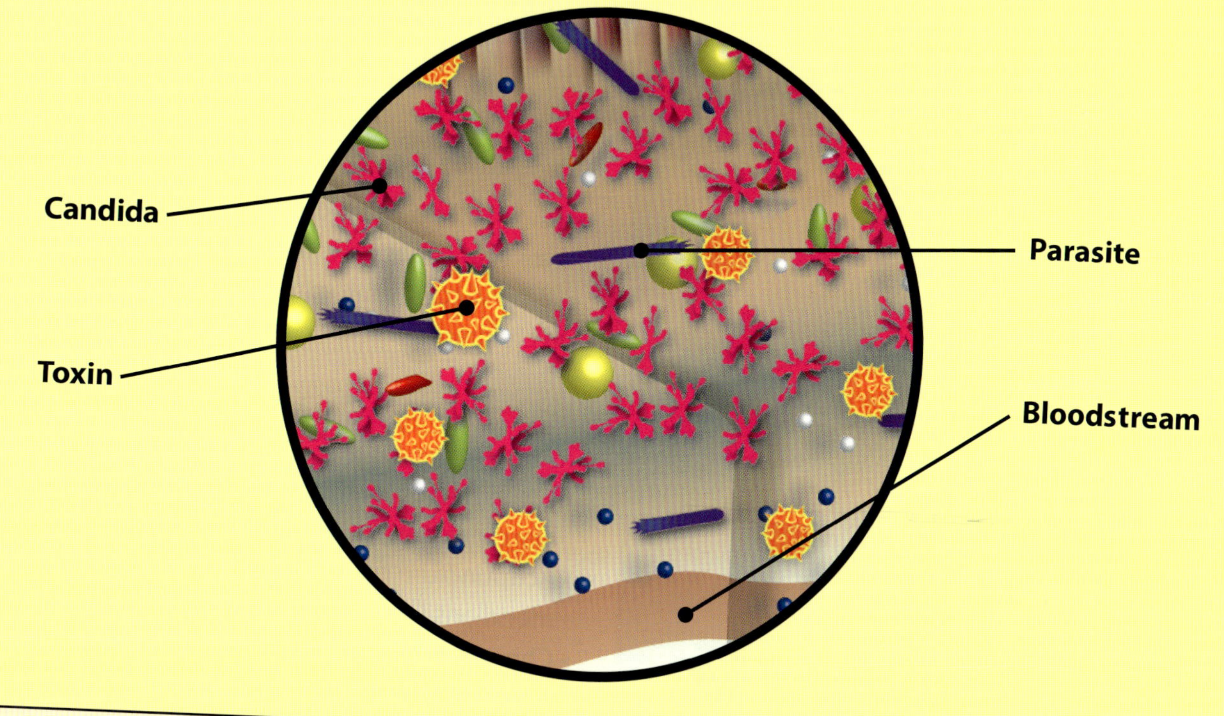

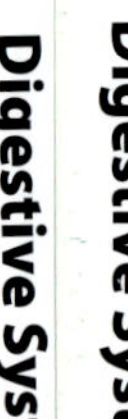

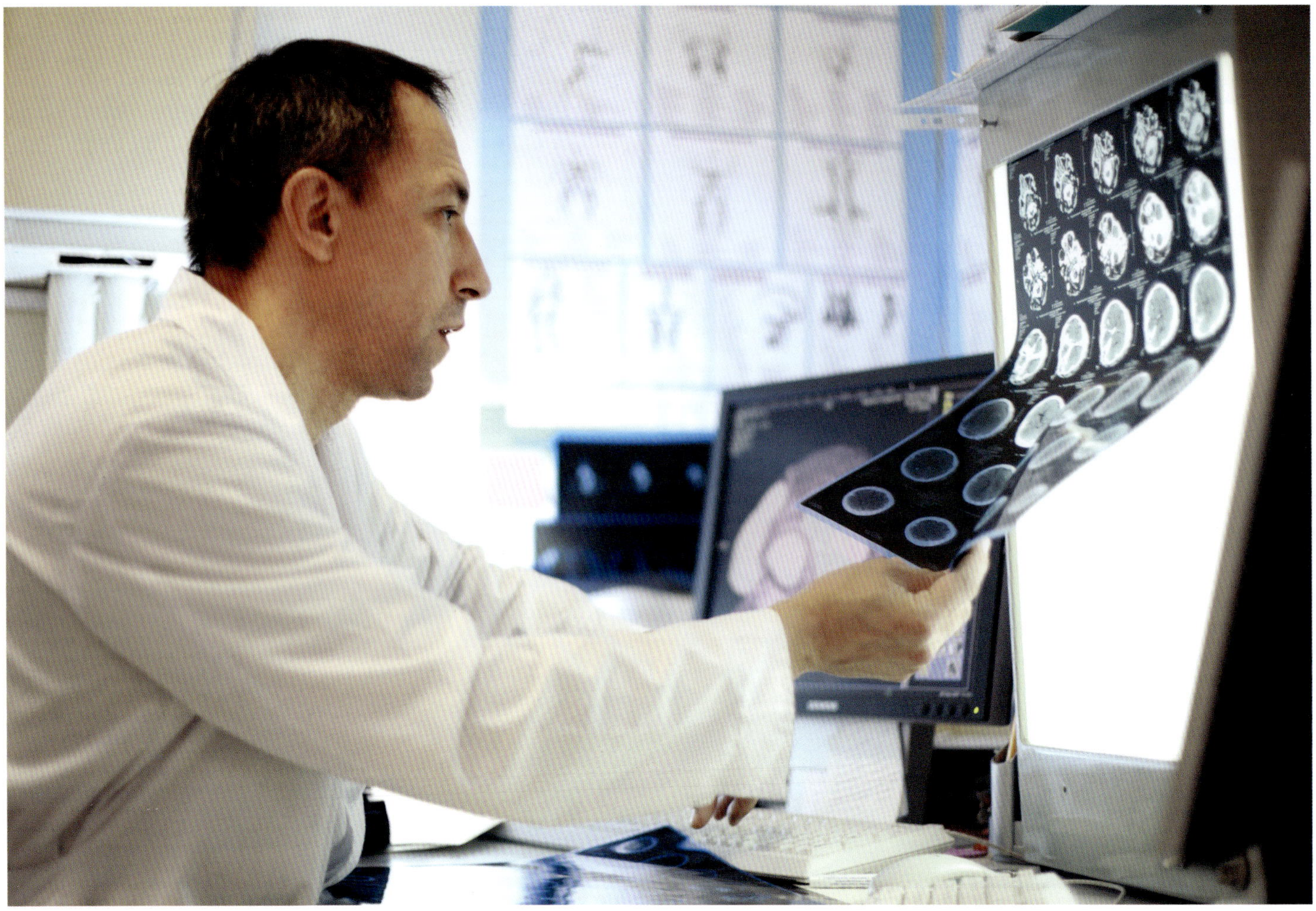

A technician viewing a CT scan

blood vessel to rupture. Abdominal distress may increase after eating.

The mere presence of diverticular pouches is not a problem requiring treatment; only when the pouches become inflamed is action needed. While diverticulosis may be asymptomatic, a person with diverticulitis will definitely know that something is amiss. The symptoms will probably move a sufferer to seek immediate medical attention, which is a correct course of action, since this disease can lead to potentially life-threatening consequences. A person who has developed diverticulitis may experience any of the following symptoms:

- Abdominal pain, cramping, tenderness (usually left-sided)
- Fever
- Chills
- Bloating
- A change in bowel habits (constipation or diarrhea)
- An almost continual need to eliminate
- Blood in the stool
- Elevated white blood cell count (an indication of infection)
- Nausea
- Vomiting

Serious complications, including intestinal obstruction and perforation, may develop. With obstruction, there is blockage of the flow of fecal material out of the body. In perforation, a tear or hole in the wall of the colon develops allowing colon bacteria to spill over into other areas of the body. If the person is lucky, the body will seal off the infection with the surrounding tissue. If the inflammation does not seal this perforation, the colon bacteria can infect the peritoneal abdominal cavity, a very serious condition called peritonitis. If the infection gains systemic access through the bloodstream, septicemia (infection of the bloodstream) results. Such infections are very serious, and can lead to death if not promptly treated.

Infection can spread to other areas of the body in the form of a fistula, which is an abnormal passage between two organs or between an organ and the skin. Most commonly this occurs between the colon and the bladder when colonic bacteria invade the bladder and cause infection there.[10] Formation of a fistula is a serious medical problem usually requiring surgical intervention.

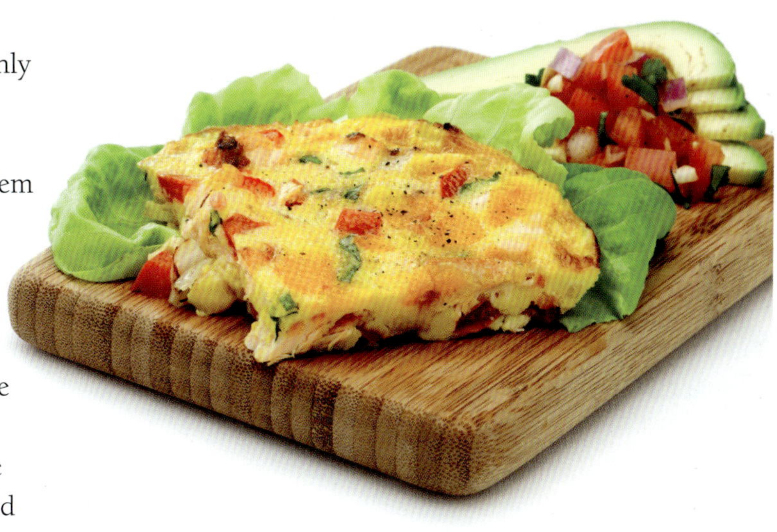

A breakfast recipe from the Fiber 35 Eating Plan

How Is It Diagnosed?

Many times, diverticular pockets are found in the course of routine diagnostic procedures, such as x-rays or endoscopy, done for other purposes. Since many people with diverticulosis have no symptoms, they are surprised to learn of the presence of the condition.

Abdominal palpation will give the examining physician a clue regarding the correct diagnosis. Even with mild diverticulitis, discomfort tends to increase as pressure is applied. Routine blood tests can be helpful because an elevated white blood cell count will indicate infection, a common sign of diverticulitis. An ultrasound examination or computerized tomography (CT) scan can provide more information if diverticulitis is suspected.

A barium enema may be used to confirm the diagnosis, but some doctors caution against using this procedure during acute episodes since it involves filling the colon (or a portion of it) with liquid barium.[11,12] The reason for concern is, if the bowel has already perforated, there will be spillage of barium, which is quite irritating, into the abdominal cavity.

A sigmoidoscopy or a colonoscopy may also be performed. In these procedures, the doctor is also able to take tissue samples for later analysis. As with the barium enema, some doctors feel that an endoscope may be a dangerous instrument to pass into an inflamed colon.[13] It may be prudent to hold off on any invasive diagnostic procedures until inflammation has subsided. In some cases the patients own clotted blood can be mixed with clotting agents and injected into the identified bleeding site which may obviate the need for surgery.

Where bleeding is present, a bleeding scan is employed as an initial screen. An isotope (a mildly radioactive material) is injected into an arm vein and allowed to circulate in the body. To confirm the site of bleeding, a special X-ray, called an angiography, is done. In this procedure, a dye is injected into an artery that goes into the colon so the site of bleeding can be located. This is very helpful in the event that emergent surgery is needed to locate the general problem area.

In the rare instance where inflamed diverticular pouches occur in the ascending colon (right side of the abdomen) distinguishing diverticulitis from appendicitis can be

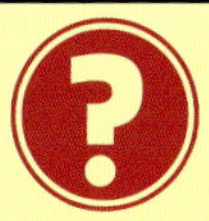

Did You Know

- Diverticulosis is more prevalent as people age. For example, it is estimated that half of the people in the United States ages 60 to 80 have diverticulosis, but only one person in 10 develops it by age 40. It is equally common in women and men.
- About 10 to 25 percent of people with diverticulosis develop diverticulitis. This occurs when the diverticula become inflamed or infected.
- People who eat high-fiber diets are less likely to develop diverticular disease. The American Dietetic Association recommends 20 to 35 grams of fiber a day, preferably from fruits, vegetables and grains. Natural health practitioners recommend eating between 35 and 50 grams of fiber per day.
- Physical activity also may lower the risk of diverticulosis.

problematic for the physician. It is also significant that soft tissue, abdominal, muscular or ovarian problems can mimic diverticular disease.[14] Additionally, the inflammation of diverticulitis can resemble the segmental inflammation characteristic of Crohn's disease, and the symptoms of diverticulitis may mimic those of colon cancer and other conditions. Differential diagnosis in these situations becomes extremely important.

What Is the Standard Medical Treatment?

Where diverticula are found, but no symptoms or inflammation is present, treatment is not recommended, though the patient may be counseled to increase the amount of fiber in the diet as a preventive measure. One very large study has found that insoluble fiber is of particular importance.[15] A good diet, one that is free of processed foods and high in fiber, can help keep existing diverticula free of infection. There is no known way to get rid of diverticula once they have formed, but individuals can take steps to prevent more of them from forming, and to avoid their development into diverticulitis by following the Fiber 35 Eating Plan in the Appendix of this book.

In the acute stages of an episode of diverticulitis, whether it is a mild or severe case, there are two critically important steps that must be taken to successfully treat the condition:

1. Rest the bowel – bowel rest is accomplished through elimination of solid foods and adhering to a clear liquid diet during the initial phases of the episode. If the condition is severe, the patient may be placed strictly on intravenous fluids, and hospitalization may be required. As symptoms subside, a soft, low-fiber diet is initiated. Keeping fat intake low may also help in reducing pressure inside the colon.[16]

2. Control the infection[17] – infection control is traditionally accomplished through the use of antibiotics. These will be administered intravenously to the patient whose condition is severe enough for him/her to be hospitalized. Total bed rest will be required. In milder cases, bed rest is still advised, though the patient need not be hospitalized. The patient will be given oral antibiotics and put on a clear liquid diet initially, then a soft, low-fiber one. The Fiber 35 Eating Plan can be initiated within a month of recovery from the acute episode of diverticulitis. The majority of patients recover without surgery.

Once a normal diet is resumed, in addition to emphasizing high-fiber foods, the patient is often counseled to avoid tiny seeds and nuts as it is believed that these may get trapped in diverticula causing inflammation. These are healthy foods, though, and can be ground in a coffee grinder before eating without having a harmful effect on the intestine. Although diverticulitis is a serious condition, it is encouraging that diverticula do not predispose a person to colon cancer, or even to precancerous polyps.[18]

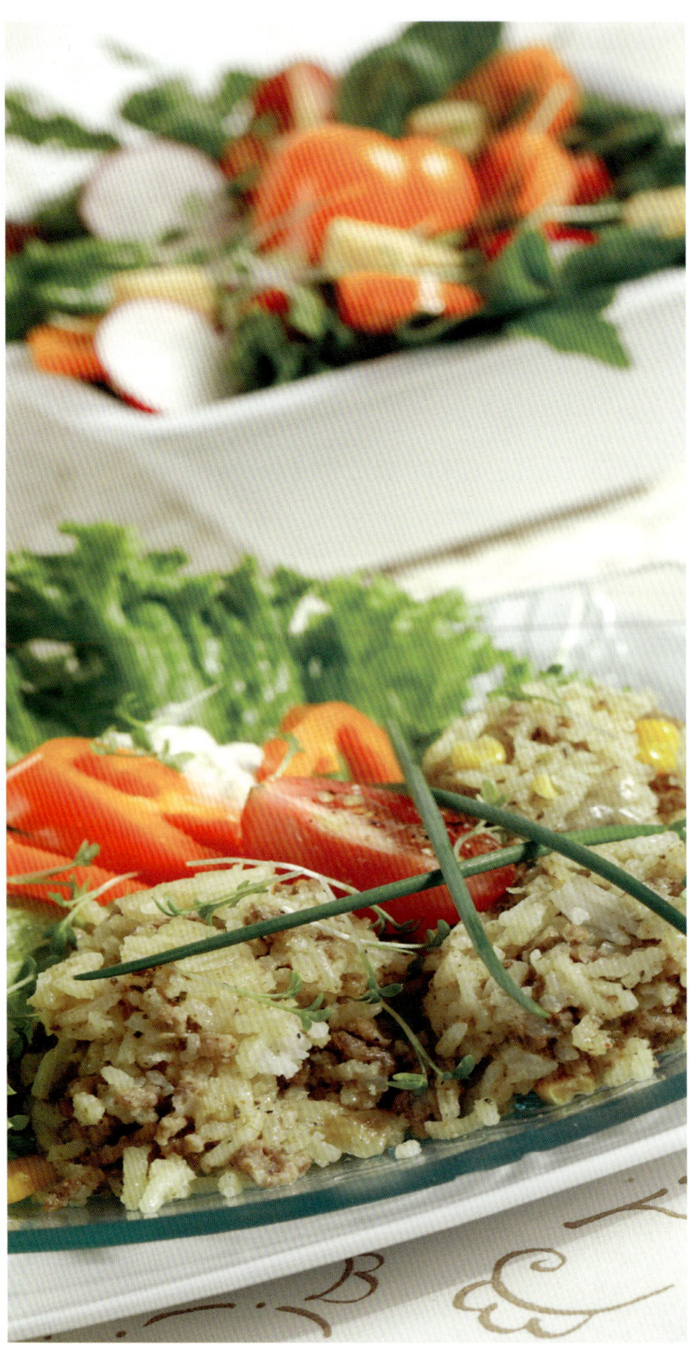

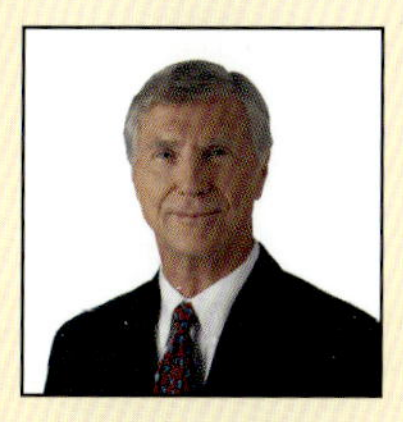

Dr. Smith's Comments

In my own personal experience I have treated many patients with acute diverticulitis but have not found it necessary to operate on but a small percentage. With bed rest, IV fluids, antibiotics, and even in some cases hyperalimentation, it was surprising how many patients recovered without surgery. Furthermore, on long-term follow up, a percentage of these patients did not appear to develop recurrent diverticulitis. This was most likely the outcome in people who were willing to follow a prescribed program which included hydration, and the HOPE program – High fiber, Omega oils, Probiotics and digestive Enzymes. In addition, supplements with multivitamins, minerals and antioxidants were recommended.

The sad part of early surgical intervention for diverticulitis is that it invariably results in two, if not three operations. Typically, the first operation will be drainage of an abscess and a diverting colostomy; the second operation being resection of the area of the diverticular perforation, often with much of the surrounding area that includes diverticuli; and third, closure of the colostomy. When all three operations are necessary, it often takes at least three to six months for the patient to recover, and at great expense. However, sometimes all of this is necessary.

We now know that at least SCAD (segmental colitis associated with diverticula) may occur due to dysbiosis, or microfloral imbalance.[19] Therefore, in order to prevent diverticulosis/diverticulitis, good hydration, exercise, daily bowel movements, good nutrition, fiber and probiotics should be used on a regular basis as part of a wise health program.

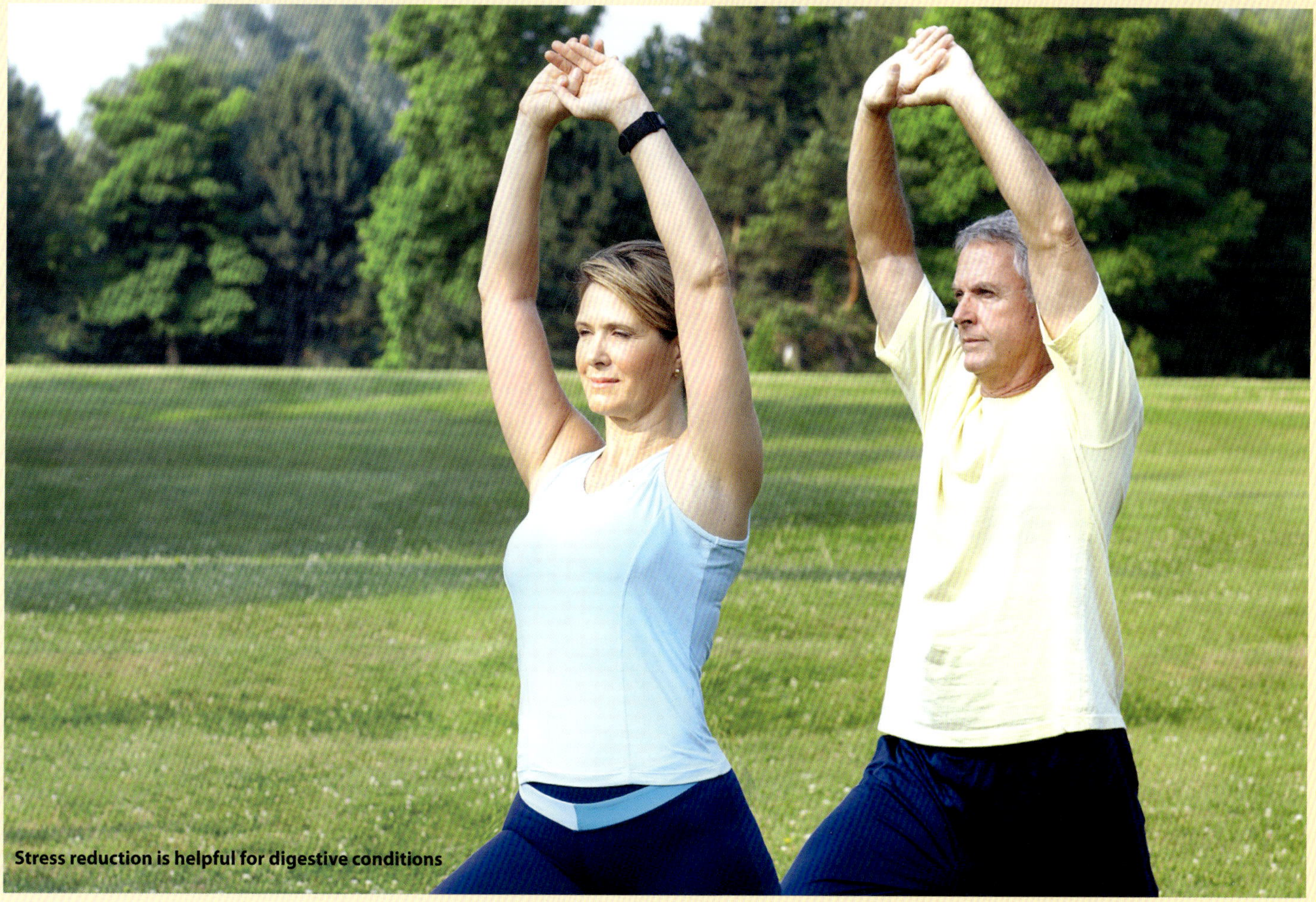

Stress reduction is helpful for digestive conditions

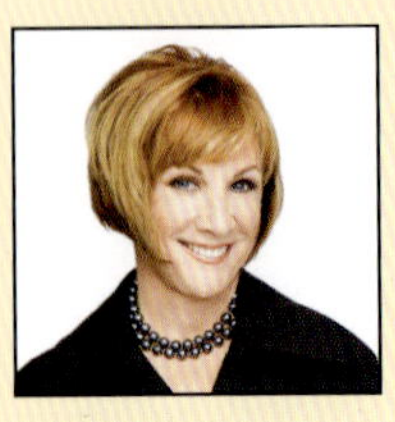

Brenda's Bottom Line

Diverticulosis is clearly due to a lack of dietary fiber. A high-fiber diet is protective against the development of diverticulosis, as well as protective of the inflammation of diverticulitis in people who already have diverticulosis. Follow the Fiber 35 Eating Plan (see the Appendix) as an important part of maintaining health with diverticulosis.

Diverticulitis can be a dangerous condition, especially if a ruptured diverticula is involved, which can poison the whole body. A medical doctor should be consulted in the case of diverticulitis. For those who have been treated by a doctor, are coming out of an attack of diverticulitis, and are allowed to eat food, the following suggestions will be helpful.

Diet

- Active diverticulitis may require a total liquid diet and/or intravenous fluids under hospital supervision.
- If you are recovering from a recent attack, and have been approved to eat soft foods, follow the Fiber 35 Eating Plan in the Appendix until feeling better.
- When using nuts and seeds, soak them overnight, and then grind with a high-speed blender or coffee grinder before eating.
- Use fresh garlic liberally as it is a great natural antibiotic, and can help prevent recurrent infections.
- Cook whole grains with twice the recommended water and for twice as long.

Lifestyle

- Exercise, such as walking or light jogging, has been shown to be helpful to protect against diseases of the colon.
- Avoid constipation by using stool softeners or natural laxatives.
- Use the LifeStep, a toilet step that will help raise your feet, so you are in natural squatting position for better elimination.
- Eat slowly and chew foods well to mush before swallowing.
- Drink plenty of clean, purified water.

Complementary Mind/Body Therapies

- Periodic colon hydrotherapy can be extremely helpful with diverticulosis as part of your preventive measures. Colon hydrotherapy should NOT be used during a diverticulitis attack.
- Yoga and/or pilates could be beneficial as there are exercises to strengthen the abdominal area. The colon is a muscle and, just like any other muscle, needs to be toned.

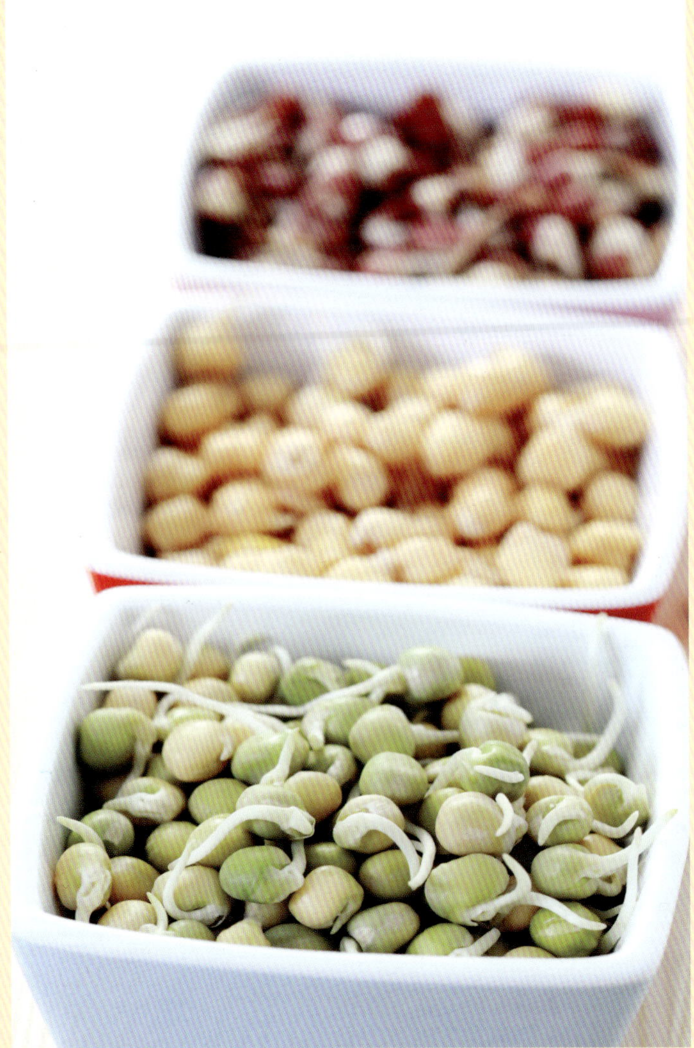

Recommended Nutraceuticals	Dosage	Benefit	Comments
Critical Phase	Daily maintenance recommendations should also be taken during this phase unless otherwise indicated.		
Follow daily maintenance protocol below.	In the case of diverticulitis, medical intervention is necessary. Always follow your doctor's suggestions and care. The following recommendations are for maintenance of diverticulosis and reduction of the likelihood of infection and inflammation.		
Helpful			
Natural Laxative Formula	Use as directed	Reduces straining and pressure due to constipation.	Use products based on magnesium with mild herbs. Avoid purgative herbs like cascara and senna.
Antioxidant Supplement	Use as directed	Protects tissue from damage.	Look for a high-potency antioxidant formulation.
Daily Maintenance			
Probiotics	50 billion culture capsule 1-2 times daily	Maintains and restores bacterial ecology and pH of the colon.	Look for one with high amounts of bifidobacteria. This is the main bacteria in the colon.
Fiber	10-15 grams twice daily	Adds bulk to strengthen the colon wall. Reduces the chance of waste getting into diverticula.	Extremely important to the prevention of diverticulitis and the further development of diverticula.
L-Glutamine Powder with Gamma Oryzanol	5-10 grams daily	Helps maintain health and integrity of intestinal lining. Reduces inflammation.	Best taken in loose powder form.
Omega-3 Fatty Acids	At least 2 grams daily of EPA/DHA combination	Helps reduce inflammation.	Look for a concentrated, enteric coated fish oil.
Digestive Enzymes	Take with meals	Helps digest and absorb nutrients from food.	Look for one that includes protease, lipase, amylase and lactase.

See further explanation of supplements in the Appendix

GAS

What Is It?

The presence of excessive gas in the stomach is known as eructation, or belching, and in the intestines it is known as flatulence. Flatulence, when paired with other gastrointestinal symptoms, can be a sign of a serious GI disorder such as: malabsorption, bacterial imbalance in the intestines (dysbiosis), parasitic infection, irritable bowel syndrome (IBS), colitis, gallbladder disease, Candida overgrowth, gastroesophageal reflux disease (GERD) or even a pancreatic tumor. At the very least, excessive gas production is a signal of incomplete digestion. In and of itself, the passing of gas is not considered a medical problem unless it is excessive. Trapped gas can cause a great deal more distress than that passed either through the rectum or by belching.

Certain gases are normally present in the GI tract and have no odor. These include nitrogen, oxygen, carbon dioxide and hydrogen. It is other gases, like hydrogen sulfide and byproducts of anaerobic bacteria (like indole, butyric acid, cadaverine, putrescine and skatole) that give off the foul-smelling odor of flatulence. People who pass excess gas have more sulfate-reducing bacteria in their feces. These bacteria cause high levels of sulfides in the feces, which is associated with disease of the colon.[1]

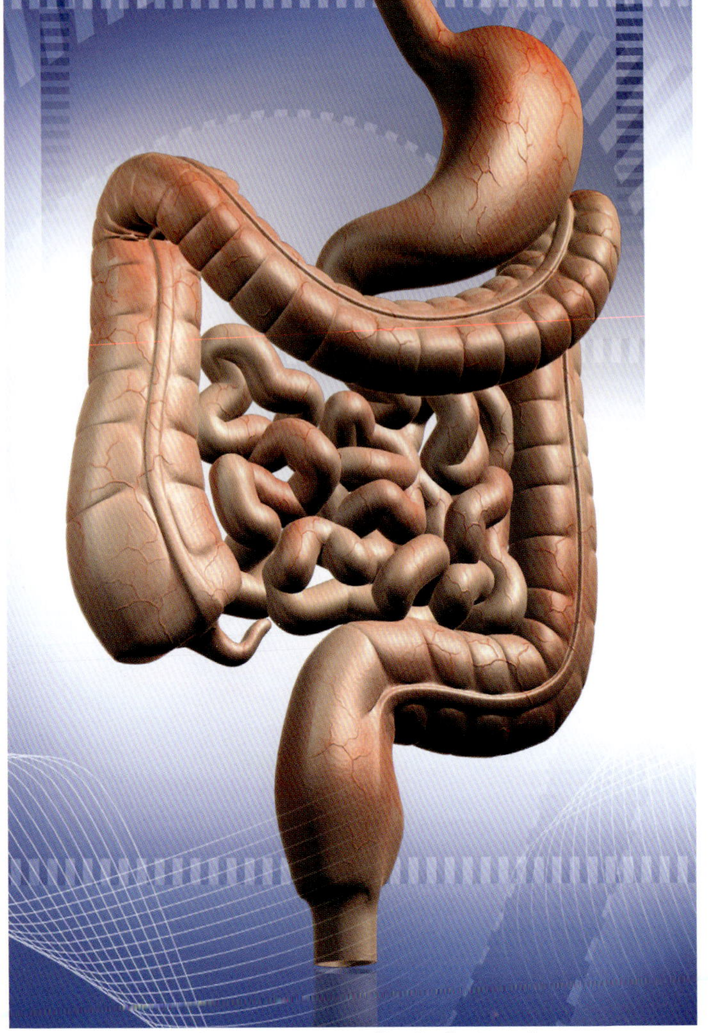

Gas can develop in the upper gut as well as in the intestines.

What Causes It?

There are five major reason gas could create problems:

- A person may be hypersensitive to trapped gas and react to this gas in a similar way as irritable bowel syndrome (IBS)
- Carbon dioxide gas that is formed in the duodenum by a chemical reaction of hydrochloric acid from the stomach and the bicarbonate of the pancreatic secretions[2]
- Incomplete digestion of protein, carbohydrates or fats
- Candida overgrowth causing yeast fermentation
- Dysbiosis causing bacterial fermentation

When bacteria in the colon or distal small bowel act on undigested food not absorbed in the small intestine, sulfide gases are generated by the bacteria resulting in an unpleasant odor.

Excessive gas can be the result of swallowing too much air. This can happen when: talking too much while eating, eating too rapidly, drinking carbonated beverages, chewing gum, smoking, or sucking on hard candies. Postnasal drip and ill-fitting dentures can also cause air to be swallowed due to excessive salivation.

Lactose intolerance is another cause of excessive gas. People who are lactose intolerant lack the enzyme lactase needed to break down the lactose (milk sugar) present in milk. The milk, therefore, is not properly digested, and undergoes fermentation in the large intestine causing gas. (See the Lactose Intolerance section for more information.)

Some people are intolerant to other sugars and sugar substitutes also due to a deficiency in the enzymes that digest those sugars.

Some foods that may give rise to gas production include:

- Cauliflower
- Brussels sprouts
- Legumes (peas, beans, lentils)
- Broccoli
- Cabbage
- Dried and sulfured fruits
- Cucumbers
- Celery
- Apples
- Carrots
- Onions
- Garlic
- Rutabaga
- Cantaloupe
- Kohlrabi
- Radishes
- Grapes
- Raisins
- Prune juice
- Bananas

Not all of these foods will cause excess gas in all people, but any of these can be a potential problem. The cruciferous vegetables—kale, collard greens, broccoli, cauliflower, cabbage, brussels sprouts and turnips—contain a special type of carbohydrate (stachyose) that is poorly absorbed by the body, but is quickly digested by bacteria in the intestines.[3]

Overeating can also result in excess gas production due to incomplete food chewing and digestion.

Did You Know

The average person will pass gas, or flatus, emitted from the rectum approximately 13 times a day.

Healing HOPE Testimonial

"I recently began taking the probiotics, and digestive enzyme for gas, both with foods that normally give me gas. I ate a whole pile of coleslaw one night, a soy protein shake another morning, and I had no problems with gas! I am so excited that these supplements are working so well. I should have tried this years ago."
– Brenda

Over-consumption of the irritants caffeine, alcohol, salt, refined sugar, carbohydrates and processed oils can be particularly problematic.

Nutritional deficiencies of digestive enzymes, hydrochloric acid, B vitamins (needed for carbohydrate combustion) and food allergies or sensitivities may also result in excessive gas production, as can too much vitamin C.

Poor food combining may result in excess gas production for some people. Improper food combining results primarily from mixing starchy foods, like grains, potatoes or fruits; with protein foods, like meat, eggs or cheese. Starchy foods and fruits are relatively low in protein and fat, and are more quickly absorbed and digested when eaten alone (especially raw fruit with its high enzyme content). It is believed that when protein and fat are combined with starch or fruit the slower overall absorption allows for more bacterial fermentation of the starch and sugars, thereby creating more gas. The total digestive need for more enzymes then becomes a factor, particularly with aging.

Everyone passes gas. The average person passes it approximately 13 times a day.[4] About 30 percent of the U.S. population have bacteria in the colon or small intestine that produce excessive amounts of methane and hydrogen.[5] These are the people who are likely to be the most disease-prone. Overgrowth of bacteria in the colon or small bowel can cause serious problems due to increased intestinal permeability that allows absorption of microbial toxins and partially digested food.

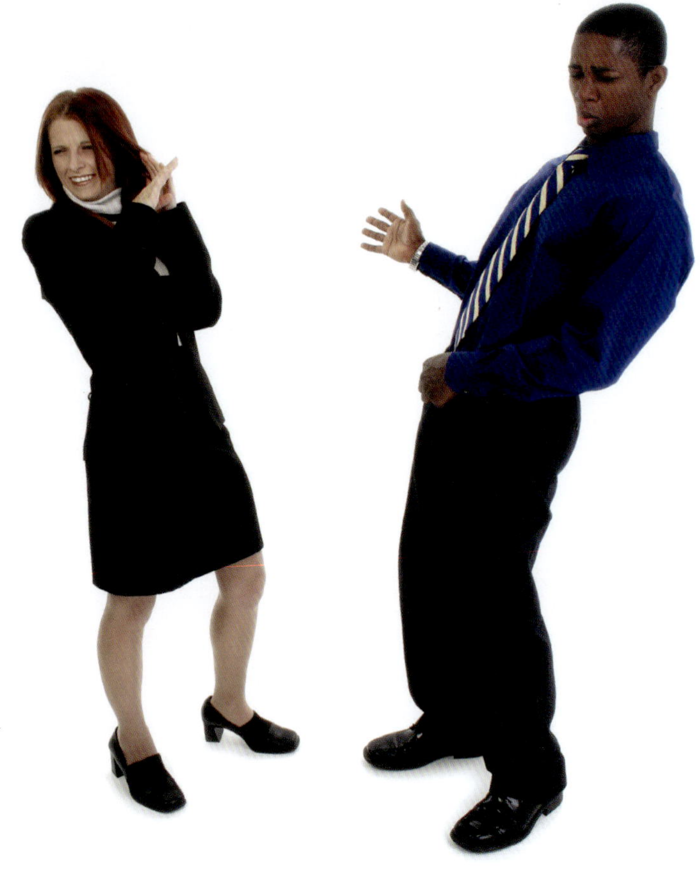

What Are the Signs and Symptoms?

Excess intestinal gas is thought to produce:

- Belching
- Bloating
- Abdominal distention and discomfort
- Bad breath
- Feeling of fullness
- Release of malodorous gas through the anus

It appears that some people who suffer from these symptoms (especially those with irritable bowel syndrome) produce normal amounts of gas and yet are hypersensitive to it.

How Is It Diagnosed?

Unless the passage of gas is chronic and accompanied by other symptoms, no special diagnostics are indicated. Taking a thorough and detailed medical history can help give the attending physician an idea of the cause of the problem.

Consultation with a physician is recommended for anyone experiencing any of the symptoms above. Further tests will then be done to rule out or confirm the suspected diagnosis.

A comprehensive stool analysis (CSA), often used by natural health practitioners, can be used to detect candidiasis and other dysbiotic imbalances. Food sensitivities, which can sometimes be spotted by keeping a food diary, may be determined through testing. (See the Appendix for information on these tests.)

What Is the Standard Medical Treatment?

Recommended treatment is aimed primarily at:

- Altering lifestyle elements so that air swallowing is reduced
- Suppressing symptoms through use of drugs
- Altering the diet

The following measures may help to reduce air swallowing:

- Eat slowly and chew thoroughly with the mouth closed.
- Avoid chewing gum.
- Quit smoking.
- Eliminate carbonated beverages.
- Make sure dentures fit properly.
- Seek treatment for any disorder (such as peptic ulcer) that may cause reflex hypersalivation.
- Don't talk excessively while eating.
- Drink iced-cold beverages in moderation, if at all.
- Eliminate or reduce sorbitol and xylitol, undigestible sugars that may cause gas.
- Exclude dairy products if lactose intolerant.
- Reduce or eliminate medications (under a doctor's supervision) that may cause excessive salivation.
- Try biofeedback and relaxation therapy.
- Eliminate antacids if associated with belching.

Several drugs incorporating simethicone, an agent that breaks up small gas bubbles, have been used (with variable results) to treat gas. Anti-cholingergic drugs have been used with similar results. These affect the nervous system.

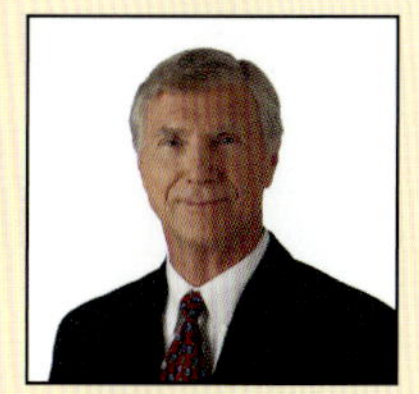

Dr. Smith's Comments

Since excessive intestinal gas at times may be associated with increased microbial fermentation in the lower intestine, a test known as the lactulose tolerance test can be done. This involves giving the patient a standardized dose of the poorly-absorbable sugar lactulose. After a given period of time expired air is measured for both methane gas and hydrogen gas. It is generally considered that excess fermentation is present if the test is positive test for hydrogen or methane. This indicates a condition known as small intestinal bacterial overgrowth (SIBO), a form of dysbiosis which is usually remedied with the 4R program: Remove pathogens with antimicrobials, Reinoculate with probiotics, Replace with digestive enzymes, HCl and bile salts, and Repair with glutamine, arginine, vitamin A, zinc, gamma oryzanol and N-acetyl-D-glucosamine.

Interestingly, in applying the lactulose breath test to patients with IBS, those with IBS constipation tend to have higher levels of methane whereas patients with IBS diarrhea tend to have higher levels of hydrogen, which would support the fact that different bacteria may cause different problems.

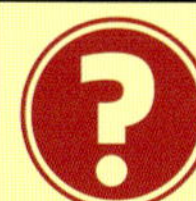

Did You Know

- Almost half of Americans (46 percent) claim to have been embarrassed by intestinal gas in public.
- According to the Canadian Society of Intestinal Research, careful analysis of intestinal gas has shown that about 90 percent is ingested air, and only 10 percent is actually formed in the intestine.
- Gas occurring within one to one and a half hours after eating may suggest poor digestion of food which is being delivered undigested to the lower intestines.
- There are some people who lack the enzyme that is needed to digest lactose, the sugar in milk, resulting in the production of gas in the large intestine.

A positive lactulose breath test result may also be found in patients with other conditions such as fibromyalgia. In one study 42 out of 42 patients were positive with elevated hydrogen, suggesting that the SIBO led to increased intestinal permeability (leaky gut) with immune upregulation contributing to fibromyalgia.[6]

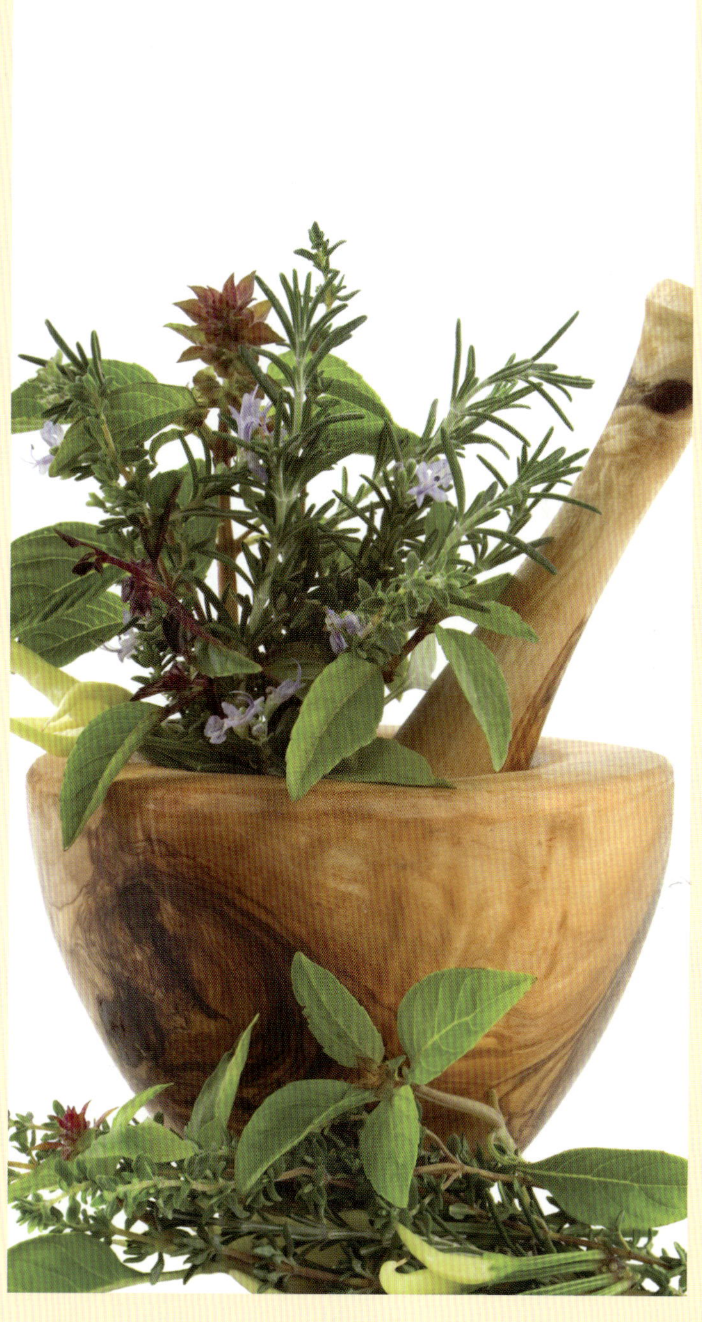

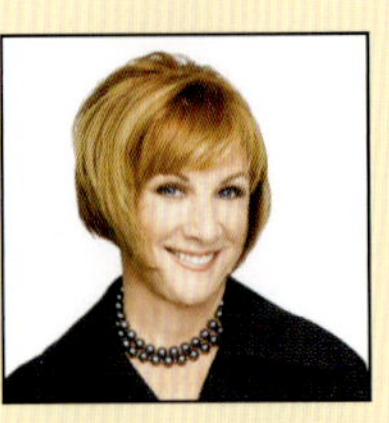

Brenda's Bottom Line

Gas is a broad symptom that can be a part of different conditions. It is important to determine just where the gas occurs, and if it is associated with other symptoms. Many times people simply say, "It's in my stomach," or "It's in my belly," but they are not clear on just where the gas and bloating occur. Figure out where in the body the gas is located. If the gas involves belching, bloating or discomfort that feels higher up towards the ribs, you are dealing with something different than if your lower abdomen is bloated and you are experiencing flatulence.

After pinpointing just where the gas occurs, then determine whether there are other accompanying symptoms. Do you also have diarrhea? Constipation? Heartburn? Does your gas occur after eating certain foods? If your gas involves the lower intestines, you may have over-fermentation in the lower small intestine. This can involve bacterial or Candida overgrowth, and can lead to a more serious condition known as nonalcoholic fatty liver disease (NAFLD). (See the NAFLD section for more information.)

If you are able to rule out the possible underlying conditions (see below), follow the suggestions below to help minimize or eliminate your gas and bloating.

Rule Out:

After you have really investigated your symptoms, it is important to rule out the following possible underlying conditions:

- Candida overgrowth (See the Candidiasis section.)
- Parasites (See Parasitic Disease section.)
- Food sensitivities (See Allergies or Gluten Sensitivity sections.)
- Lactose intolerance (See the Lactose Intolerance section.)

Recommended Testing

- Comprehensive stool analysis (CSA) (See the Appendix.)
- Lactulose breath test (See the Appendix.)

Diet

Follow the Candida Diet (see the Appendix) if you think that different foods are triggering your gas. This diet is also helpful for people who experience over-fermentation in the gut due to sugary foods and simple carbs. From there, you can begin to introduce certain foods and move toward the Fiber 35 Eating Plan, keeping out any foods that you determine to be gas-producing.

Lifestyle

- Check with your doctor to see if any medications you are taking could be causing gas.
- Do not eat late at night; stop eating a few hours before bed to give your body enough time to digest the food you have eaten.
- Exercise to help stimulate the passage of gas through the GI tract.

Complementary Mind/Body Therapies

- Colon hydrotherapy sessions could be helpful in removing excess gas from the colon.
- Abdominal massage can be helpful in moving out trapped gas.

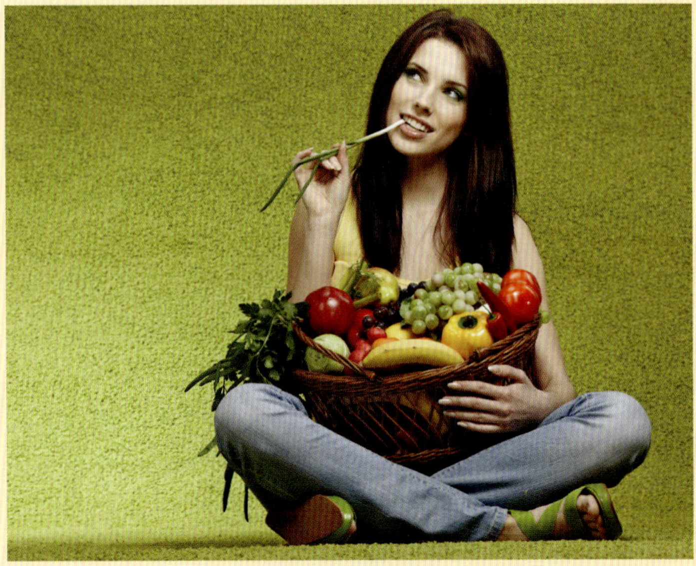

Recommended Nutraceuticals	Dosage	Benefit	Comments
Critical Phase	**Daily maintenance recommendations should also be taken during this phase unless otherwise indicated.**		
Enzyme Formula specific for gas	Take with meals	Helps digest gas-forming foods.	Look for formula with alpha galactosidase, phytase, cellulase and fennel seed.
Bentonite clay / Apple pectin / Charcoal Formula	Use as directed	Absorbs bacterial toxins from over-fermentation and improves regularity.	Take with plenty of water.
Helpful			
Fennel or Peppermint Tea	2-3 cups daily or when needed	Has long history of relieving gas and bloating.	Either use the prepared tea bags or seeds of fennel.
Daily Maintenance			
Digestive Enzymes	Take with meals	Helps digest and absorb nutrients from food.	If low stomach acid is found find a formula that contains hydrochloric acid.
Probiotics	30 - 80 billion cultures daily	Re-establishes bacterial balance in intestine.	May need to start with lower dosage and increase over time to avoid excess flatulence as bacteria rebalance.
Omega-3 Fatty Acids	At least 2 grams daily of EPA/DHA combination	Helps restore moisture to the intestinal tract and reduces inflammation.	Look for a concentrated, enteric coated fish oil.
Fiber	4-5 grams twice daily	Helps produce healthy bacteria levels and good elimination.	Use in conjunction with high fiber diet to reach 35 g daily.

See further explanation of supplements in the Appendix

Gluten Sensitivity / Celiac

What Is It?

Gluten is the insoluble protein constituent of wheat and other grains, a mixture of gliadin, glutenin and other proteins.[1] It is the gluten in grains that makes the rising of flour possible.

Gluten sensitivity is an inflammatory reaction to eating foods containing gluten. It occurs mainly in the lining of the small intestine where an immune response is triggered against the gluten proteins. The degree of gluten sensitivity can be minor to life threatening. Thus, there are numerous terms, encompassing several different conditions, that involve some degree or form of gluten or grain sensitivity. This can be very confusing for those not acquainted with this subject.

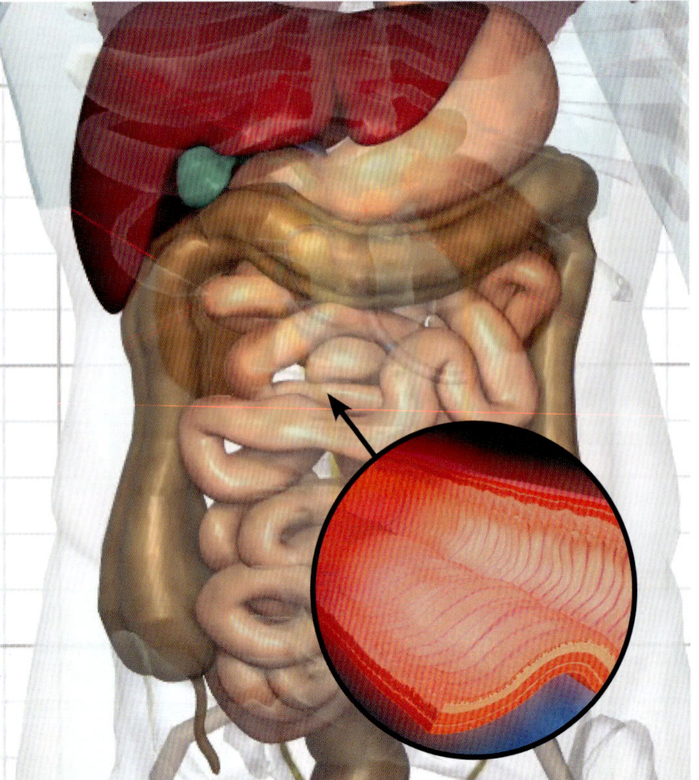

Illustration of small intestinal inflammation in someone suffering from gluten sensitivity

Celiac disease, which is the most severe form of gluten sensitivity, can, in fact, go by six different names: sprue, non-tropical sprue, celiac sprue, gluten-induced sprue and gluten-induced enteropathy. These are terms for true celiac disease.

Due to the fact that many people are gluten sensitive, there has been a paradigm shift, and the new term for this condition is "non-celiac gluten sensitivity" or, simply, "gluten sensitivity."

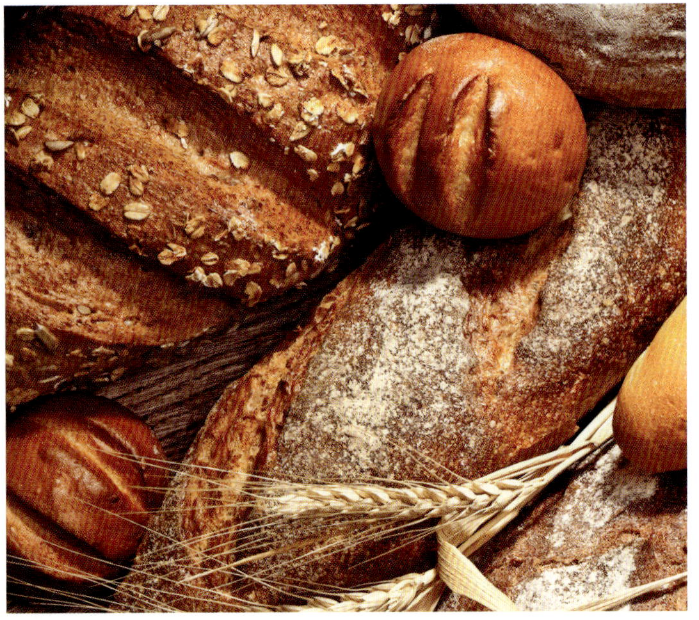

Until 200 years ago, the wheat used to make bread had two sets of chromosomes (made up of DNA) in its molecular structure. This is also known as 2N, or diploid chromosome structure. With the development of agricultural hybridization, which combines different varieties and even species of plants to "improve" crop production, the wheat plant has drastically changed over time, so that it no longer has a 2N structure.

Wheat plants of today have from six to even 12 or more sets of chromosomes. This means that wheat has a much more complex DNA structure than it did originally. One particular amino acid sequence in modern wheat, known as 33-mer, not present in wheat before agricultural progress, is unable to break down in the digestive tract. In patients with celiac disease, 33-mer is acted upon by an enzyme that initiates an inflammatory immune response in the small intestine creating the intestinal damage found in these patients.[2]

What Causes It?

There are several causes of gluten sensitivity. They include: bacterial, viral or fungal infections, other food sensitivities, stress, chemotherapy or anything that would cause a chronic increase in leaky gut or intestinal permeability. Gluten sensitivity is a chronic disorder caused by an inability to properly digest foods that contain gluten. These foods include:[3]

- Wheat
- Rye
- Barley
- Possibly oats

The failure to properly digest these foods results in damage to the cells lining the small intestine, which results in malabsorption of nutrients from food. Gliadin is the main protein component in wheat that causes difficulty for those suffering from gluten sensitivity. However, similar proteins in other grains may cause the same reaction such as: hordein in barley, secalin in rye and avidin in oats.

Current research suggests that the gliadin is absorbed between cells, and certain fragments of gliadin induce intense immune inflammatory reactions that injure the bowel lining further exacerbating the injury. In addition, antibodies produced in the immune reaction can cross react with other tissues leading to a wide array of autoimmune diseases. Interestingly, gliadin that has been completely broken down by digestion does not activate gluten sensitivity in susceptible individuals. This suggests that gluten sensitivity may arise from a deficiency of enzymes that break down gliadin or other factors involved with protein digestion.[4]

The inflammatory immune response typical of celiac disease eventually destroys the villi of the intestines through which nutrients are absorbed into the bloodstream. The result is malabsorption.

In addition, the inflammation can break the junctions between the cells of the intestinal lining through which larger toxins can be absorbed. Through this increased intestinal permeability, or leaky gut, toxins enter and directly interact with the immune system located within the intestinal wall (gut-associated lymphoid tissue, or GALT). These toxins trigger antibodies that go into the bloodstream where they circulate throughout the body. **It is important to realize that not everyone with gluten sensitivity has full blown celiac disease.** Some people simply lack the enzymes needed to properly break down gluten that can cause leaky gut and inflammation even if it doesn't create the full immune response of celiac disease.[5]

The stage may be set for development of celiac disease in infancy. The early introduction of cow's milk is believed to be a major causative factor in celiac disease.[6] Early introduction of cereals appears to be another factor. In fact, research has indicated that delayed administration of [both] cow's milk and cereal grains are the primary preventive steps that can greatly reduce the risk of developing celiac disease.[7] Interestingly, these are often the very first foods introduced in an infant's diet. Another study showed the protective effects of introducing gluten-

Healing HOPE Testimonial

"I had all the symptoms for Candida, parasites and leaky gut, probably the result of taking antibiotics for over three years as a teen. My list of symptoms went on and on. Over the past year, after reading **Gut Solutions, Detox Strategy** and **The Fiber35 Diet** books, I followed the recommendations arduously. I did the Steps to Cleansing (Total Body Cleanse, Candida Cleanse, Parasite Cleanse and Liver Detox) and took the HOPE supplements daily (High Fiber, Omega oils, Probiotics and Enzymes), as well as eating organic fresh foods and eliminating sugar. After a year I felt much better, but still felt like something was missing.

At Brenda's recommendation, I did the gluten sensitivity testing. I am so amazed! I did not realize that I had celiac disease. I stopped eating gluten and in a few weeks, I felt like a new person.

Not a week goes by that I am not talking to someone about this topic. I pray that Brenda Watson is encouraged to continue in the quest to educate on this most vital topic. May Brenda Watson become a household name!"
– Tina

containing products before the child was weaned from breast milk.[8] This is likely due to the increased immune benefits that come from breast milk, highlighting the importance of breastfeeding for longer periods of time.

Celiac disease, in some cases, has a hereditary component. Therefore, many family members may be affected. The disease is usually identified in early childhood, but may disappear in adolescence and reappear later in adulthood.[9] It can also make its first appearance in adult years. Celiac disease occurs twice as often in females as in males,[10] and primarily affects Caucasians and people of European descent.[11] It rarely occurs in people of African, Jewish, Mediterranean or Asian descent.[12] The highest incidences of the disease occur in northern and central Europe, the northwestern Indian subcontinent and any other areas where wheat cultivation is a relatively recent development.[13] Estimates of the frequency of the disease in the United States vary widely from source to source, often ranging from one in 1,000 to one in 5,000 people. However, recent studies show that silent, or subclinical, celiac disease affects many more people than previously thought.[14] For every celiac patient diagnosed, there are eight more who have not been diagnosed.

There are many other factors which may contribute to gluten sensitivity. While genetics plays a role; so do factors such as other food sensitivities, intestinal infections (including viral infection), surgery, extreme stress, child birth[15] and the consumption of the Standard American Diet (SAD). Others who have an elevated risk of developing celiac disease are those with Down's syndrome, Type 1 diabetes or chronic arthritis in childhood.[16]

What Are the Signs and Symptoms?

Some people with gluten sensitivity have no symptoms, while others become quite ill experiencing:

- Weight loss
- Gas and bloating
- Diarrhea (which is typical of malabsorption)
- Abdominal pain
- Nutritional deficiencies
- Anemia (due to iron deficiency)
- Edema (fluid accumulation in the extremities due to a decrease in blood protein)
- Steatorrhea (gray or tan, fatty, greasy, foul-smelling stools that float)
- Dermatitis herpetiformis (a chronic skin condition)
- Weakness
- Lack of appetite
- Early satiety (feeling full after eating a small amount of food)
- Nausea/vomiting
- Depression
- Fatigue
- Irritability
- Muscle cramps and wasting
- Joint and/or bone pain

The first five listed are usually the first to develop. Celiac disease may cause slow growth in children, and suppress the onset of menses in adolescent girls. Also, children may exhibit behavior changes, develop blisters and sores, or a red rash all over their bodies; they may also develop mouth ulcers.[17] On the other hand, symptoms in children may be mild and are likely to be dismissed as a simple stomachache.

The immune response that is produced with gluten sensitivity may also occur in other organs. The central and peripheral nervous systems are particularly vulnerable.[18] In fact, in one recent study, neurologic disorders or findings were found in 51 percent of celiac patients.[19] There are many conditions in which gluten sensitivity is an underlying factor. Some of these include:

- Inflammatory bowel disease (IBD)
- Nonalcoholic fatty liver disease (NAFLD)
- Pancreatic disease
- Infertility
- Insulin-dependent diabetes
- Thyroid disease
- Lupus
- Rheumatoid arthritis
- Chronic fatigue syndrome
- Dementia
- Depression
- ADD/ADHD
- Autism
- Schizophrenia

Bear in mind that, while symptoms of gluten sensitivity and celiac disease may be severe, they may also be absent.

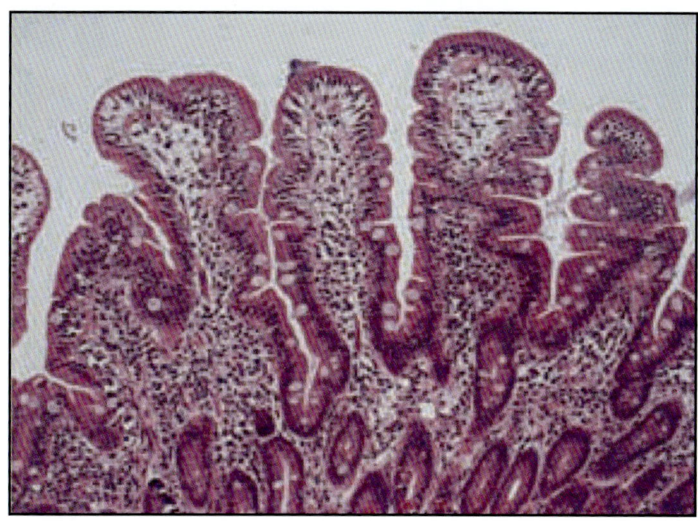

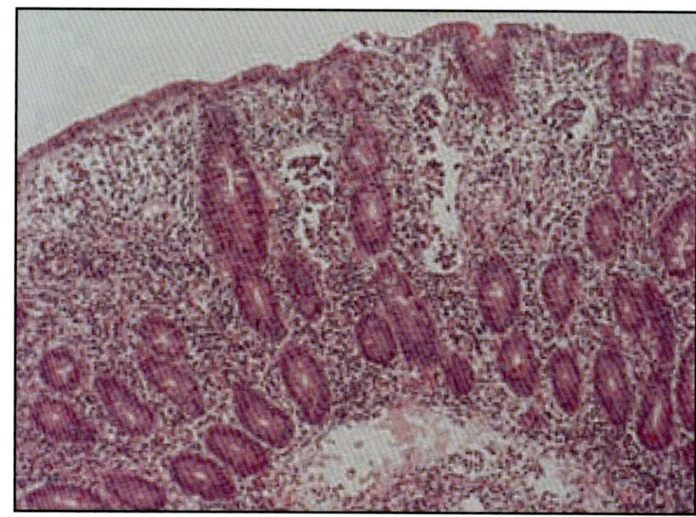

On the left, microscope image of healthy intestinal villi. On the right, villous atropy, or degradation of the villi due to intestinal inflammation in response to gluten.

New research shows that traditional gastrointestinal symptoms may be delayed for up to eight years in some adults with the first clinical signs being iron deficiency anemia, bone disease and sterility in women.[20]

A person with mild wheat intolerance may not have the inflammation in the cells lining the intestine, but nevertheless may experience such symptoms as gas and bloating, distention and even diarrhea.[21]

How Is It Diagnosed?

Diagnosis of celiac disease by symptoms alone is not possible with any degree of accuracy because of its similarity to aspects of other disorders: irritable bowel syndrome, gastric ulcers, anemia, intestinal infection, food allergy, gastroesophageal reflux disease, ulcerative colitis, Crohn's disease, lactose intolerance, HIV-related diseases and certain cancers.[22-24] It is common, therefore, to run certain tests to rule out or confirm the celiac disease diagnosis.

Traditionally, a blood test to check for IgA and IgG antibodies to gliadin (a subfraction of gluten) and to tissue transglutaminase antibody is often done. The transglutaminase antibody is most specific (found in 95 percent of cases of celiac) and is related to destruction of the intestinal lining. However, it has been determined that this test is ineffective for detecting most patients with subclinical or silent gluten sensitivity.[25] If these tests yield a positive result, they would ideally be followed by a biopsy of the small intestine that would reveal if damage to the villi is present, giving a definitive diagnosis. The biopsy is typically done in conjunction with endoscopy. Some doctors may choose to forego the biopsy, basing their diagnosis instead upon blood-test results and symptoms.

Recently, a more sensitive anti-gliadin stool antibody test has been developed by EnteroLab (see the Appendix). In hundreds of tested patients EnteroLab found only nine percent had anti-gliadin antibodies present in the blood, while 79 percent had the antibodies present in stool.[26] This is possible because the very first immune response occurs inside the intestine where the intra-epithelial lymphocytes are located. They release antibodies in the intestine that are then carried out of the body with stool. What does this mean? It means that it is now possible to detect gluten sensitivity before it has damaged the intestine. If anti-gliadin antibodies are detected in the blood, it is likely that the intestine has already been damaged, and that the antibodies may also be damaging other tissues in the body. By detecting the first stages of gluten sensitivity, with the stool test, the patient can then remove gluten and related grain proteins from the diet before the intestine becomes damaged.

Another test that is available is a saliva test for IgA antigliadin and transglutaminase antibodies. In patients with active celiac disease, this test has been shown to be reliable.[27]

Many people find that, once they implement a gluten-free diet, their health greatly improves. This alone can be a simple tool for those who believe that they may have a gluten sensitivity.

Lactose intolerance is common in people with celiac disease due to the fact that the damaged intestinal cells temporarily lose their lactase enzyme activity making it impossible to digest the lactose in dairy products. Some doctors may therefore choose to also test for lactose intolerance using a lactose breath test (see the Appendix), in addition to using the tests described above for celiac disease.

A patient who is making antibodies to gluten, but has no intestinal damage, would be diagnosed with gluten sensitivity rather than celiac disease, which is a more progressed form of gluten sensitivity. With either diagnosis, there is a probability of increased intestinal permeability (leaky gut). Physicians who are aware of this condition may elect to order intestinal permeability screening. (See the Appendix.) It is also useful to assess digestive efficiency with a comprehensive stool analysis (CSA).

What Is the Standard Medical Treatment?

Once diagnosed, prompt and thorough treatment of celiac disease is essential, for without treatment, the disease can result in malnourishment that will adversely affect the entire body. There is no known cure for celiac disease, but it can be controlled by a lifelong adherence to a totally gluten-free diet. The removal of gluten-containing grains and other gluten-containing foods from the diet eliminates irritation, giving the intestine a chance to heal. Strict adherence to a totally gluten-free diet results in the disappearance of symptoms, prompt healing of the intestinal lining and the gaining back of lost weight.

The problem is that it is not always easy to identify—much less avoid—all gluten-containing food products, particularly when there is such an abundance of processed and genetically modified foods that are wheat-based or wheat-containing. It has been shown that the closer a grain is related to wheat, the greater its ability to activate celiac disease.[28] There has been some controversy as to whether those with celiac disease can safely eat oats. Although several studies suggest that people with the disease can safely eat them, since oats are often processed along with other grains, cross contamination may occur.[29]

The list in the chart on this page is by no means comprehensive, but it gives a good idea of how much hidden gluten there is in commonly consumed foods. Add to this the fact that celiac disease patients may also need to avoid dairy products, as well as any foods to which they may be allergic, it is easy to see how food selection and preparation can be quite problematic.

The good news for the patient with gluten sensitivity is that there are many supportive organizations (see Resource Directory), periodicals and products to help make life easier. The magazine "Living Without" (www.livingwithout.com) carries current information about many lines of gluten-free products of all types. These including baked goods and pastas made with safe grains: rice, soy, potato, corn, quinoa, millet, amaranth, sorghum and buckwheat (which is not actually wheat).

Some people with a severe or long-standing case of celiac disease may not respond to dietary management. In other words, their symptoms may not subside when they eliminate gluten. In such cases, doctors often prescribe corticosteroids to bring down the inflammation in the intestine. If damage to the small intestine is extensive, affected sections of tissue may have to be surgically removed.

Hidden Sources of Gluten

- **Modified food starch**
- **Caramel coloring**
- **MSG**
- **Malted milk**
- **Flavored and instant coffees**
- **Soy sauce (some brands)**
- **Hydrolyzed vegetable proteins**
- **Packaged rice mixes**
- **Creamed vegetables**
- **Some non-dairy creamers**
- **Prepared meats (like sandwich meats, hot dogs)**
- **Salad dressings**
- **Vodka, ale, whiskey, beer, gin, wine, malt**
- **Ovaltine**
- **Ice cream**
- **Soup or bouillon cubes**
- **Chocolate**
- **Catsup**
- **Pie fillings**
- **Baking powders**
- **Chewing gum**
- **Dry seasoning mixes**
- **Processed cheeses**
- **Vanilla and flavorings made with alcohol**

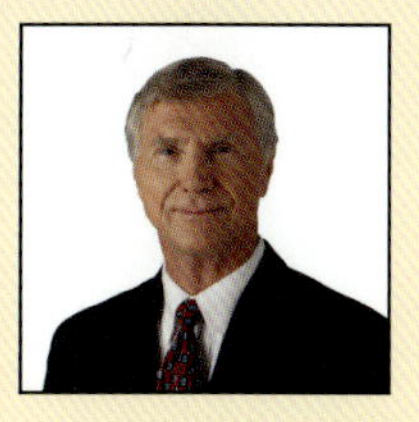

Dr. Smith's Comments

I have personally seen patients with a wide variety of conditions in which gluten sensitivity has been implicated. One case was a 19-year old college student with a gradual history of pressure sensations in the back of his head and visual difficulties, especially precipitated by exercise. His MRI scan and neurologic exams were normal. ELISA food-sensitivity testing showed a 2-3+ sensitivity to wheat and dairy, and he was a blood type O. Strict removal of gluten and dairy foods, while adding antioxidants and fish oils, decreased his symptoms considerably over several months.

Another case involved a 52-year-old truck driver, who, over a period of several years, noted increasing abdominal cramping and diarrhea, especially after eating pizza. He could relieve the symptoms somewhat if he took a probiotic product before eating pizza. He presented to the hospital with massive bloody diarrhea and toxic megacolon. He improved somewhat on strict hospital treatment; however, on colonoscopy, he had severe ulcerative colitis. He eventually had to have a subtotal abdominal colectomy.

What is the common link in these cases, as well as the many others with conditions ranging from childhood type 1 diabetes, to multiple sclerosis to colon cancer? I believe it begins not with a sensitivity to wheat, but with leaky gut or increased intestinal permeability. There are many causes of this that have nothing to do with wheat. Some common causes are:

- Excessive sugar and simple carbohydrates in the diet, which can promote an overgrowth of yeast, especially Candida, and pathogenic bacteria.
- Stress, dehydration, poor mucus production, poor nutrition, antioxidant status and genetics
- Alcohol consumption and food sensitivities

It is known that a protein produced in the intestine called "zonulin" can, under certain conditions, increase the paracellular permeability. When this happens, the gliadin gets by the lining into the submucosal area, and it is here that a variety of severe immune events can take place. It could be that when children have a gastrointestinal flu syndrome with diarrhea, the resultant transient increased permeability may set the stage for serious sensitivities to wheat and dairy if they are introduced back into the diet before the intestinal tract has healed. This could be as long as three to five days during which time soups and cooked vegetables should be the diet of choice. Similarly, over-consumption of alcohol while eating commonly sensitive foods, such as wheat and dairy, could be the start of a sensitivity to a previously tolerated food.

There is data in the pediatric literature showing that pre-treating of wheat- and dairy-sensitive children with sodium chromoglycate (a histamine blocker) will actually prevent the expected increase in intestinal permeability. In addition, there is data suggesting that the herb quercetin can block histamine release and prevent leaky gut as well. Any symptoms suggestive of gastrointestinal dysfunction, particularly in combination with inflammation in the body, such as arthritis or fibromyalgia, should warrant food sensitivity testing and elimination of sensitive foods as a starting point.

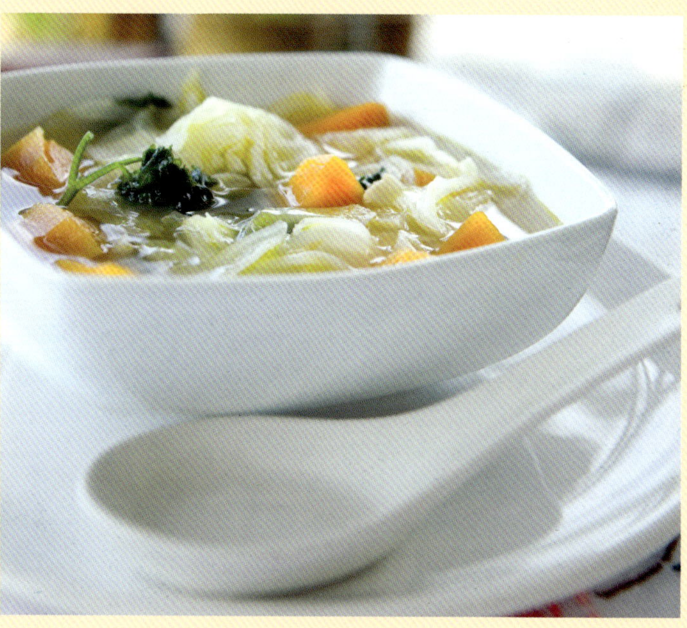

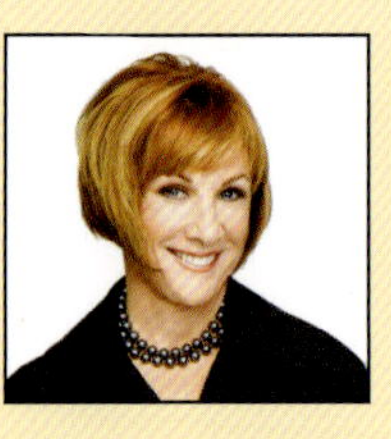

Brenda's Bottom Line

In this chapter, two conditions are addressed: gluten sensitivity and celiac disease. With both conditions, the solution is the same: take gluten out of your diet.

I am glad to see that the science behind detecting gluten sensitivity and celiac disease has really progressed since I first started practicing in a clinic 20 years ago. During my years of helping others, I encountered many people with terrible health problems who never knew that they had gluten sensitivity. The methods of testing for this in the past have been inaccurate. Unfortunately, these same inaccurate methods are used by traditional medicine still today.

At EnteroLab, Dr. Fine has developed a stool test that is able to detect gluten sensitivity where it happens first—in the gut! The testing used by traditional doctors looks for gluten sensitivity markers only in the blood, but the markers make their way into the bloodstream only after there is considerable damage to the intestine allowing them to get through. By the time these gluten-sensitive or celiac markers have entered the bloodstream, the condition is quite progressed. The beauty of the stool test is that it can detect if you are reacting to gluten in the gut before too much damage is done to the intestine.

For years I followed a diet that was very low in gluten, but did not exclude it entirely. Then one day, recently, I woke up with pain and inflammation in the joints of my hand. I went to the doctor who told me that it was arthritis—just a normal part of getting older. I did not accept this as my final answer. Because I know that many health conditions are rooted in gut health, I did the gluten sensitivity stool and gene test from EnteroLab. (See the Appendix.) I discovered that I have two genes that make me more likely to develop gluten sensitivity or celiac. I also had elevated levels of the IgA immune markers, indicating an immune response to gluten in the gut.

After that I was very careful to avoid all gluten, but it still took six months of the diet and supplementation before my hand pain completely healed. For more complex health conditions that are triggered by gluten sensitivity it can take a while for the body to heal. It takes a high level of commitment, and the results can be amazing.

Rule Out:

- Candida overgrowth (See the Candidiasis section.)
- Parasites (See the Parasitic Disease section.)
- Dairy (casein) sensitivity

Recommended Testing

- Gluten sensitivity test (See the Appendix.)

Diet

- Follow either the Candida Diet or the Fiber 35 Eating Plan minus any gluten-containing foods. (See the Appendix.)
- Gluten sensitivity is much more common than most people are aware. Most of us can benefit from a gluten-free diet whether we have celiac disease or not.
- Remember that most beer, ale, gin, whiskey and vodka are distilled from grain.

Lifestyle

- Learn to read labels carefully. Educate yourself on the many foods, other than wheat, that may contain gluten such as luncheon meats, grain vinegars, condiments and seasonings.
- When dining out, inquire about sauces or "secret" ingredients. Let the waiter and cook know that you are on a no-wheat or gluten-free diet restriction.
- Join support groups, which usually offer food ideas.

Complementary Mind/Body Therapies

- Colon hydrotherapy can be helpful in removing toxins from the colon.
- Massage, yoga, biofeedback and meditation can help you relax and assist in the healing process.

Recommended Nutraceuticals	Dosage	Benefit	Comments
Critical Phase	Daily maintenance recommendations should also be taken during this phase unless otherwise indicated.		
Follow daily maintenance protocol below			
Helpful			
High Potency Multi-vitamin/mineral	Use as directed	Provides needed nutrients that may be deficient in people who are gluten sensitive or celiac.	Powder formulation would be helpful as it is easier assimilated and absorbed.
Antioxidant Supplement	Use as directed	Protects tissue from damage.	You can purchase a high-potency antioxidant formulation from most health food stores.
Daily Maintenance			
Probiotics	50 to 200 billion cultures daily	Numerous benefits to intestinal health, helps reduce gut permeability and food sensitivities.	For celiacs: 200 billion powdered formulation For sensitivity: 50-80 billion capsule
Digestive Enzymes	Take with meals	Helps break down proteins and other nutrients, possibly reducing reactions to undigested food.	Make sure it has high amounts of protease, amylase, lipase and cellulase.
Omega-3 Fatty Acids	At least 2 grams daily of omega combination	Helps restore moisture to the intestinal tract and reduces inflammation.	Best combination is flax, fish and borage oils.
Fiber	4-5 grams twice daily	Helps keep food moving through bowel, reduces toxic colon and accumulation of wastes.	Look for a flax-based fiber with added ingredients such as glutamine, probiotics and healing herbs.
L-Glutamine Powder with Gamma Oryzanol	5,000-10,000 mg daily in divided doses	Helps repair the intestinal lining, reducing permeability and severe reactions to foods.	Best if taken in powder form.

See further explanation of supplements in the Appendix

HEMORRHOIDS

What Is It?

Hemorrhoids (also known as piles) are swollen blood vessels in the anal area that stretch under pressure. They are much like varicose veins in the legs and may develop either inside the lower rectum (internal hemorrhoids) or under the skin around the anus (external hemorrhoids).

What Causes It?

There are two basic causes of hemorrhoids:

(1) A genetic weakness in the wall of the veins and/or
(2) Excessive pressure on those veins.[1]

The pressure is often due to chronic constipation or straining during bowel movements, but may also be caused and aggravated by chronic diarrhea. The most frequently recognized cause of constipation is a low-fiber diet; however, other factors such as: lactose intolerance, inadequate water intake, low-thyroid function and magnesium deficiency may also cause or contribute to the condition. (See the Constipation section for more information on the subject.)

Excess pressure on the veins can also result from abdominal muscle strain stemming from heavy or improper lifting, or from pushing during childbirth, thus placing a great deal of pressure on the anus. Pregnancy itself, due to the accompanying hormonal changes that cause blood vessels to expand, may cause hemorrhoids. The increased intra-abdominal pressure present in pregnancy as the fetus grows can also lead to development of hemorrhoids. This same type of increased intra-abdominal pressure can result from:[2]

- Defecation
- Violent coughing
- Sneezing
- Vomiting
- Physical exertion
- Portal hypertension due to cirrhosis of liver

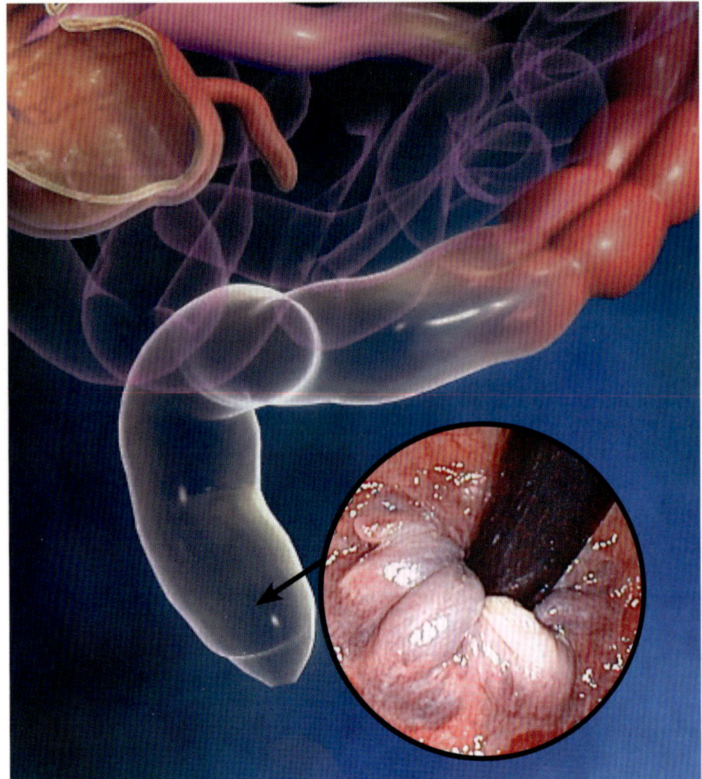

Illustration of the end of the digestive system (anus area) with a zoomed in photo of hemorrhoid in this area

Prolonged sitting or standing also exerts excessive pressure on veins that can cause them to weaken and herniate.

Other factors that can cause or contribute to development of hemorrhoids include: obesity, lack of exercise, liver damage, food allergies or sensitivities, and nutritional deficiencies.

About 89 percent of Americans will develop hemorrhoids at one time or another in their lives.[3] It is interesting to note that the incidence of hemorrhoids increases up to age 70, after which it decreases.[4] While they primarily affect older people, hemorrhoids can develop at any age. Those younger individuals who are most affected are pregnant women and women with children. Heredity can also play a role in the development of hemorrhoids.

While hemorrhoids are a very common complaint in the U.S. and in other industrialized nations, the condition is non-existent in indigenous cultures that have no access to processed foods. The processing of our foods results in removal of fiber and important nutrients causing constipation and digestive problems.

What Are the Signs and Symptoms?

Not everyone who has hemorrhoids will have symptoms. When present, hemorrhoids may cause or display any or all of the following signs and symptoms:

- Rectal bleeding
- Rectal pain
- Burning
- Swelling of tissue/inflammation
- Protrusion of tissue (prolapse)
- Painful bowel movements
- Engorgement with blood
- Sensation of incomplete evacuation
- Mucous discharge
- Itching

When bleeding occurs, it is generally bright red (a sign of fresh blood) and usually indicative of internal hemorrhoids that occur in the anal canal out of view. This may be the only symptom displayed with internal hemorrhoids. Some bleeding should not be cause for alarm unless the bleeding is dark and/or lasts for more than a few days, in which case medical help should be sought. Bleeding can also be a sign of other conditions such as polyps, ulcerative colitis or even rectal or colon cancer, and so should be thoroughly investigated.

When straining to pass stools, internal hemorrhoids can cause a great deal of pain when they herniate (prolapse or collapse) and protrude below the anal sphincter. A mucous discharge and itching may accompany the prolapsed hemorrhoid. This is generally the only time that itching is experienced as a result of hemorrhoids.

External hemorrhoids are visible to the eye since they occur in veins outside the anus. These ballooned, skin-covered veins often appear as hard, bluish lumps. There is generally no pain with an external hemorrhoid unless it ruptures and forms a blood clot (thrombus). This clotting can also occur with prolapsed internal hemorrhoids. In

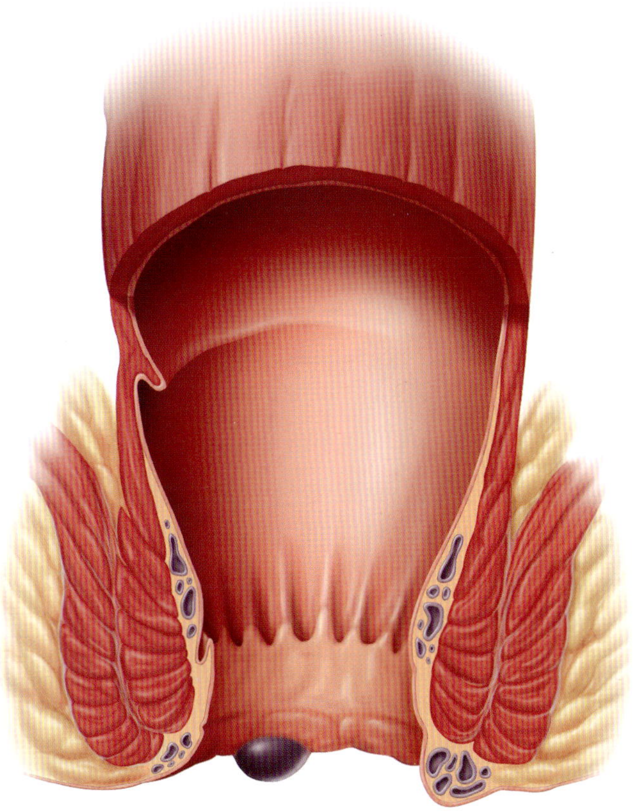

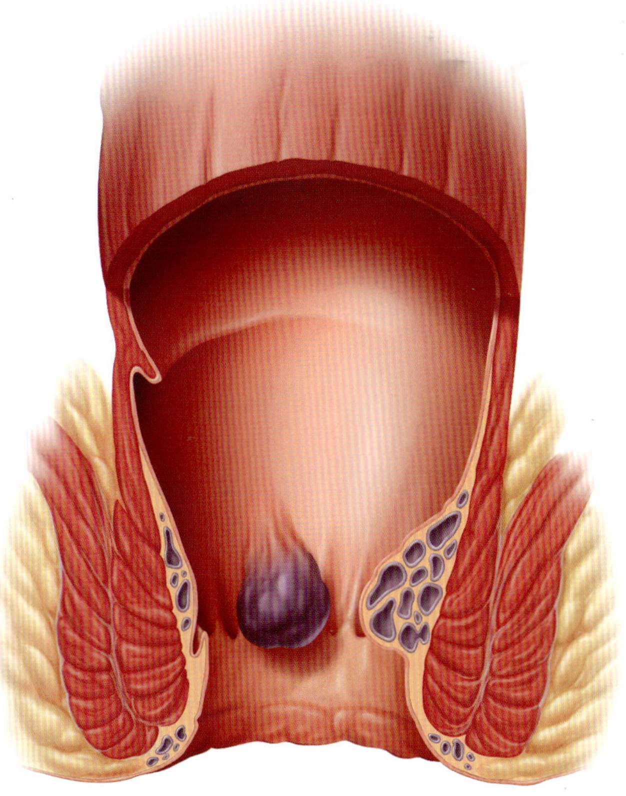

Hemorrhoids, a mass of dilated veins in swollen anal tissue. On the left, an external hemorrhoid, and, on the right, an internal hemorrhoid.

time, the clot is replaced by fibrous connective tissue, and the hemorrhoid may shrink and not be detectable.

How Is It Diagnosed?

Diagnosis is based upon the doctor's examination of the anus and rectum for signs of swollen blood vessels. He or she will also do a digital rectal exam using the fingers of a gloved hand. Closer inspection of the rectum is possible with the aid of an anoscope, a flexible lighted tube. The tube is inserted in the rectum, and internal hemorrhoids may be viewed. A proctoscope is used for a more extensive examination of the entire rectum, if needed. A sigmoidoscopy or colonoscopy may be performed to rule out gastrointestinal bleeding or find its source. If necessary, tissue may be cauterized to stop the bleeding.

What Is the Standard Medical Treatment?

Standard treatment of hemorrhoids consists of relieving pain and preventing irritation through such measures as:

- Tub or sitz baths (in three to four inches of warm water) for ten minutes several times daily (baking soda or one-fourth cup Epsom salts may be added to the water)
- Local applications of creams, suppositories, ointments or anorectal pads sold over-the-counter for temporary relief of pain (Note: these do not shrink hemorrhoids.)
- High dietary fiber intake (fruits, vegetables, whole grains and bulk fiber supplements) to promote peristalsis and soften stools
- Adequate water consumption – six to eight glasses per day
- Local application of ice packs to reduce swelling of hemorrhoids
- Use of stool softeners
- Frequent cleansing of anal area with warm water (no soap)
- No sitting on hard surfaces; use a soft cushion
- Use of proper lifting technique – exhale while lifting; don't hold the breath
- No heavy lifting
- No use of rough toilet paper; use damp toilet paper
- Regular exercise
- No sitting on the toilet for long periods of time (over ten minutes), as blood will pool in the hemorrhoidal veins.

Although some cases of hemorrhoids may be successfully treated using the above conservative methods, at times doctors will elect to use more aggressive treatments aimed at shrinking and destroying hemorrhoidal tissues. These treatments may include:[5]

- Rubber band ligation – a rubber band is placed around the base of an internal hemorrhoid to cut off its circulation. The result is that the hemorrhoid withers and drops off within a few days. Although ligation is the most common treatment used today, it can be painful and may require repeat treatments.
- Infrared photocoagulation – involves the use of infrared heat to treat minor internal hemorrhoids. It is less painful than ligation, but is not always as effective.
- Bipolar electrocoagulation – uses intermittent electrical current to shrink hemorrhoids, and is comparable to infrared photocoagulation in terms of pros and cons.
- Sclerotherapy – involves injection of a solution containing either quinine and urea or phenol directly into the hemorrhoid for the purpose of shrinking it and stopping any bleeding that may be present.
- Laser – heat (laser coagulation) is used to burn off hemorrhoidal tissue. This is the easiest and least painful way of medically dealing with internal hemorrhoids. However, there is controversy about its use, with some researchers believing that more study to improve the effectiveness of the technique is needed before it is routinely recommended.
- Hemorrhoidectomy – The surgical removal of hemorrhoidal tissue is occasionally used in severe cases. Although the surgery is considered completely effective in 95 percent of cases, additional surgery is needed should the hemorrhoids reoccur.
- Circular stapled hemorrhoidopexy[6] – excess mucosal tissue around the entire circumference of the anal canal is removed pulling the hemorrhoids back up into place. The tissue above and below this ring is then stapled. This procedure is less painful than a closed hemorrhoidectomy.

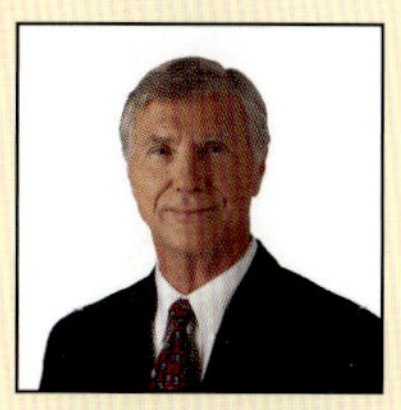

Dr. Smith's Comments

I would have to say that most patients whom I have treated for hemorrhoids are women who have had children and patients with a history of constipation associated with a low-fiber diet and inadequate water intake.

Stress is another important factor. I have seen healthy young college students present with acute prolapsed or thrombosed (clotted) hemorrhoids and anal fissures (cracks in the anal lining) due to tight anal sphincters (very similar to a chapped lips), especially near the time of their final exams. Often, people who are chronically anxious with tight jaw muscles and teeth grinding will also have tight anal sphincters that impede venous drainage and result in hemorrhoids. These can, at times, be treated with gentle self-anal dilation with aloe gel, muscle relaxants or anti-anxiety medications. With time, lifestyle changes and patience, many of these people can avoid surgery.

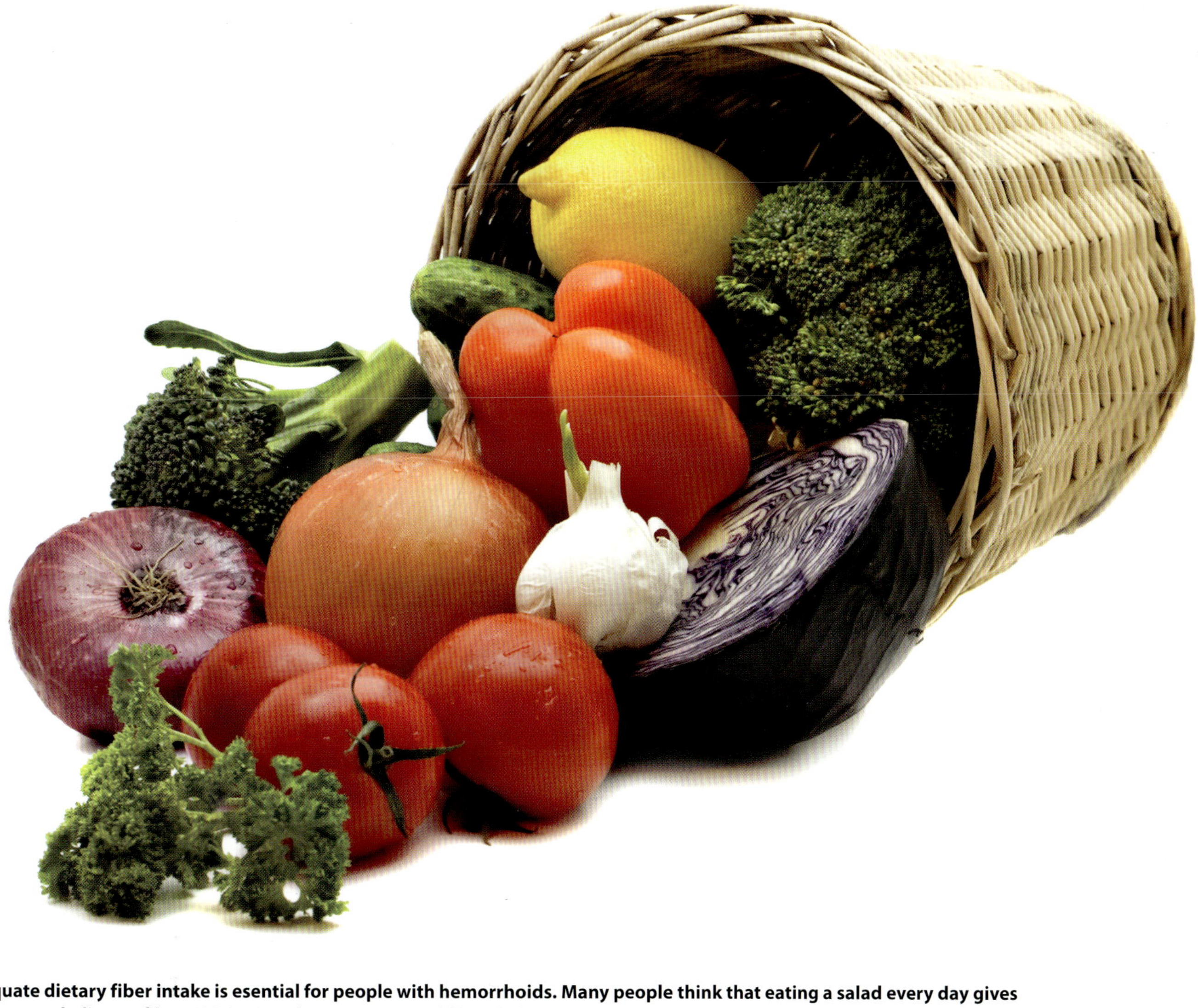

Adequate dietary fiber intake is esential for people with hemorrhoids. Many people think that eating a salad every day gives them enough dietary fiber. WRONG! At least 35 grams of fiber daily must be consumed.

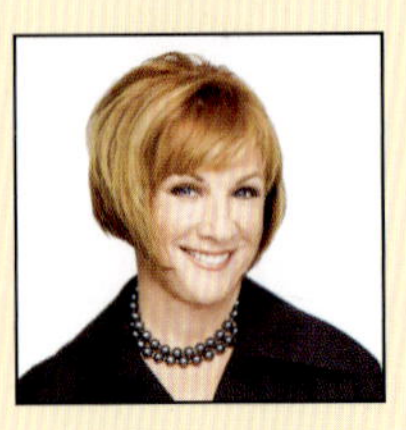

Brenda's Bottom Line

Over the course of many years, I performed thousands of colonics and saw many cases of hemorrhoids. The main reason hemorrhoids form is because of a lack of dietary fiber consumption. Most Americans do not have a clue about the amount of fiber needed in their diet. Most people think they consume enough fiber. This is especially true in people who have daily bowel movements. Even those people are usually not getting enough fiber.

Take one or two days to count your daily fiber intake. If it is not at least 35 grams per day, you're not getting enough. The Fiber 35 Eating Plan (see the Appendix) is a great plan that helps you obtain enough dietary fiber. If followed, this can help, even if hemorrhoids have already developed.

If you have an acute problem, you can make a poultice out of a powder containing L-glutamine and gamma oryzanol. (See the Appendix.) This poultice can help with inflammation when directly applied to the area.

One seemingly strange folk remedy that I have seen relieve the inflammation of hemorrhoids involves coring the center of a potato and placing it in the rectum. This could be helpful to relieve some of the pain of the hemorrhoid.

Sometimes hemorrhoids are internal, and people will notice bright red blood when wiping. Certainly blood in the stool needs to be checked out by a doctor because it can indicate a more serious problem, but in most cases with hemorrhoids it is caused by hard stool passage and can be relieved by increasing dietary fiber intake. If there is rectal itching and burning it will also be necessary to rule out the following:

- Parasites, especially pinworms (See the Parasitic Disease section.)
- Candida overgrowth (See Candidiasis section.)

Diet

- Follow the Fiber 35 Eating plan found in the Appendix of this book. A high-fiber, less processed diet is one of the best treatments and preventions for hemorrhoids.
- Juicing of fresh vegetables, especially green ones, can be helpful in maintaining digestive health and keeping small veins healthy.
- Include lots of flavonoid rich foods such as berries, citrus and cherries.

Lifestyle

- Follow the lifestyle suggestions under the Standard Medical Treatment section, and eat slowly, chew foods well and drink plenty of water.
- Avoid wearing tight-fitting clothes that constrict the abdomen.
- Assume a squatting position during bowel elimination. This will help prevent hemorrhoids or keep them from reoccurring. To do this, use a device that elevates the feet when sitting on the toilet, such as the LifeStep. (See the Appendix.)
- After hemorrhoids have healed, start an exercise program.

Complementary Mind/Body Therapies

- Colon hydrotherapy is indicated for hemorrhoids as it decreases abdominal pressure. Use as part of your biannual detox program.

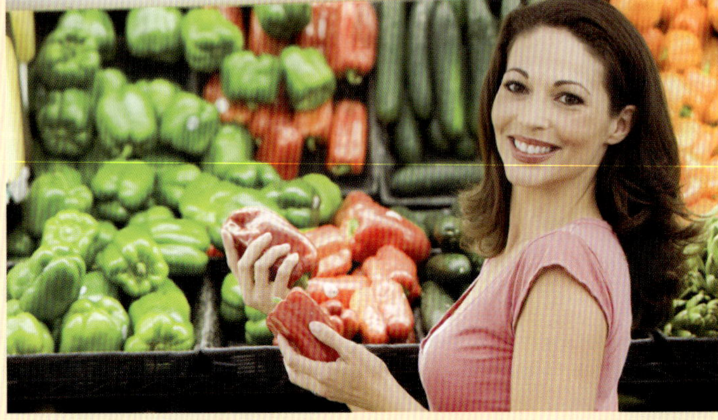

Recommended Nutraceuticals	Dosage	Benefit	Comments
Critical Phase	Daily maintenance recommendations should also be taken during this phase unless otherwise indicated.		
Fiber	6-8 grams twice daily for two weeks	Try to obtain 45 grams of fiber daily in the diet.	One that provides both soluble and insoluble is best, such as flax, acacia and oat blend.
Natural Laxative Formula if constipated	Use as directed	Softens stool to reduce straining and pressure.	Look for gentle ingredients such as magnesium, aloe and rhubarb.
Vitamin C with bioflavonoids	3,000 to 5,000 mg vitamin C daily with at least 100 mg bioflavonoids per dose.	Aids in healing and strengthening the veins and capillaries.	Divided doses throughout the day.
L-Glutamine Poultice	Use as directed	Helps to heal the digestive lining, which includes hemorrhoids.	See Appendix for instructions.
Helpful			
Herbal Formulation Pilexim	Use as directed	Helps shrink hemorrhoids and stop bleeding.	Make sure it is the trademarked Himalaya formula.
Antioxidant Supplement	Use as directed	Protects tissue from damage.	Look for a high-potency antioxidant formulation.
Daily Maintenance			
Omega-3 Fatty Acids	At least 2 grams daily of EPA/DHA combination	Helps restore moisture to the intestinal tract and reduces inflammation.	Look for a concentrated, enteric coated fish oil.
Fiber	4-5 grams twice daily as part of a 35 gram daily fiber diet after critical phase	High-fiber diet best treatment and prevention of hemmorhoids.	Diet that provides both soluble and insoluble is best, such as flax, acacia and oat blend.
Probiotics	30 - 80 billion culture count twice daily	Restores bacterial balance and pH of colon and promotes regularity.	Look for high amount of bifidobacteria, the main beneficial bacteria in colon.
Digestive Enzymes	Take with meals	Helps to digest foods and absorb nutrients.	If low stomach acid is found find a formula that contains hydrochloric acid.

See further explanation of supplements in the Appendix

IBD-Crohn's Disease

INFLAMMATORY BOWEL DISEASE (IBD)

What Is It?

Crohn's disease is an inflammatory bowel disease (IBD) that can affect tissue anywhere along the gastrointestinal tract from mouth to rectum, but it most commonly involves the intestines, particularly the last section of the small intestine, the ileum. Crohn's disease causes the bowel wall to thicken, and may cause a narrowing of the bowel channel. Unlike ulcerative colitis and some other intestinal conditions, all layers of the bowel wall are usually affected not just the inner lining. Adjacent organs can be affected as well since ulcerated lesions may spread by forming unnatural tunnels called "fistulas." The inflammation characteristic of Crohn's tends to develop in a skip pattern (i.e., it is not continuous, but may skip areas of tissue).

Dr. Burrill Crohn, for whom the disease is named, is generally credited with first describing Crohn's disease in 1932. He called it regional ileitis because, at that time, it was considered to be a localized disease. When it was later discovered that any portion of the GI tract could be affected by Crohn's disease, new names for it cropped up. These names often described the disease by location:

- Enteritis (intestinal involvement)
- Ileitis (ileum involvement)
- Proctitis (rectum involvement)
- Colitis (colon involvement)
- Ileocolitis (involvement of both the ileum and the colon)
- Granulomatous ileitis or granulomatous colitis

Granulomas are clusters of inflammatory cells. They appear as small nodules in the intestinal wall giving it a cobblestone appearance. They form as the affected tissues go through cycles of inflammation, damage and healing. These cycles are common, characterized by periods of remission and flare-ups. Of those who suffer from Crohn's disease, 35 percent have only the ileum affected, 20 percent have only the colon affected and 45 percent have both ileum and colon affected,[1] making it primarily a disease of the right side of the body.

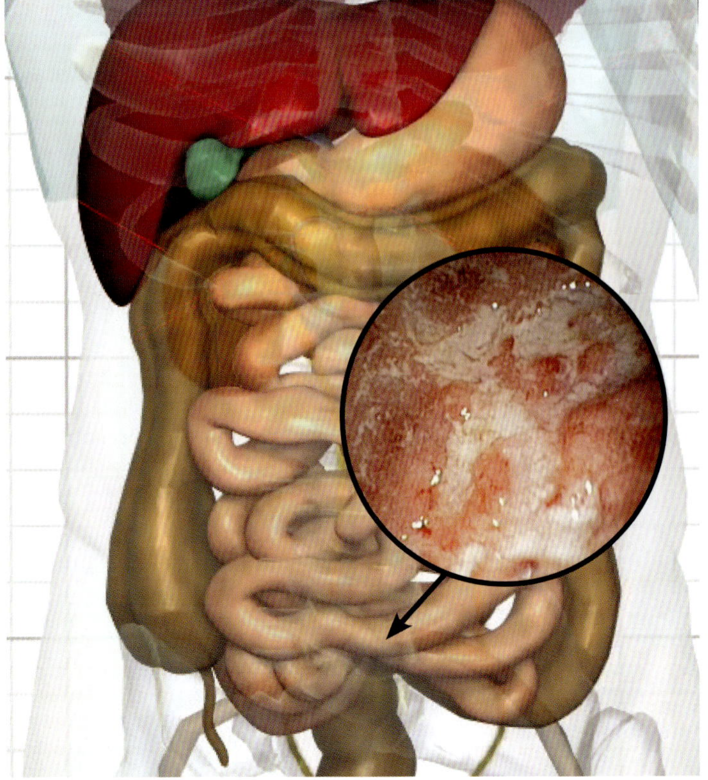

An endoscope image of Crohn's disease

What Causes It?

It is known that infections cause flare-ups of Crohn's disease. Recent findings identify infectious agents involved in the development of the disease, affirming that the inflammation of Crohn's disease is the body's reaction to the presence of a foreign agent—a virus, bacteria, fungus or parasite. That inflammation is then accelerated when the immune system attacks its own tissues where the microorganism resides.[2]

The genetic component to Crohn's disease is known as the NOD2 gene mutation. This mutation has been found in up to one-third of Crohn's patients.[3] It is possible that this genetic mutation is activated by the presence of a pathogen.[4] It is also possible that the NOD2 mutation reduces antimicrobial activity in the gut mucosa thereby creating a pathogen-friendly environment.[5] It is known that bacteria can stimulate the production of cytokines (proteins that cause inflammation).[6] There is some compelling evidence that a particular bacterium, mycobacterium paratuberculosis, may be the culprit.

Mycobacterium paratuberculosis, also known as Mycobacterium avium subspecies paratuberculosis (MAP), affects cattle giving them Johne's disease which produces symptoms that are virtually identical to Crohn's disease in humans. People with Crohn's disease are seven times more likely to have MAP present in the blood or gut tissue compared to people who do not have Crohn's.[7] It is no longer a question of whether MAP is associated with Crohn's. MAP triggers a massive immune reaction against the body's affected tissue in the gut, but cannot be detected using standard testing procedures. It is the only one of all the pathogens once believed to be associated with Crohn's disease that, when directly cultured from cattle, is capable of causing pathologically indistinguishable diseases in other animals.

This information raises the possibility that humans may become infected with MAP by drinking cow's milk or eating beef. This suspicion seems to be confirmed by the fact that Crohn's disease is only seen in milk-drinking areas of the world. Since the bacterium is extremely heat-resistant, it is not destroyed by pasteurization. It seems to be no coincidence that the U.S. has the worst MAP problem in the world, and also has the highest incidence of Crohn's disease. Unfortunately, since MAP is not considered a human pathogen, there are no efforts to keep dairy products from infected cattle out of the food supply.[8]

With regard to diet and lifestyle factors, the following have been found to contribute to Crohn's disease:

- Low-fiber diets[9]
- Fast foods[10]
- Cigarette smoking[11]
- Birth control pills[12]
- High consumption of refined carbohydrates and sugar[13]
- High intake of animal protein[14]
- Low intake of omega-3 fatty acids (found in flaxseed oil and fish oil)[15]

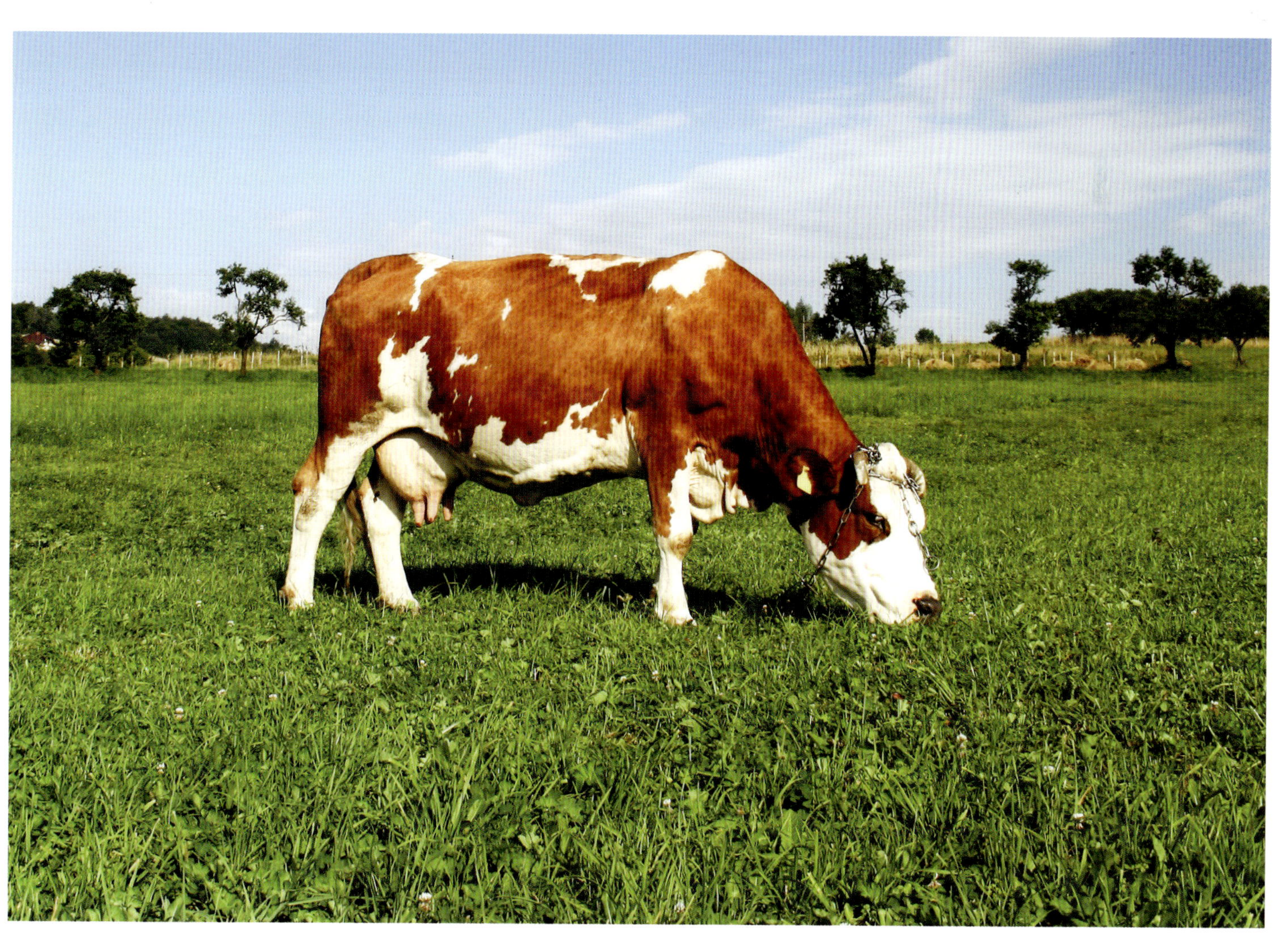

- Antibiotic use (The annual increase in prescriptions for antibiotics parallels the annual increase in the incidence of Crohn's disease.)[16]
- Food allergies and sensitivities (especially to wheat and dairy)[17]
- Low vitamin D levels (inadequate sun exposure or lack of supplementation)
- Leaky gut

Many of the factors listed above contribute to leaky gut syndrome prevalent in IBD sufferers.[18] With leaky gut syndrome, the bowel wall becomes hyper-porous allowing undigested food particles, toxins and microorganisms to pass into the bloodstream. Interestingly, intestinal permeability (leaky gut), has been found to be associated with relapses in Crohn's disease, and indicates subclinical (silent) disease.[19] This suggests that leaky gut is involved in the development of Crohn's. (See the Leaky Gut Syndrome section for more information about this condition.)

Food allergies can develop when the body launches an immune reaction in response to the presence of undigested food particles or microbial toxins in the blood because these particles are seen as foreign bodies. As such, food allergy, highly implicated in Crohn's disease, is considered to be an autoimmune disease as is Crohn's disease itself.

Not surprisingly, friendly flora (good bacteria) are found to be significantly out of balance in IBD patients.[20] This imbalance can be caused by antibiotic use, a diet high in refined sugar and carbohydrates and/or by the presence of an infectious agent.

Carrageenan, a compound extracted from red seaweeds, is often used to induce ulcerative colitis (another form of IBD) in experimental animals.[21] This compound is also used widely in the food industry as a stabilizing and suspending agent, most particularly in dairy products to stabilize the protein in milk.

It is thought that the presence of a particular bacterium is needed in order for carrageenan to cause the inflammatory lesions typical of ulcerative colitis.[22] The bacterium that has been linked to facilitating the carrageenan-induced damage in animals is a strain of Bacteroides vulgatus[23] an organism that is six times more prevalent in people with ulcerative colitis than in healthy people. Although evidence from animal models has demonstrated that degraded carrageenan causes ulcerations and malignancies in the gastrointestinal tract, there is no Food and Drug Administration restriction on the use of the substance in the food supply in the U.S.[24]

People with both forms of inflammatory bowel disease, Crohn's disease and ulcerative colitis, show an increase in the synthesis of inflammatory compounds called leukotrienes. Like histamines, leukotrienes respond to allergens in the body. Therefore, they can be reduced by eliminating or reducing consumption of foods to which the body is sensitive, such as meat and dairy products.

Increasing consumption of omega-3 fatty acids (found in ocean fish, chia seed and flaxseed oil) is also effective in managing leukotrienes.[25] This fact, coupled with

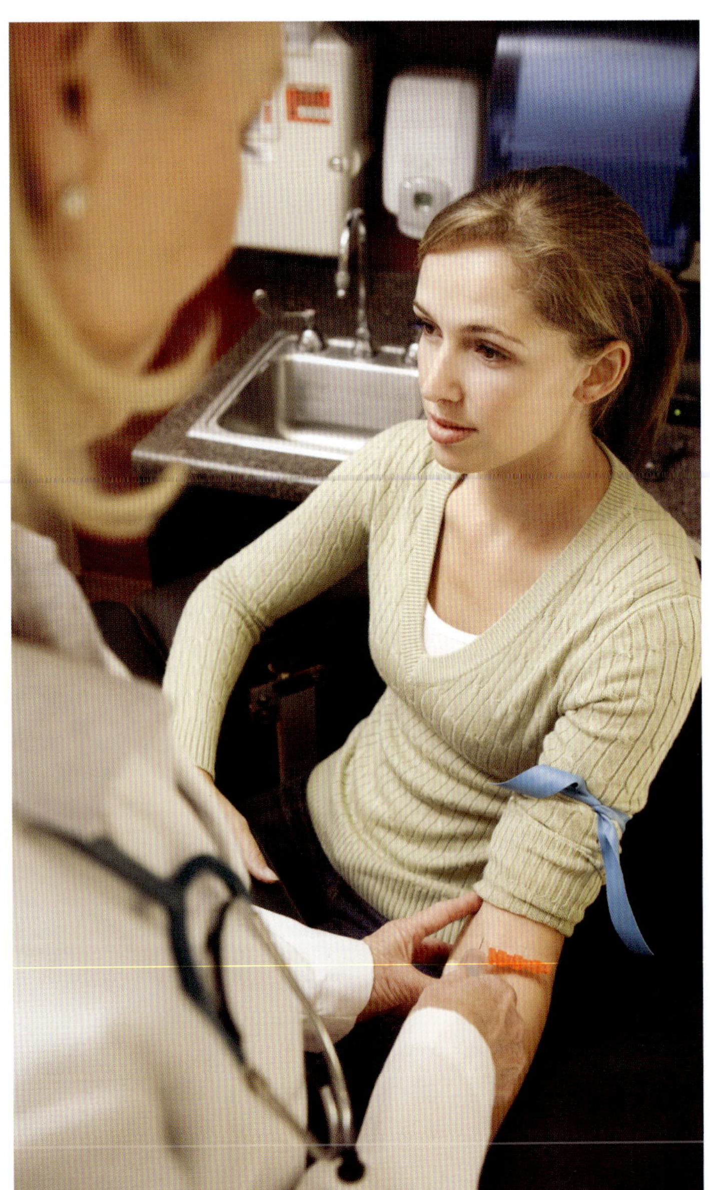

knowledge of the high allergic potential of dairy products and the possible presence of pathogens that could trigger inflammatory reactions in the gut, would seem to give the IBD sufferer ample reason to eliminate dairy products and reduce or eliminate red meat consumption.

IBD is not just about what is put in the body, but, also, what is taken out of it. Several studies have shown reduced antioxidant concentrations (vitamins A, C and E and the minerals selenium and zinc) in patient groups with both active and inactive Crohn's disease compared to control groups.[26] This may be both a result of and a contributing factor to the disease because inflammation increases the production of free radicals that consume the antioxidants. Lower tissue antioxidant levels negatively affect cell functions, and hasten tissue damage if inflammation continues unabated.

Crohn's disease is thought to affect somewhere between 400,000 and 600,000 Americans.[27] Crohn's disease is concentrated in developed countries, particularly in urban rather than rural areas. Although it affects all age groups, onset of the disease generally occurs between the ages of 15 and 30 and, less often, after age 50.[28]

Of all people with Crohn's, 20 percent have a close blood relative with the disease.[29] People who have a relative with Crohn's have at least 10 times the risk of developing it compared with the general population.[30]

People who smoke cigarettes, have other autoimmune diseases, eat processed foods and/or have a high intake of animal proteins and sugar-containing products are also at increased risk for developing Crohn's disease.

What Are the Signs and Symptoms?

The symptoms of Crohn's disease are similar to those of other intestinal disorders, especially ulcerative colitis. They generally occur intermittently—every few months to every few years in some people. However, in rare cases, symptoms may appear once or twice and never return.[31] Symptoms range from mild to severe. Gastrointestinal signs and symptoms of Crohn's disease include:

- Abdominal pain (usually right-sided)
- Diarrhea (may alternate with constipation)

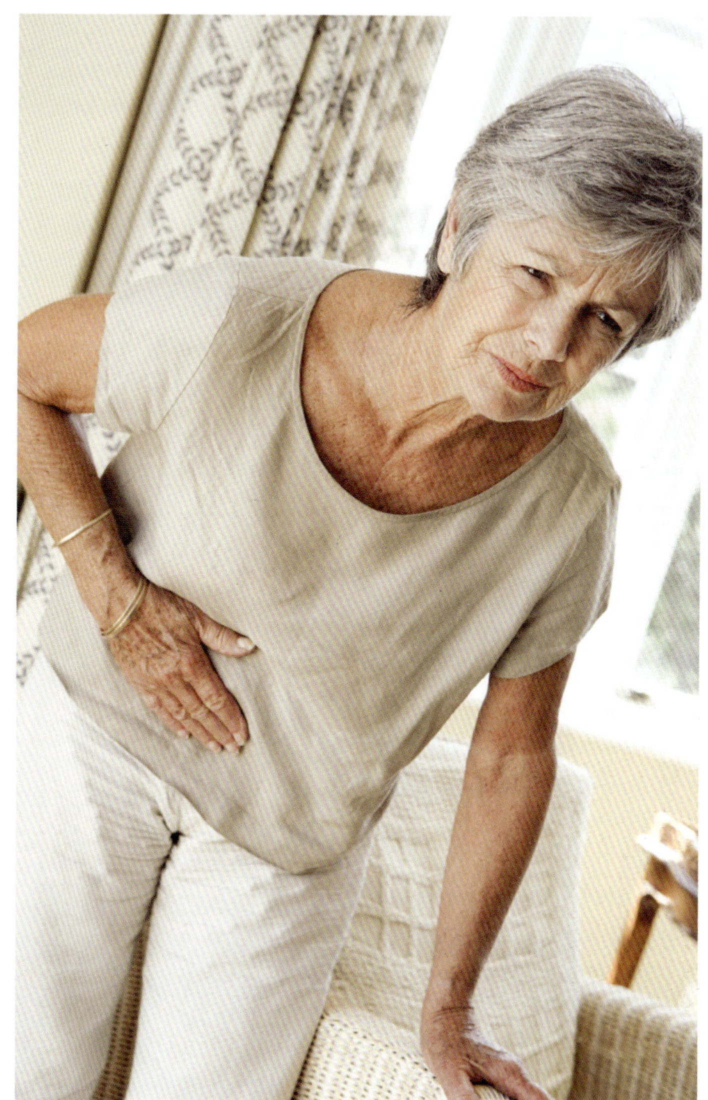

- Loss of appetite
- Weight loss
- Nausea/vomiting
- Blood in stool
- Mucus in stool
- Fever
- Flatulence
- Malaise
- Bouts of severe fatigue
- Delayed development/stunted growth in children
- Steatorrhea (excess fat in feces) from fat malabsorption

Fat malabsorption occurs due to a loss of bile salts seen in Crohn's disease. Normally, 95 percent of bile salts are reabsorbed in the ileum, particularly in the terminal ileum. In Crohn's disease, a much smaller portion of bile salts are reabsorbed. The unabsorbed bile acids in the colon can contribute to the diarrhea that occurs with Crohn's. To make matters worse, since the majority of bile salts are not being absorbed in the ileum and recycled through the liver, the fat in the diet is not well absorbed. The fat passes into the stool undigested creating further diarrhea, or steatorrhea, in addition to malabsorption of fat-soluble vitamins.

Systemic complications often occur as a result of Crohn's disease. In fact, there are more than 100 systemic disorders that may result from inflammatory bowel disease.[32] The most common of these is arthritis, occurring in 25 percent of Crohn's disease patients—usually found in those with colon involvement.[33] Fifteen percent will develop skin lesions, while three to seven percent will have serious liver disease.[34]

Other systemic complications may include:

- Inflammation of blood vessels
- Impaired blood flow to fingers and toes
- Kidney stones
- Gallstones
- Inflammation of eyes or mouth
- Inflammation of spine
- Inflammation elsewhere in the body

The nutritional deficiencies caused by Crohn's may also result in such problems as osteoporosis, neurological dysfunction and Alzheimer's disease.[35]

How Is It Diagnosed?

As stated, symptoms of Crohn's disease are similar to those of other gastrointestinal disorders, especially ulcerative colitis. When inflammation is also present elsewhere in the body—often in the joints, skin or eyes—the doctor will most likely suspect Crohn's disease. Accurate diagnosis may be difficult especially early in the disease process. It may be necessary to watch and wait until the course of the disease makes it possible to differentiate between Crohn's disease and ulcerative colitis. Endoscopic evaluation of the colon with tissue biopsy may be necessary. A telltale sign of Crohn's disease is the presence of patches of inflamed tissue with a cobblestone appearance.

A lower GI series (barium enema) of X-rays may be ordered to help distinguish between ulcerative colitis and Crohn's disease. An upper GI series of X-rays with small bowel study may be ordered to see if the ileum is involved.

These tests will, of course, be preceded by a thorough physical examination, including a rectal exam, to rule out cancer of the rectum and a health history. Proctoscopy, an in-office procedure, may also be performed allowing the doctor to examine the mucosal lining of the rectum if necessary.

Blood tests are typically done to find clues in the body's chemistry. These tests allow physicians to detect anemia based on iron levels, to assess protein status, and to spot inflammation based on an elevated erythrocyte

Side Effects of Corticosteroids

- Depression of protein synthesis
- Inhibition of calcium absorption (by increasing excretion of vitamin C in the urine)
- Bone thinning
- Skin problems
- Muscle deterioration
- Infections
- Pancreatic damage
- Neurological problems
- Stimulation of protein breakdown
- Decreased absorption of phosphorus
- Urinary excretion of vitamin C, vitamin K, calcium and zinc
- Increased levels of blood glucose, serum triglycerides, and serum cholesterol
- Increased requirements for vitamin B6, vitamin C, folate and vitamin D
- Impairment of wound healing
- Electrolyte imbalances
- Cataracts
- Weight gain
- Bone-mineral depletion
- Ulcers
- Congestive heart failure
- Diabetes
- Hypertension
- Facial hair growth
- Obesity of the upper torso

sedimentation rate and white blood cell count. Stool analysis can be useful to detect the presence of hidden (occult) blood as well as bacteria and parasites. To detect parasites with any degree of accuracy, specialized tests (see the Appendix) are needed. Many holistic physicians will use an extensive stool analysis that will give helpful information on the patient's digestive and absorptive capabilities as well as intestinal flora balance (or imbalance).

Further tests that may be ordered (typically by nutritionally-oriented doctors) are:

- Food sensitivity test (See the Appendix.)
- Comprehensive stool analysis (CSA) (See the Appendix.)
- Intestinal permeability screening (See the Appendix.)
- Nutritional analysis (of blood and/or hair)

What Is the Standard Medical Treatment?

Exact treatment protocol depends upon the severity of the Crohn's disease, the phase of the disease and its location in the body. Medical treatment goals ideally would be to:

- Control inflammation
- Relieve symptoms
- Control infection if present
- Prevent stimulation/irritation of the GI tract
- Correct nutritional deficiencies

The first three of these goals would generally be addressed through drug therapy that may include use of:

- Mild anti-inflammatory drugs (often salicylates like sulfasalazine) to prevent flare-ups
- Corticosteroids (like prednisone or hydrocortisone) to treat flare-ups
- Antibiotics (Flagyl and Cipro) are often used in serious cases especially if abscess or fistula is present.
- Immunosuppressive drugs – (like methotrexate, cyclosporine and Remicade) based on the theory that IBD is an autoimmune disease
- Anti-spasmodic drugs (opium derivatives to slow down diarrhea)
- Pain killers

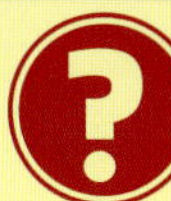

Did You Know

Crohn's disease is a chronic condition associated with inflammation and injury of the intestines. It typically begins in young adulthood, most often between 15 and 50 years of age.

The most commonly used drugs, sulfasalazine and corticosteroids, have a host of side effects. Sulfasalazine inhibits the transport of folic acid (a B vitamin) and iron, causing anemia;[36] increases urinary excretion of vitamin C; and may cause nausea, vomiting, weight loss, heartburn and/or diarrhea among other side effects.[37] Corticosteroids have a host of side effects. (See chart for a partial list of these side effects.) Crohn's disease patients typically take a lot of prescription drugs. It is not unusual for them to take 10 or more daily.[38]

Most drugs cause some degree of nutritional deficiency or imbalance. For the Crohn's disease patient, who may already be suffering from malnutrition as a consequence of the disease process itself, the added nutritional depletion of constant drug therapy can create serious nutritional deficiencies. For these reasons, nutritional supplementation along with a balanced and appropriate diet is absolutely vital.

Unfortunately, the nutritional awareness and knowledge of the traditional medical doctor may be limited to advising the patient to eat whatever can be tolerated. The doctor will be aware of the most important aspect of nutritional therapy—that is to provide adequate caloric intake—and will probably be aware of the need to increase protein intake (because of blood loss and damaged intestinal mucosal tissue). He may even be aware of the probability of secondary lactose intolerance with Crohn's disease. Unfortunately, his awareness of nutritional matters may not extend any further; though he will likely counsel his patient to avoid alcohol, tobacco and caffeine, or to use them moderately. Some doctors may recommend an increase in dietary fiber and a fiber supplement to control diarrhea; most will rely on anti-diarrhea medications.

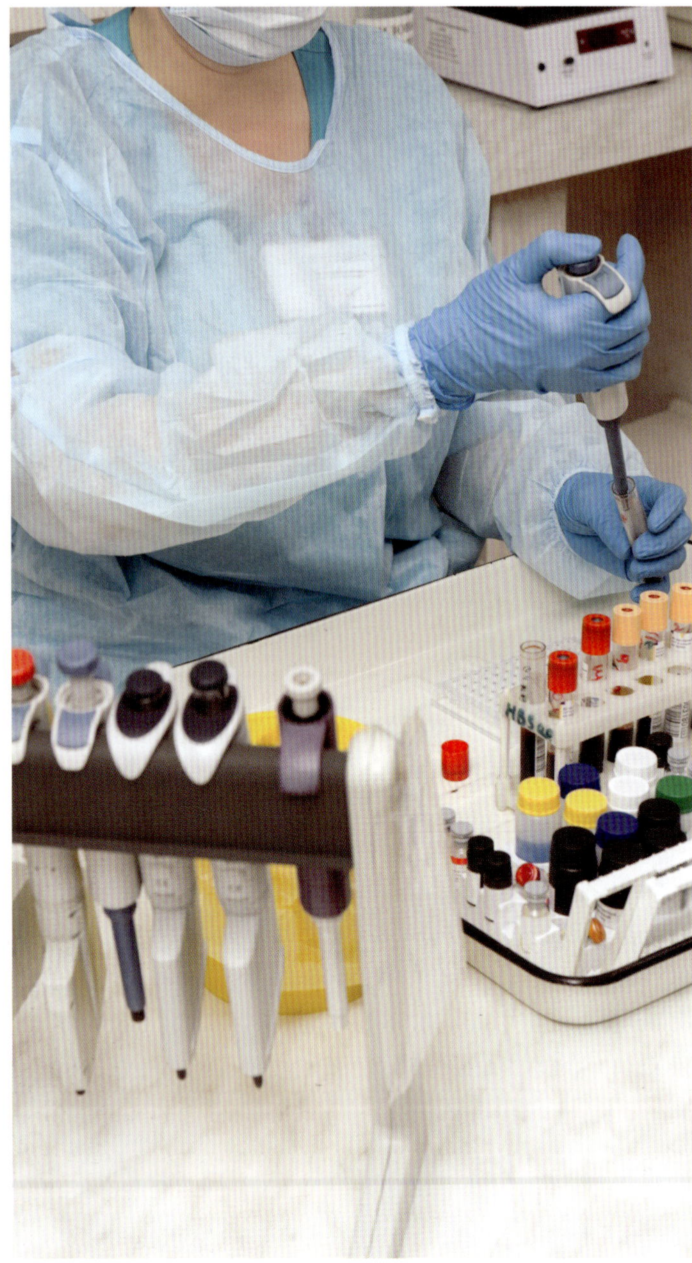

In severe cases, patients may require surgery (a bowel resection) where inflamed segments of the intestine are removed and the remaining segments connected. Surgery, like drug therapy, cannot cure Crohn's disease. It is typically done when blockages, perforation, abdominal abscesses or fistulas are present. Once a resection is done, the possibility exists of an adjacent area of the intestine being affected by the disease requiring another resection. When repeated resections are done on the small intestine, short bowel syndrome, a condition in which absorption of nutrients declines even further, develops. This is a critical situation; in fact, it is unlikely that the patient will survive when as much as 75 percent of the small intestine is removed.[39]

Preventing stimulation and irritation of the GI tract is generally done through total bowel rest at the onset of a flare-up. If it is severe and the patient is hospitalized, all food and beverages will be withheld for a short time, with fluids, electrolytes and glucose being administered intravenously to prevent dehydration. At the appropriate time, food will be either introduced orally through a tube (enteral nutrition) or intravenously (parenteral nutrition) depending upon the condition of the patient. Parenteral or IV feedings deliver nutrients directly into the bloodstream. They are generally used when a fistula or obstruction is present, and the patient is malnourished. Enteral tube feedings are used if the patient is not strong enough or well enough to drink. Nutrients are provided in a predigested (elemental) or partially hydrolyzed form. As healing progresses, the patient will move to a liquid diet, then to a soft diet and then on to regular eating.

Those patients experiencing mild flare-ups, who do not require hospitalization, will still need to rest the bowel initially, then ease into regular eating as described above. Some people benefit from drinking enteral formulas. The use of elemental diets has been found to be effective in delaying the time between onset of Crohn's disease and the first bowel resection. In addition, such a diet reduces the need for a second resection.[40] The benefits seen from such a diet may be attributable to the fact that it has a very low allergenic potential, and is an easily digestible form that is absorbed in the upper small bowel. Still, this approach isn't perfect. While enteral formulas provide readily utilized nutrients, they are costly and unpalatable.

Patients with steatorrhea (fat loss in stools) may benefit from a decreased intake of dietary fat as well as supplementation with medium-chain triglycerides, a form of fat that does not require emulsification and requires minimal digestion to be absorbed.[41]

As Crohn's disease patients recover from flare-ups, they will need to adhere to a low-fiber diet for a time to reduce gastrointestinal stimulation. Once able to return to normal eating, however, a high intake of dietary fiber is recommended to optimize bowel function.

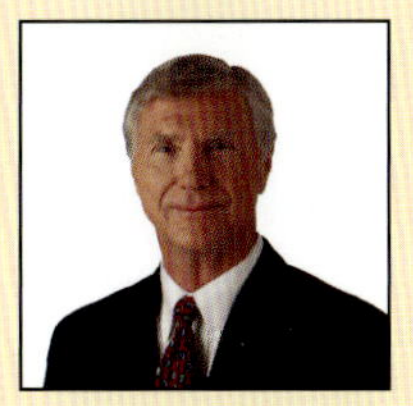

Dr. Smith's Comments

The gut connection in Crohn's disease (CD) is obvious, since it can occur in most any part of the gastrointestinal tract but predominatly in the terminal ileum and the right colon. Involvement may include: gastroduodenal area (five percent), right colon (35 percent), distal ileum (35 percent), small bowel alone (five percent), and colon alone (20 percent).[42] In addition, there can be "skip areas" which involve different sections of the GI tract, such as the right colon and peri-rectal fistulas with duodenal involvement, all at the same time.

The etiology of Crohn's disease is not clear but can involve many factors. In some ways CD is a classical example of how to use a systems biology approach to medicine. This means the causes are multifactorial including genetic, epigenetic, environmental, immunologic, infectious and psychoemotional components. The widespread bodily effects of CD can involve not only the gut but also the eyes, joints, bones, teeth, blood vessels, biliary tract, liver, mouth, and kidneys, to name a few.

It is well known that genes play a role in CD. The genetic defects occur on several chromosomes, but the main one seems to be chromosome 16. They have even identified the specific gene known as NOD2 (nucleotide-binding oligomerization domain containing 2), which is responsible for many of the problems seen in CD.

There are at least 30 variations of this gene, which make a protein by the same name, NOD2 protein, which is produced in the Paneth cells found in the bottom of the intestinal villi. Certain substances produced by bacteria get into the villi, enter the cell and cause activation of another gene known as NF kappa B, leading to an increase in the production of inflammatory cytokines such as TNF alpha.

This excessive inflammatory response, often to non-pathogenic bacteria, is responsible for many of the relapses people have with CD. The mainstream medical approach is to block inflammation with pharmaceutical drugs like Remicade, which is a TNF-alpha blocker. This works very well for short periods of time, and can allow the patient to go into remission, but long-term use of Remicade (like so many pharmaceuticals), can have serious side effects associated with immune over-suppression.

Chronic disease management is a very different approach. There will likely still be a need for some pharmaceutical medications such as the immunomodulators azothioprine, or mercaptopurine, the anti-inflammatory drugs like prednisone or budesonide, or even oral Remicade for some period of time (in many cases indefinitely). Ideally, if a patient is continuing to improve there are many other therapies that can be instituted.

It has been shown that an ideal diet (partly based on food sensitivity testing), exercise in moderation, fish oil, vitamin D, glutamine, fiber, probiotics, multivitamin/antioxidant/mineral supplements, quality sleep, good elimination, and an effective lifestyle management with stress reduction program will keep many of the patients in long-term remission. I have had several patients who were students at the University of Florida doing quite well until finals, when a flare-up would begin. With testing (lactulose/mannitol intestinal permeability test), doctors can often predict sometimes a month or more in advance that a relapse is coming. These patients will be symptom free but have an increase in intestinal permeability (leaky gut) which may be the earliest indication that a relapse is on the way. Is this recurrent leaky gut due to diet, lifestyle, lack of sunshine and exercise, or stress? I would say most often it involves all of these.

So it is pretty clear that the relationship between your microflora and intestinal lining is the foundation of the problem. There is research that now shows when people are under stress it can effect the gut lining, and the bacteria sense this and attach more tightly, reproduce quicker and may liberate chemicals to defend themselves against cathelicidins and other antimicrobial substances produced by the gut lining. In fact, many commensal or neutral bacteria, under stressful conditions, can begin to act as pathogenic (disease-producing) bacteria, taking a stressful situation and making it even worse.

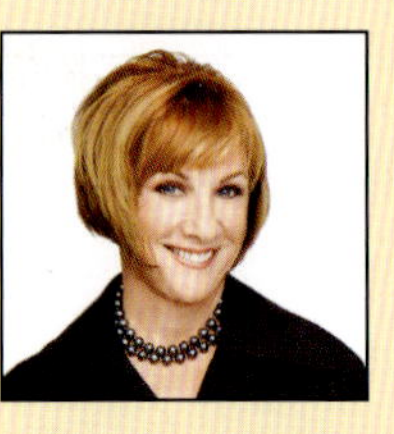

Brenda's Bottom Line

A very important component of dealing with Crohn's disease is finding the contributing factors to the inflammation. Alternative functional testing is a critical part of this process. A comprehensive stool analysis or CSA (see the Appendix) is a great way to take a look at what is happening in the digestive tract. In addition, a food sensitivity test (see the Appendix) can determine if certain foods (often gluten and/or dairy) are creating a reaction in the gut. From there, correcting the gut imbalance by following the suggestions below will go a long way to helping heal the gut.

In my experience, many people who develop Crohn's are still in their teenage years. This is a difficult age for parents to convince children to change their diets, but I cannot express strongly enough the importance of making the diet an important part of the program for getting this condition under control.

Many times people take gluten, dairy or yeast out of the diet for a week or two, maybe even a month, and do not get relief of symptoms. This leads them to assume that these foods are not part of the problem. I recommend following these diets for at least three months because it can take the body quite a while to respond to the diet and heal.

This is a serious condition that requires a focused effort and attention to symptoms so that the gut can be rebalanced and begin to heal.

Recommended Testing

- Food sensitivity test (See the Appendix.)
- Comprehensive stool analysis (CSA) (See the Appendix.)
- Intestinal permeability screening (See the Appendix.)

Diet

- Some people with Crohn's do well on a Candida Diet, which eliminates wheat, dairy, and many other foods that may irritate the digestive tract.
- During active phase, avoid processed, fatty and spicy foods, red meats, caffeine, alcohol and carbonated beverages until feeling better. Steam vegetables until soft before eating.
- Consuming raw foods can be beneficial but must be blended in a mixer and taken with digestive enzymes.
- Drink herbal teas like chamomile, slippery elm and fennel. Avoid artificial sweeteners.
- When dining out, try to call ahead for menu options suitable for you. Try to choose an entrée that is either steamed, baked or broiled rather than fried.

"A very important component of dealing with Crohn's disease is finding the contributing factors to the inflammation."

Lifestyle

- Exercise is very important and can help reduce pain levels. Low-impact walking, swimming and weight training are good.

Complimentary Mind/Body Therapies

- Stress can be a major component of this disease; so find ways to reduce it with therapies such as meditation, yoga, deep breathing, massage, biofeedback or music therapy.
- Acupuncture may be helpful as it targets the meridians associated with the digestive system, and it is also a stress reducer.
- Colon hydrotherapy is contraindicated in Crohn's disease, unless constipation is a major issue. If in remission, consult with your doctor before proceeding with this therapy.

Recommended Nutraceuticals	Dosage	Benefit	Comments
Critical Phase	Daily maintenance recommendations should also be taken during this phase unless otherwise indicated.		
Follow daily maintenance protocol below			
Helpful			
Powdered or Liquid Multi-vitamin/mineral Formula	Use as directed	Supplies nutrients lost from malabsorption.	Powdered or liquid formulas verses tablets are best for those with Crohn's.
Zinc	Additional 25-30 mg daily for 3 months.	Low zinc levels associated with inflammatory bowel disease.	You could choose to continue zinc at 15 mg per day after 3 months.
Mucilaginous herbs such as slippery elm, marshmallow, cranesbill and aloe vera	Use as directed	Soothes irritated and sore intestinal tract.	Take one or two separately or look for a formula that includes several.
Anti-inflammatory herbs such as tumeric, aloe, and boswellia	Use as directed	Helps reduce inflammation of the intestinal tract.	Take one or two separately or look for a formula that includes several.
Daily Maintenance			
L-Glutamine Powder with Gamma Oryzanol	5 grams twice daily	Essential for maintaining the health and integrity of the intestinal lining.	Added gamma oryzanol may help relieve pain associated with gastrointestinal complaints.
Probiotics	200 billion culture count twice daily	Shown to help reduce severity and relapse of IBD.	Look for high amount of bifidobacteria in powder form for higher culture counts.
Omega-3 Fatty Acids	At least 2 grams daily of EPA/DHA combination	Helps restore moisture to the intestinal tract and reduces inflammation.	Look for a concentrated, enteric coated fish oil.
Fiber	4-5 grams twice daily	Helps produce healthy bacteria levels and good elimination.	Use as part of the maintenance protocol, avoid during acute attack of Crohn's.
Digestive Enzymes	Take with meals	Can be helpful to digest foods and absorb nutrients.	If low stomach acid is found find a formula that contains hydrochloric acid.
Vitamin D_3	At least 1,000 to 2,000 iu daily	Helps heal leaky gut, decrease inflammation, increase overall health.	Research is showing many health complications as a result of low vitamin D levels.

See further explanation of supplements in the Appendix

IBD-Ulcerative Colitis

INFLAMMATORY BOWEL DISEASE (IBD)

What Is It?

Ulcerative colitis is an inflammatory bowel disease (IBD) generally affecting the rectum (proctitis) and the lower left portion of the colon (the sigmoid colon) though it may spread throughout the entire colon (pancolitis). In this chronic condition, there are ulcers along with inflammation. Also, there is usually blood in the stool as well as diarrhea and cramping. Unlike Crohn's disease, which involves the entire thickness of the bowel wall, the inflammation of ulcerative colitis is generally confined to the first layer of the colon lining, the mucosal membrane. It spreads in a continuous fashion rather than in patches like Crohn's disease. Ulcerative colitis does not involve the small intestine—except in those few cases when it backs up into the ileum (lower portion of the small intestine).[1]

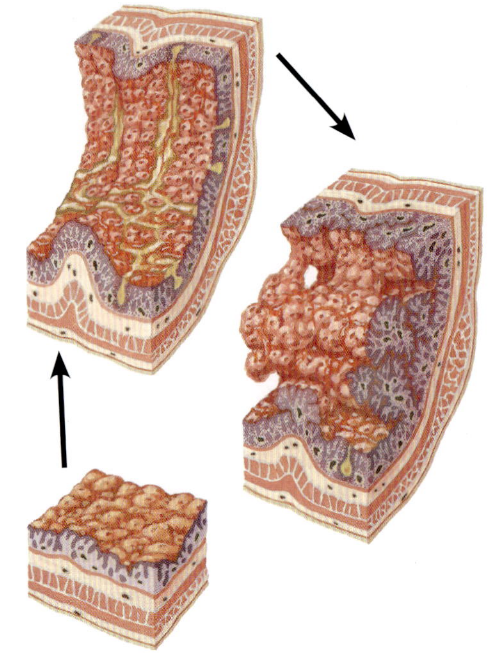

Progression of inflammatory bowel disease (IBD)

What Causes It?

While the cause of ulcerative colitis is unknown, many theories have been put forth, and a number of contributing factors have been identified. Among the proposed contributing factors are poor eating habits, stress, food allergies and infectious agents.[2] Involvement of microbes, like pathogenic bacteria, is often associated with the use of antibiotics, which alter the normal bacterial balance in the intestines permitting microorganisms normally held in check to proliferate.[3]

A dominant theory about the cause of ulcerative colitis is that the immune system overreacts to the presence of microbes, toxins or other stress factors (like irritating or allergenic foods) in the gut. What is unknown is whether the immune system disturbances found in the disease are the cause or the result of ulcerative colitis.[4] For a more in-depth discussion of possible microbial involvement in IBD see the previous section on Crohn's disease.

Like Crohn's disease, ulcerative colitis symptoms generally first appear between ages 15 and 30, with a second peak between ages 50 and 70.[5] Like Crohn's, ulcerative colitis affects men and women equally, and the disease appears to run in families. Most studies show that ulcerative colitis is more common than Crohn's disease.[6] In the United States, 10 to 12 Americans out of 100,000 develop ulcerative colitis.[7]

What Are the Signs and Symptoms?

The symptoms of ulcerative colitis often resemble those of Crohn's disease or irritable bowel syndrome. Microscopically, however, the superficial inflammation of ulcerative colitis gives a different appearance than the deep lesions of Crohn's disease. Still, ulcerative colitis, like Crohn's disease, usually lasts a lifetime, but may go into remission for long periods of time. Those with ulcerative colitis may experience any of the following symptoms:

- Diarrhea, which is often bloody, and may lead to iron-deficiency anemia
- Pain in the low abdomen (especially in the lower left quadrant)
- Weight loss
- Fever
- Fatigue
- Nausea
- Fissures
- Hemorrhoids
- Abscesses

Like Crohn's disease, the diarrhea of ulcerative colitis can lead to dehydration and electrolyte disturbances. Unlike Crohn's, the malnutrition that may result from ulcerative colitis is not directly due to malabsorption (because the small intestine is not generally involved) but rather due to loss of appetite and fear of eating stemming from the discomfort of the symptoms.[8]

Another similarity between ulcerative colitis and Crohn's disease is that both may produce systemic problems such as inflammation of the joints, eyes, spine, liver or gallbladder. This inflammation is usually mild and disappears when the colitis is treated.[9] Having ulcerative colitis also increases the risk of developing other serious conditions such as osteoporosis and kidney stones.

A rare but serious complication of ulcerative colitis is toxic colitis which can develop into a condition known as toxic megacolon. Toxic megacolon is a condition in which the entire colon is damaged and loses its ability to contract. In time, it will dilate or expand due to loss of muscle tone. Toxic megacolon can lead quickly to perforation, a life-threatening complication. Another possible complication of ulcerative colitis is the development of dysplasia, abnormal cell changes that increases the risk of cancer.

Healing HOPE Testimonial

"I suffered from crippling diarrhea and cramping that made it difficult to have a normal life. I was diagnosed with bleeding hemorrhoids and colitis. I learned about the benefits of taking probiotics and L-glutamine powder to heal and rebalance the gut. Within three days, I was symptom-free! I stopped the products for a while, but my symptoms came back. I went to my gastroenterologist who scheduled a colonoscopy for six weeks later. On my way home from that appointment, I made the decision to commit to the use of these products that had made such a difference.

I stuck to the daily supplementation and was symptom free when I had the colonoscopy. Before the procedure, I told my doctor about the supplements I was taking, but he didn't give much response. After the colonoscopy, he came back into the room with images of my healthy colon and began to ask about what I had been taking. I told him about Brenda Watson and Dr. Leonard Smith and he requested more information about them.

I continue to live free of crippling symptoms that once controlled me and my life."
– Tammy

How Is It Diagnosed?

In addition to physical examination and thorough health history, a colonoscopy with biopsy can help doctors to diagnose ulcerative colitis and assess its severity. A sigmoidoscopy may alternatively be used if complaints are confined to the rectal area. These types of endoscopic exams allow the doctor to take a biopsy—tissue sample—that can later be microscopically evaluated for a definitive differential diagnosis. They also look for dysplasia. A barium enema (lower GI series of X-rays) may also be used to reveal abnormalities in colonic tissue.

In addition to endoscopic evaluation—and possibly barium enema—blood tests are normally ordered for the purposes of detecting iron deficiency anemia, signs of inflammation, and protein status. Finally, an extensive stool analysis can be helpful in detecting infection and/or parasites. Specialized testing, involving more than one stool sample, may be needed to accurately detect parasites.

Natural health practitioners may also suggest additional diagnostic testing such as a comprehensive stool analysis (CSA), intestinal permeability test, food sensitivity testing, or a Heidelberg stomach pH test to determine stomach-acidity levels. (See the Appendix for information about these tests.)

What Is the Standard Medical Treatment?

Treatment depends upon the severity and extent of the ulcerative colitis. It would ideally be tailored to meet the individual needs of the patient. Most doctors will recommend the avoidance of irritating substances that may include highly seasoned foods, alcohol, caffeine and sugar.

Interestingly, nicotine patches may help induce remission, or at least reduce symptoms, in approximately 40 percent of patients who use the patch for more than four weeks.[10]

The nutrition-oriented doctor would most likely expand the list of offending foods to include those to which the patient is sensitive or allergic as established through stool (see the Appendix) or blood testing, or through a trial on an elimination diet. Even without testing, some doctors may advise the avoidance of milk and wheat since these foods have the highest allergy potential.

Traditional dietary treatment of serious cases of IBD (both Crohn's disease and ulcerative colitis) often involves use of an elemental (predigested) diet or one that is administered intravenously. These approaches, as well as the elimination diet (to treat allergies) have been quite successful in managing inflammatory bowel diseases. Medical management, however, relies very heavily on drug therapy that can be problematic.

The most widely used drugs in treatment of both Crohn's disease and ulcerative colitis are corticosteroids and sulfasalazine. The side effects of both of these medications are discussed in the section on Crohn's disease. Additionally, ulcerative colitis patients may be placed on medications to relax them, relieve their pain, suppress their immune systems (due to the suspected autoimmune nature of the disease) and to counter infection and diarrhea. All these drugs contribute to nutrient depletion, already an issue with IBD patients. Protein depletion is of particular concern due to tissue damage in the bowel that is sometimes extensive. Ongoing diarrhea raises concerns about iron and trace mineral status. Supplementation with a good multiple vitamin/mineral is therefore needed, though this need may go unrecognized by some traditional physicians whose knowledge of nutrition is limited.

Mild cases of ulcerative colitis, such as proctitis (inflammation of the rectum), may be treated with a mesalamine or steroid suppository or enema at bedtime. There is some danger of absorption of these medications into the body, however, with the accompanying side effects. (See the chart in the Crohn's disease section.)

The holistic physician would be more likely to prescribe a butyrate enema. Butyrate is a short-chain fatty acid, produced by bacterial fermentation of dietary fiber, that serves as food for the cells of the colon, helping to heal the colitis. Omega-3 essential fatty acids, found in fish oil, chia seeds and flax, are also helpful in reducing inflammation.

Hospitalization is required for those with severe cases of ulcerative colitis. Here nutrients, antibiotics and steroids are administered intravenously. If these treatments are not effective, then immunosuppressive drugs like cyclosporine may be added, first intravenously, then orally. In patients with severe colitis, anti-diarrheal drugs are generally avoided since they can precipitate the development of toxic megacolon.[11] To treat toxic megacolon, the bowel is compressed by inserting a tube through the nose into the stomach, so air and stomach contents may be aspirated on a continuous basis; a rectal tube may also be placed to decompress the colon.[12] A low-fiber diet is necessary during the initial stages of recovery in the disease process to be replaced with a higher-fiber diet later, if tolerated.

Treatment goals for the hospitalized patient are to:

- Correct malnutrition (often through administration of an elemental diet that is pre-digested)
- Stop diarrhea
- Stop blood loss
- Stop loss of fluids and minerals

If these conservative measures fail, surgery may be recommended. Although the majority of patients with ulcerative colitis will never require surgical intervention, about 20 to 25 percent will eventually require removal of part or all of their colon due to one or more of the following:[13]

- Massive bleeding
- Chronic debilitating illness
- Perforation of the colon
- Cancer risk (which may be as much as 32 times normal, especially if the whole colon is involved and the disease has been longstanding)
- Failure of drug treatment (as described above)
- Side effects of steroids (or other medications)

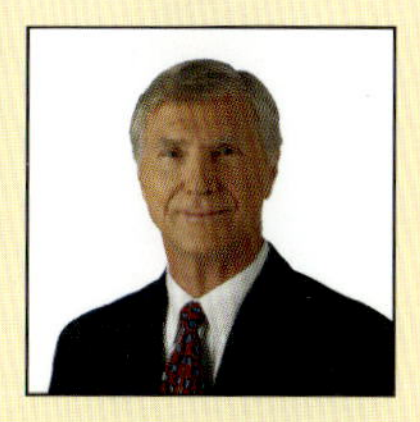

Dr. Smith's Comments

Ulcerative colitis (UC) is the other inflammatory bowel disease (IBD) which involves genetic, epigenetic, environmental, and immunological factors that create the perfect storm resulting in widespread ulceration and bleeding in the colon. Like Crohn's disease (CD), UC involves the body's inability to distinguish foreign invaders (antigens) from self.

The etiology of UC has not been clearly delineated, however there are many theories, most of which center around imbalances in the overall colonic microflora. Since there is cross-talk between the microflora, the epithelial lining and the immune system, significant imbalances in the microflora will reprogram the gut epithelial/immune system to that of a pro-inflammatory state.

There are two exciting therapeutic modalities for reprogramming the epithelial/immune imbalances: use of beneficial parasites, and human to human fecal implant.

There is much support in the literature for the use of pig whipworm (Trichirus suis) therapy in IBD for both UC and CD. A University of Iowa double-blind placebo-controlled study[14] gave 2500 pig whipworm ova (eggs) or placebo orally at two week intervals for 12 weeks to 54 patients with active colitis. Those treated with the pig ova were statistically significantly improved over the placebo group and there were no side effects.

It was the genius of Dr. Joel Weinstock, MD and others who demonstrated that using a pig whipworm is ideal since it is not a pathogenic parasite in humans and is expelled from the body within six weeks. This represents a beautiful example of how a low-grade parasitic infection can reprogram the gut epithelium and immunity as if it were reprogramming a computer. Maybe in the natural order of things we were meant to live closer to nature, and as a result would have a more natural balance of a microflora that would even include some low-grade beneficial parasitic infections.[15]

The rationale behind transplanting fecal matter from a healthy patient to a patient with IBD or even C. difficile diarrhea, is explained by work being done through the Human Microbiome Project showing that there are between 15,000 and 36,000 species of bacteria inhabiting the human gastrointestinal tract.[16] It may be that there are multiple bacteria creating the inflammation of UC, therefore, in severe cases, the more probiotics given, the better. With a fecal transplant from a healthy donor, the patient may be receiving up to 30,000 or more species of commensal bacteria, which would include many probiotics.

"The etiology of UC has not been clearly delineated, however there are many theories, most of which center around imbalances in the overall colonic microflora."

In a study published in the Journal of Clinical Gastroenterology and Hepatology, severe UC patients were treated with antibiotics and cathartics and then received fecal transplant. Some patients were completely free of UC up to 13 years later! This is a small study, but there have been many more like it in the past seven years. In fact, fecal therapy is also now being used for irritable bowel syndrome (IBS) and chronic constipation.[17]

There are other novel natural therapies for IBD, including aloe vera. In one double-blind randomized placebo-controlled trial, patients receiving oral aloe vera gel for four weeks had a statistically significant positive clinical response and reduced histological disease activity compared to the placebo.[18]

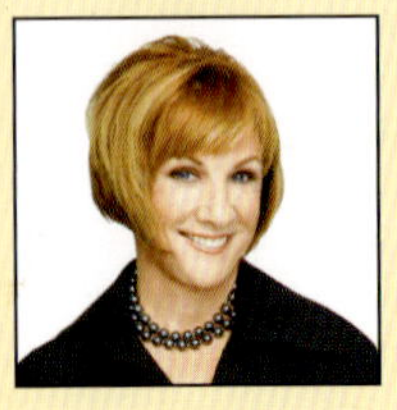

Brenda's Bottom Line

Ulcerative colitis usually involves the descending colon, which is on the left side of the abdomen. Diarrhea is often present with ulcerative colitis. Suggestions for this condition are similar to those for Crohn's disease since the two conditions are so similar in nature. Getting to the root cause of the intestinal inflammation is important, and this can be done by looking at what is occurring in the gut. A comprehensive stool analysis, or CSA (see the Appendix), is a great test that lets you do just that.

Another important component is the diet. In many cases, food sensitivity—often to wheat or dairy—is causing inflammation in the gut. This should be ruled out when dealing with ulcerative colitis. (See the Gluten Sensitivity and Allergies sections.) If food sensitivity is suspected or discovered, adherence to a diet which eliminates the offending foods for at least three months is necessary. This is an important point because it can take quite a while for the body to stop reacting and begin to heal. A strong commitment and determination are needed here. A comprehensive diet and supplement program, as outlined below and further described in the Appendix, can help you on your way to healing your gut.

Rule Out:

- Candida overgrowth (See the Candidiasis section.)
- Food sensitivity (See the Gluten Sensitivity and Allergies sections.)

Recommended Testing

- Comprehensive stool analysis (CSA) (See the Appendix.)
- Food sensitivity test (See the Appendix.)

Diet

- During active phase, avoid processed, fatty and spicy foods, red meats, caffeine, alcohol and carbonated beverages until feeling better. Steam vegetables until soft before eating.
- Consuming raw foods can be beneficial, but must be blended in mixer and taken with digestive enzymes.
- Drink herbal teas like chamomile, slippery elm and fennel.

Lifestyle

- Exercise is very important and can help reduce pain levels. Low impact walking, swimming and weight training are good.

Complimentary Mind/Body Therapies

- Stress can be a major component of this disease, so find ways to reduce it with therapies such as meditation, yoga, deep breathing, massage, biofeedback, or music therapy.
- Acupuncture may be helpful as it targets the meridians associated with the digestive system, and it is also a stress reducer.
- Colon hydrotherapy should be performed only under a physician's supervision in cases of ulcerative colitis

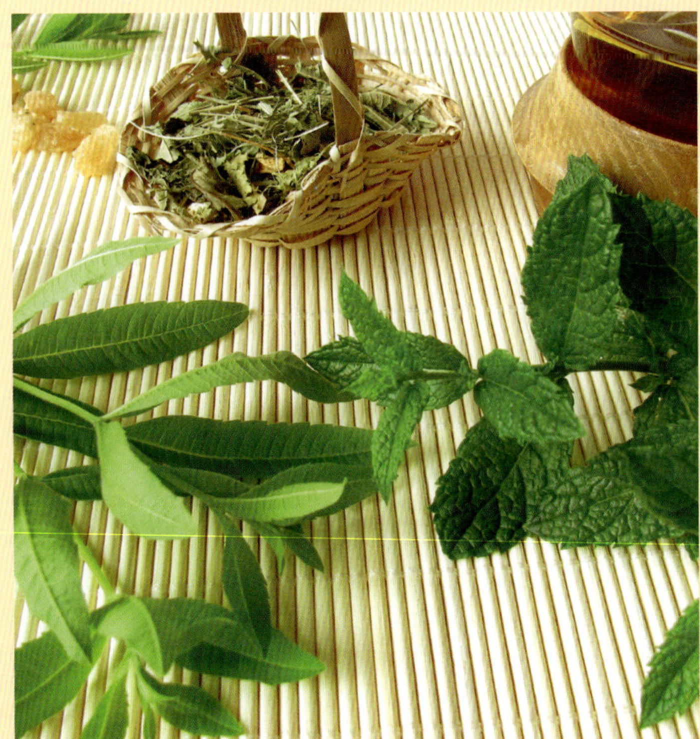

Recommended Nutraceuticals	Dosage	Benefit	Comments
Critical Phase	Daily maintenance recommendations should also be taken during this phase unless otherwise indicated.		
Vitamin D_3	2,000 to 4,000 iu daily for 6 months	Low levels associated with autoimmune diseases.	Research is showing many health complications as a result of low vitamin D levels.
Helpful			
Powdered or Liquid Multi vitamin/mineral Formula	Use as directed	Supplies nutrients lost from malabsorption.	Powdered or liquid formula verses tablets is best for those with ulcerative colitis.
Zinc	Additional 25-30 mg daily for 3 months	Low zinc levels associated with inflammatory bowel disease.	You could choose to continue zinc at 15 mg per day after 3 months.
Mucilaginous herbs such as slippery elm, marshmallow and cranesbill	Use as directed	Soothes irritated and sore intestinal tract.	Take one or two separately or look for a formula that includes several.
Daily Maintenance			
L-Glutamine Powder with Gamma Oryzanol	5 grams twice daily	Essential for maintaining the health and integrity of the intestinal lining.	Added gamma oryzanol may help relieve pain associated with gastrointestinal complaints.
Probiotics	200 billion culture count twice daily	Has been shown to help reduce severity and relapse of IBD.	Look for high amounts of bifidobacteria and in powder form for higher culture counts.
Omega-3 Fatty Acids	At least 2 grams daily of EPA/DHA combination	Helps restore moisture to the intestinal tract. Provides lubrication.	Look for a concentrated, enteric coated coated fish oil.
Fiber	4-5 grams twice daily	Helps produce healthy bacteria levels and good elimination.	Use as part of the maintenance protocol, avoid during acute attack of ulcerative colitis.
Digestive Enzymes	Take with meals	Can be helpful to digest foods and absorb nutrients.	If low stomach acid is found, find a formula that contains hydrochloric acid.
Vitamin D_3	1,000 to 2,000 iu daily after critical phase	Low levels associated with autoimmune diseases.	Research is showing many health complications as a result of low vitamin D levels.

See further explanation of supplements in the Appendix

Irritable Bowel Syndrome (IBS)

What Is It?

Irritable bowel syndrome (IBS), not to be confused with the more serious IBD (inflammatory bowel disease), used to be considered a functional disorder of the intestines. That is to say that the small and large intestine are not functioning properly though there is little or no evidence of damage or structural abnormality. Irritable bowel syndrome is usually identified by a group of symptoms. This condition is often determined more by what it is not than by what it is. It is characterized by the predominant symptoms of abdominal pain, bloating and change in bowel habit, which alternate between diarrhea and constipation.

Recent research, however, is revealing a clearer picture of irritable bowel syndrome. Dysbiosis, or, more specifically, small intestinal bacterial overgrowth plays a large role in IBS and provides a unifying explanation for the diverse and variable symptoms that accompany it.

Another inaccuracy of IBS is that it is a psychological disorder. To the contrary, IBS is a very real physiological disorder—not a psychosomatic ailment as once believed.[1] That is not to discount the emotional stress component, however. Some think IBS is a disorder of the enteric nervous system, involving the nerve supply in the brain and in the gut, that alters normal pain perception,[2] so that the bowel becomes oversensitive to normal stimuli.

What Causes It?

The following factors may play a causative role in the development of IBS:

- Dysbiosis (imbalance in intestinal flora—too many bad bacteria, not enough good bacteria)
- Irregularities in intestinal hormones and nerves responsible for bowel motility (muscle contraction)
- Bacterial, fungal or parasitic involvement
- Stress
- Dietary inadequacies
- Food intolerances (allergies and sensitivities)

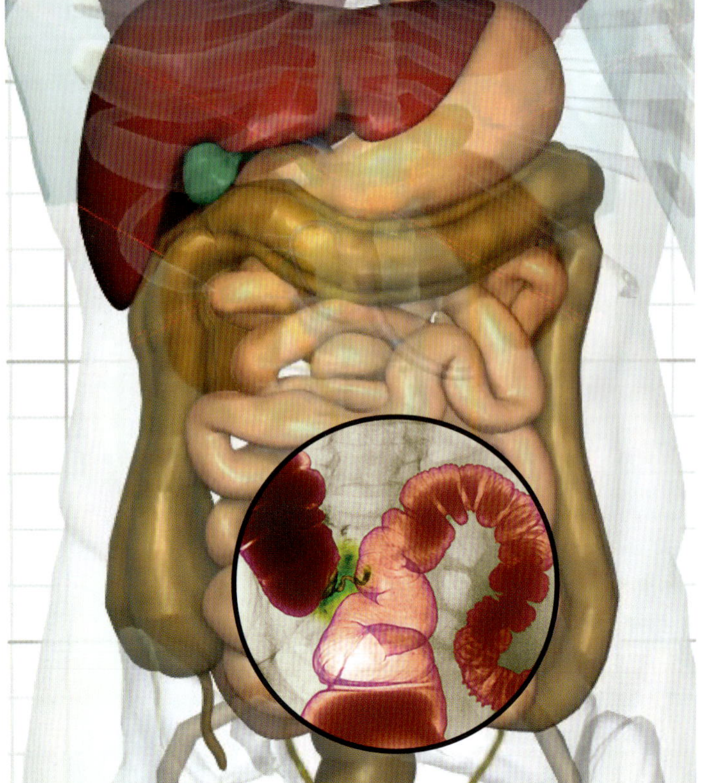

X-ray image of a bowel spasm

- Undiagnosed lactose intolerance
- Inadequate enzyme production
- Reaction to medications (such as antibiotics, which destroy intestinal flora)

Dysbiosis is a common feature that is often at the base of the complaints that present themselves as irritable bowel syndrome. The one symptom that is seen in 92 percent of IBS patients is abdominal bloating and pain.[3] This symptom has been identified as being caused by an increase in intestinal gas. While many IBS sufferers report increased bloating after a meal, many are still unable to identify a specific food trigger.[4] This points to the role that gut bacteria play in intestinal fermentation.

Excess fermentation can occur when there is an imbalance between beneficial and pathogenic or opportunistic gut bacteria. Excessive intestinal fermentation has been found in a large portion of IBS patients.[5] Dysbiosis explains both the diarrhea and constipation that accompanies IBS. It also explains the recently identified pro-inflammatory immune response that is seen in IBS.[6] And due to the increase in leaky gut—which is caused by dysbiosis—toxins and undigested food particles enter the bloodstream, triggering inflammation that ultimately affects the brain. This can be explained by the close communication that occurs between the immune system and the autonomic nervous system, located both in and near the intestines.[7] This gut-brain connection explains the psychological symptoms that are sometimes seen in those with IBS.

Interestingly, proton pump inhibitor (PPI) medication use is one possible cause of the dysbiosis that occurs in IBS. Many people with IBS also have acid reflux (GERD) or dyspepsia, and take PPIs to control it. PPIs lower the amount of gastric acid in the stomach, however, which can lead to an overgrowth of pathogenic or opportunistic bacteria resulting in dysbiosis.[8]

IBS is, at least partially, a disorder of intestinal motility. The normally rhythmic muscular contractions of the digestive tract become irregular and uncoordinated, and interfere with the normal movement of food and waste material. Mucus and toxins can then accumulate in the intestines setting up a partial and temporary obstruction of the digestive tract by trapping gas and stools that, in turn, cause bloating, distention and constipation.[9]

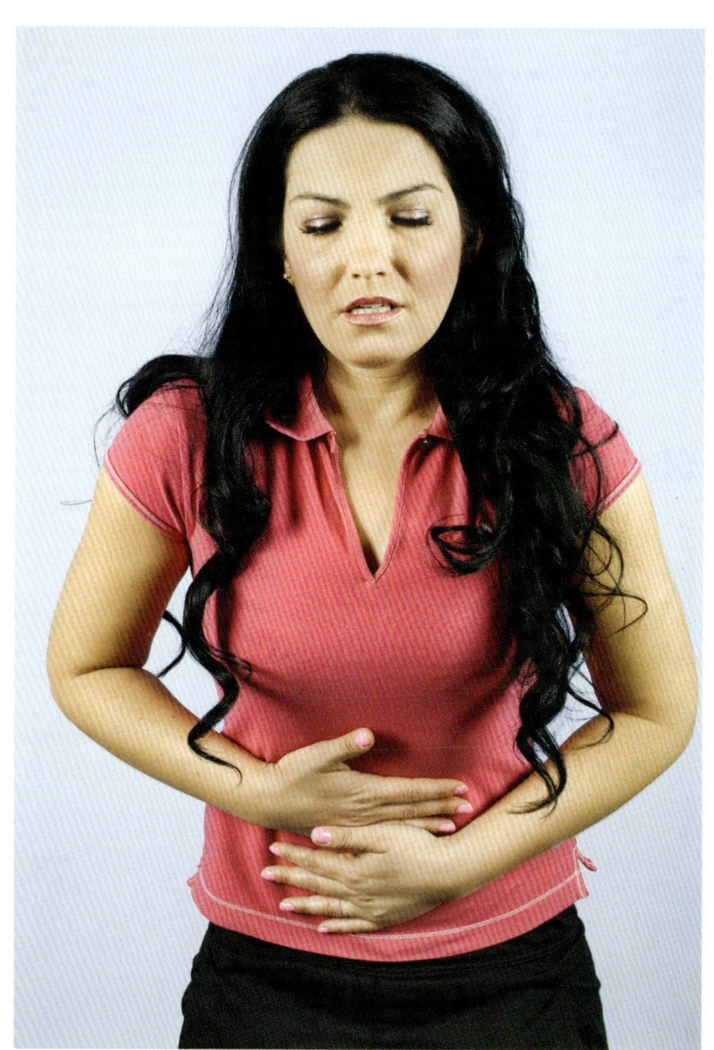

Healing HOPE
Testimonial

"I have been dealing with some form of IBS for about three years. The doctors just wanted to push medications on me and conduct invasive testing. I have always believed that if you give your body what it needs, it will repair itself. I have been taking the recommended L-glutamine powder to heal my intestines, and it began working in just two days."
– Julie

The colon of the IBS sufferer seems to be more sensitive and reactive to stimulation than that of most people. Intestinal spasms may result from ingestion of certain foods or medicines and from abdominal distention caused by gas. While these factors would not cause undue gastrointestinal stress for the average person, for the IBS sufferer they can be triggers of painful abdominal spasms.

Normally, eating causes contractions in the colon resulting in the urge to defecate within an hour after eating.For the person with IBS, however, the urge may come sooner, often accompanied by cramps and diarrhea. This is especially true if the meal is large and/or contains a high percentage of fat. Fatty foods—like meat, dairy products and oils—provide a strong stimulus of colonic contractions for the person with IBS. Interestingly, stress has a similar effect explaining its role in IBS.

There is evidence that food sensitivities and allergies may play a major causative role in IBS, for they are found in one-half to two-thirds of those afflicted with the disorder.[10] The most common allergens are dairy products and grains (especially wheat and corn). Other foods that often trigger episodes of IBS are coffee, tea, citrus and chocolate.[11] Both nicotine and caffeine in any form may serve as gut irritants.

Over-consumption of alcohol may also trigger intestinal spasms in the person with IBS. Also, meals high in sugar can contribute to IBS by decreasing intestinal motility.[12] A high percentage of people with IBS are intolerant not only to sucrose (table sugar), but also to other forms of sugar like mannitol, sorbitol and fructose.[13] Additionally, foods from the cabbage family (broccoli, Brussels sprouts, cauliflower, kale) may be irritating to the IBS sufferer because of their tendency to cause gas.

Lactose intolerance is also associated with IBS. The two sometimes coincide, and may even be difficult to distinguish. Other factors that appear to play a role in IBS include hormonal changes (women tend to have flare-ups that coincide with their menstrual cycle), low-fiber diets and infection. Many patients have reported the onset of symptoms during or soon after recovery from gastrointestinal infection (such as an episode of food poisoning), abdominal surgery or treatment with antibiotics.

The true cause of IBS symptoms may, in some cases, be an undetected parasitic infection, especially Blastocystis hominis, giardiasis or amebiasis. Because of the similarity in symptoms, it is not uncommon for Blastocystis infection to be mistaken for IBS.[14] There may also be an underlying problem with overgrowth of the yeast Candida albicans.[15]

An estimated one out of five Americans suffers from irritable bowel syndrome (IBS).[16] The average age of onset is between 25 and 45, with prevalence of the disease declining with age. It is not uncommon for IBS symptoms to surface during teen years, and the disease may even be present from infancy.[17] At least twice as many women as men are diagnosed with IBS.[18] More men may suffer from the disease than reported, however, for many with IBS (an estimated 90 percent) never consult a physician—at least in Western cultures. Interestingly, the incidence of IBS is reversed in India (twice as many men affected as women) where men are more apt than women to seek medical care.[19] Although once thought to be a disease of the white middle class, recent studies have established that the prevalence of IBS seems to be independent of race, with Japanese, Chinese, African Americans and Hispanics having the same incidence of the disease as Caucasians.[20]

IBS is the most common gastrointestinal disorder seen by physicians, and makes up 40 percent of all visits to gastroenterologists (GI disorder specialists).[21] Three and a half million office visits are made to doctors every year for IBS in the United States making it the seventh leading diagnosis overall.[22]

Did You Know

- According to the National Institute of Diabetes and Digestive and Kidney Diseases, irritable bowel syndrome (IBS) is one of the most frequently occurring gastrointestinal disorders and accounts for 41 percent of all visits to gastroenterology practices.
- It is estimated today that one in five Americans has IBS symptoms, making it second only to the common cold as the most frequent cause of absenteeism from work and school.
- Most people with IBS have such mild symptoms that they do not seek medical care for it, and those that do are seldom hospitalized.

What Are the Signs and Symptoms?

International conferences have been held to establish agreed-upon criteria by which functional bowel disease, of which IBS is one, can be recognized. These conferences have produced the Manning Criteria (named after Adrian Manning who proposed one set of criteria) and the Rome Criteria (named for the location of one of the conferences). The Manning criteria are: [23]

- Stools that are more frequent and looser at the start of episodes of abdominal pain
- Relief of pain after defecating
- A sense of incomplete rectal evacuation
- Passage of mucus with the stool
- A sense of abdominal bloating

The Rome criteria added to the above:

- Constant presence of abdominal pain and altered bowel habits
- Presence of remaining symptoms 25 percent of the time

Although the above criteria are the official ones, in reality, patients presenting with variations of these symptoms may be diagnosed with IBS.[24] These variations may include:

- Constipation with or without pain
- Pain associated with bowel movements

- Painless diarrhea only
- Alternating constipation and diarrhea

IBS sufferers may also experience other symptoms, such as:

- Flatulence
- Nausea
- Vomiting
- Headaches
- Loss of appetite
- Anxiety
- Depression
- Poor nutrient absorption (if diarrhea is severe)

The abdominal pain associated with IBS is often triggered by eating and accompanied by abdominal spasms. The person with IBS may feel an urgent need to move the bowels but be unable to do so.

Rectal bleeding is not a typical sign of IBS. If present in an IBS sufferer (who is correctly diagnosed), it may be due to a minor disorder such as hemorrhoids or a fissure (a crack in the lining where the rectum joins the skin around the anus). If rectal bleeding is present, it should be evaluated by a doctor.

How Is It Diagnosed?

IBS is, basically, a diagnosis of exclusion largely the result of ruling out of other disorders that may have the same or similar symptoms including:

- Colon cancer
- Diverticular disease
- Infectious diarrhea
- Inflammatory bowel disease (Crohn's disease and ulcerative colitis)
- Candidiasis
- Lactose intolerance
- Laxative abuse
- Pancreatic insufficiency
- Celiac disease or gluten sensitivity
- Fecal impaction
- Adrenal insufficiency
- Diabetes
- Hyperthyroidism
- Ulcers
- Parasites
- Gallbladder disease
- Endometriosis

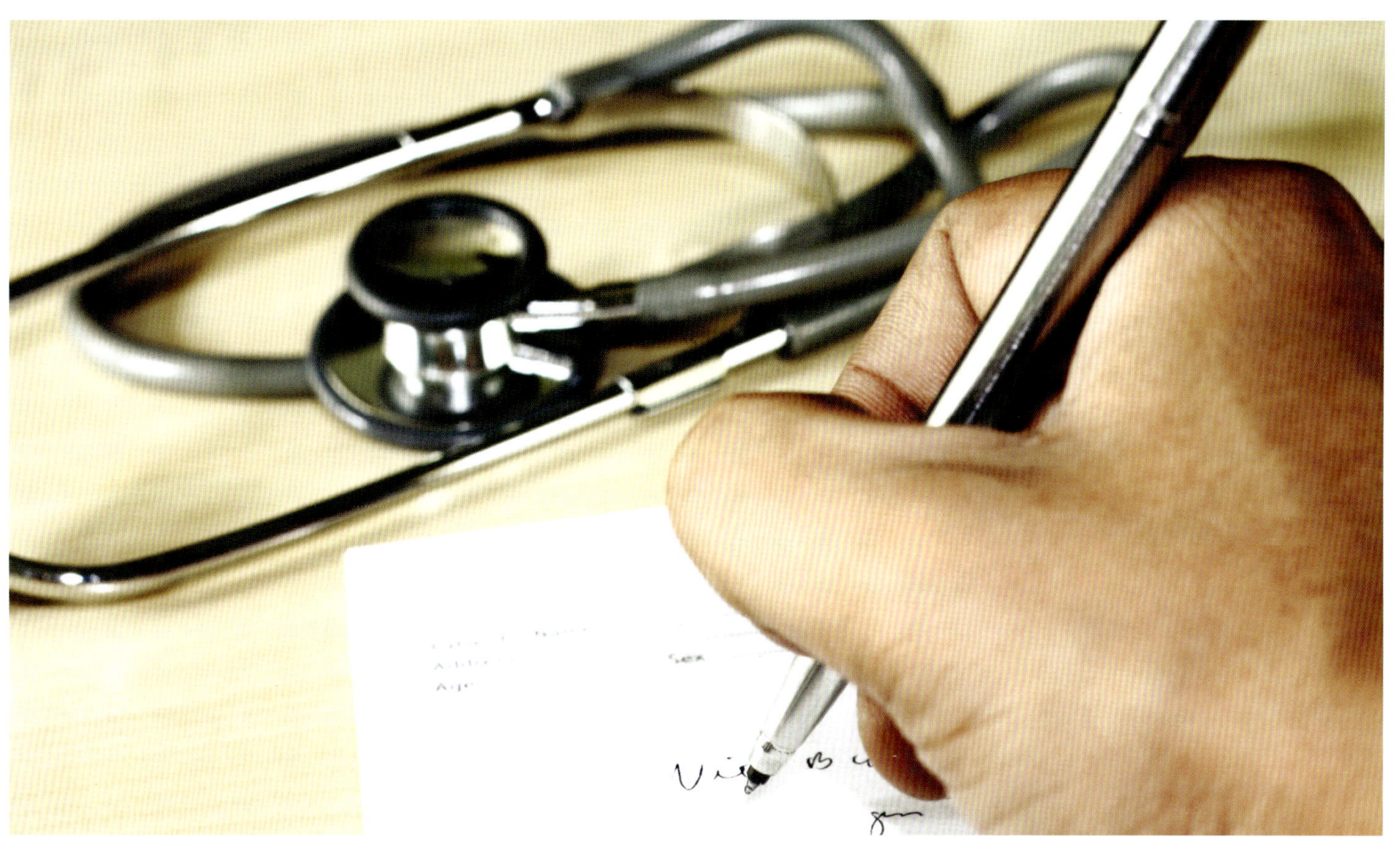

A thorough medical history and physical examination, along with appropriate laboratory tests (blood tests and stool exam), will help to rule out disorders such as those listed above. At times it may be necessary for the physician to do an endoscopic procedure in order to visually inspect the colon. A tissue biopsy may be taken in conjunction with the endoscopic procedure, and, as mentioned, a significant percentage of patients will have immunologic evidence of inflammation. Some patients with chronic diarrhea and abdominal pain may have microscopic colitis rather than IBS. A biopsy of the colon affected by microscopic colitis will show similar inflammation to patients with ulcerative colitis.[25]

Natural health practitioners may also suggest a comprehensive stool analysis (CSA) (see the Appendix) that may be helpful to determine causes of IBS symptoms such as bacterial imbalance, fungal or parasitic infection. Another test frequently suggested by natural health practitioners that may be helpful to determine causes of IBS is a food sensitivity test. (See the Appendix.)

What Is the Standard Medical Treatment?

The conventional approach to controlling IBS is through:

- Dietary restrictions
- Stress management
- Medications

Some doctors may limit their dietary advice to avoidance of caffeine-containing foods and beverages (coffee, tea, chocolate, colas), and reduced alcohol consumption. Other doctors, recognizing the role of individual food allergies (involving an immediate allergic response) and food sensitivities (involving a delayed response), may order special blood tests which measure antibodies that identify offending foods.

An alternative way of identifying food allergens and sensitivities would be through use of an elimination diet. The patient is placed on a diet of a few select foods that have a low-allergic potential, and after a time period suspected allergens back into the diet, one food at a time, as the patient observes and records the body's reaction to each. The simple act of keeping a diet journal can help identify irritating foods. Once offending foods are identified, they must be avoided for a lengthy period of time (at least two months), and then added back into the diet on a rotating basis.

Many doctors, unaware of the role that food allergies and sensitivities may play in IBS, may, nonetheless, recommend that their patients eliminate dairy products on a two-week trial basis. This recommendation is based on the recognition that lactose intolerance may play a role in the patient's symptoms. Some may also advise a trial elimination of grains based on the role that celiac disease or gluten sensitivity may play.

Most doctors, regardless of the level of their understanding of nutrition, will advise the IBS patient to increase intake of dietary fiber (whole grains, fruits and vegetables) because high-fiber diets keep the colon mildly distended and help prevent spasms from developing.[26] Doctors prescribe several types of drugs to help alleviate IBS symptoms. These include:

- Anti-cholinergic drugs to block one portion of the autonomic nerves that regulate contractions of the intestine
- Tranquilizing drugs or general relaxers
- Antispasmodics that block nerve impulses to the intestinal muscles
- Antidepressants/mood elevators to filter out painful stimuli from the gut to the brain
- Antibiotics to treat infection, if present
- Antacids – to slow the movement of food through the GI tract (See the GERD section for a discussion of the adverse effects of antacids.)
- Stool softeners/laxatives – to combat constipation if present

The above drugs all have adverse side effects (some of which may make GI symptoms worse), and they are expensive and only moderately effective.[27] Often natural dietary supplements can be used with equal benefit (and without unwanted side effects). These can be quite effective in combination with dietary management and regular exercise to help control the symptoms of IBS.

It is refreshing to see that probiotics are also becoming a standard treatment for IBS. Recent data supports the use of probiotics for many digestive complaints, IBS being one of them.

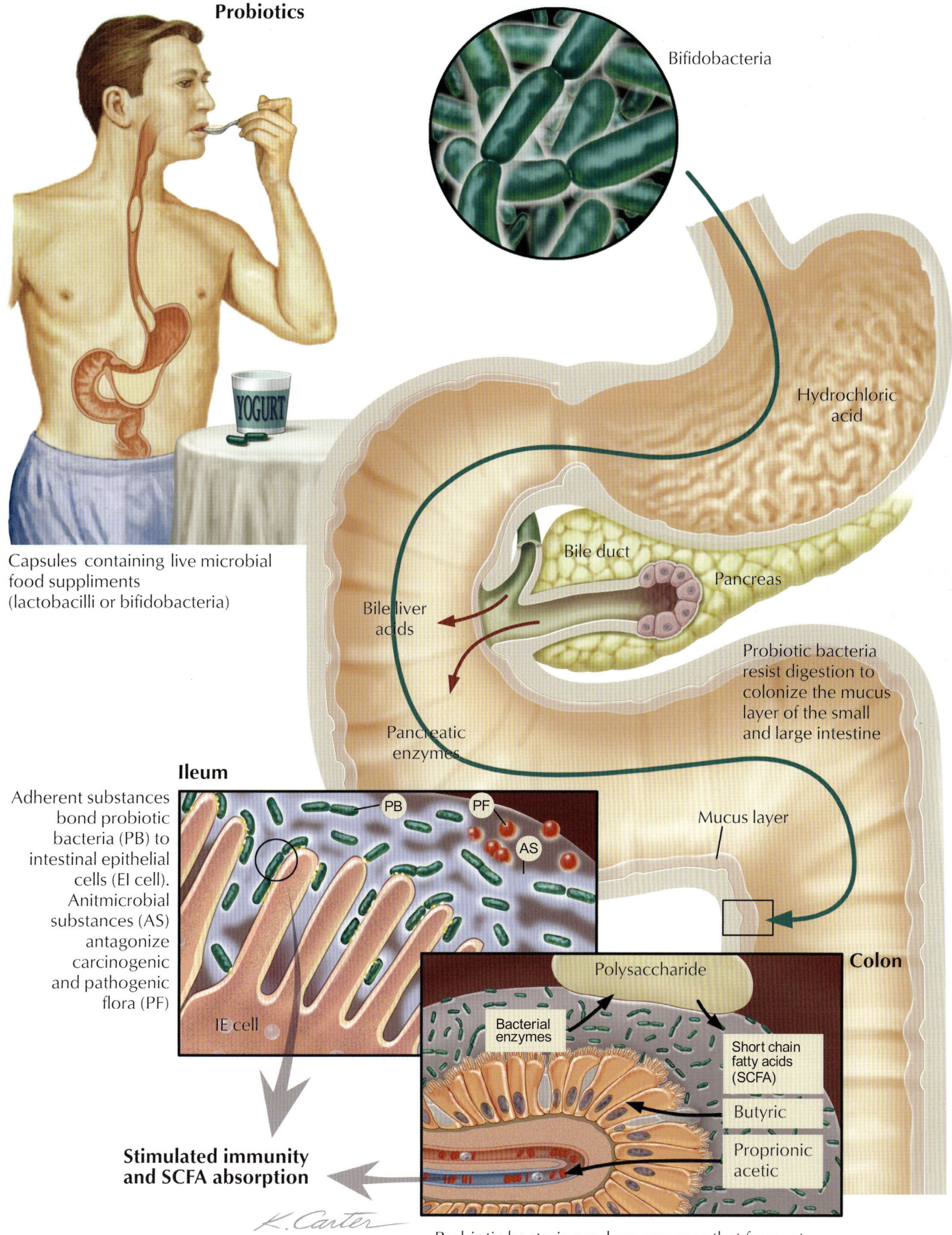

Capsules containing live microbial food suppliments (lactobacilli or bifidobacteria)

Adherent substances bond probiotic bacteria (PB) to intestinal epithelial cells (EI cell). Anitmicrobial substances (AS) antagonize carcinogenic and pathogenic flora (PF)

Probiotic bacteria produce enzymes that ferment polysaccharides

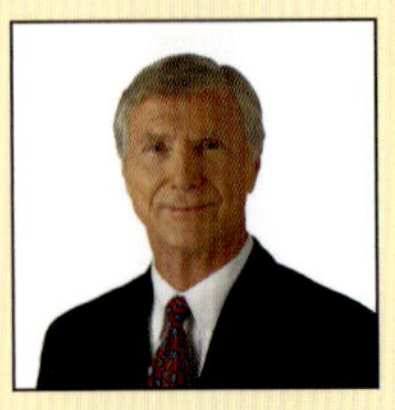

Dr. Smith's Comments

There have been long-standing beliefs that IBS is a psychological disorder. However, the physiological factors associated with IBS are becoming more plentiful in the literature.[28]

Intestinal infections can be a major factor in what is known as post-infectious IBS. Many people never have a gut problem until an episode of gastroenteritis, after which IBS-type symptoms become a way of life. In one study, IBS patients had a lactulose hydrogen breath test, and 84 percent were positive for small intestinal bacterial overgrowth (SIBO), a form of dysbiosis. One hundred and eleven subjects were given neomycin and experienced a 35 percent improvement reflected in a composite score, compared with 11.4 percent placebo. The best outcomes were observed if neomycin was successful in normalizing the lactulose breath test. This would implicate bacterial flora imbalance in IBS.

Consumption of simple carbohydrates and sugars can feed and increase the population of unfriendly bacteria and yeasts. It has been shown that toxins from Candida yeast can have an effect on the enteric and autonomic nerves of the colon, and may help promote constipation-dominant IBS. Immune deficient, carbohydrate-consuming elderly might be a set up for Candida-induced chronic constipation.

In the journal Current Opinions of Gastroenterology entitled "Inflammatory Bowel Disease and Irritable Bowel Syndrome: Separate or Unified?" several similarities between the two conditions were pointed out. Intestinal inflammation in the presence of psycho-emotional stress could constitute physiologic events that occur over time rather than being clear-cut and separate disease entities.

In the past, IBS bowel biopsy specimens appeared to be normal with routine histology. Now, using immunohistology and closer inspection, increased cytotoxic T cells, natural killer cells, colonic mast cells and increased intra-epithelial lymphocytes are seen.

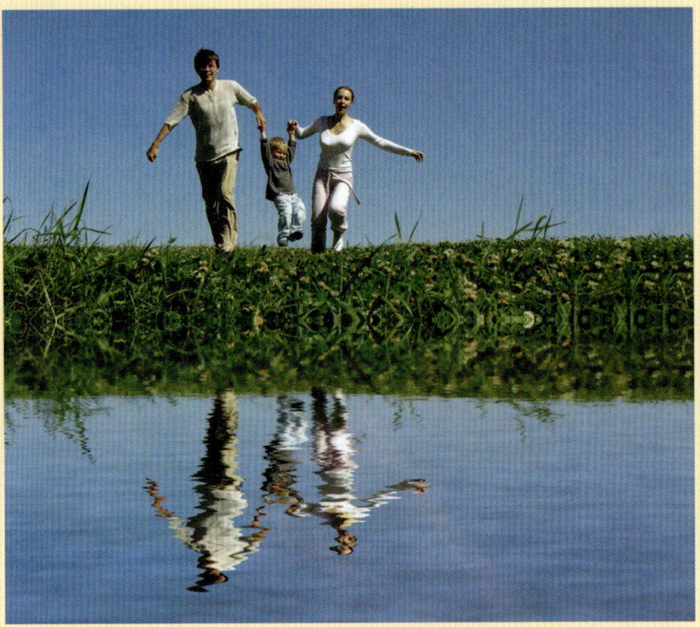

These features point to inflammatory changes in the small intestine and colon like the earliest patterns seen in IBD. Some patients with IBS, who were followed for years, had biopsy specimens with nerve degeneration in the ganglia of the bowel wall, with infiltration of CD3+ lymphocytes and longitudinal muscle hypertrophy. These are findings that begin to look more like Crohn's disease. According to current symptom criteria (Rome criteria), once organic changes like these are made, a diagnosis of the functional syndrome of IBS can no longer be used. It is easy to see why the process of labeling can lead to oversimplification confusing both practitioners and patients.

There are at least eight shared pathophysiologic mechanisms in common with IBS and IBD (which includes Crohn's, ulcerative colitis and microscopic colitis):

- Altered mucosal permeability
- Altered interaction of the luminal flora with the mucosal immune system
- Persistent mucosal immune activation
- Altered gut motility
- Sustained severe life stressors

- Histological similarities, especially with regard to inflammatory cells and cytokines
- Positive responses to probiotics, antibiotics and anti-inflammatory agents
- Genetic factors (one known factor is a genetic predisposition to enhanced immune reactivity)

One genetic predisposition, known as a SNIP (single nucleotide isolated polymorphism) which can be detected in people who are predisposed to developing IBS, is located on chromosome 2 as a change from cytosine to thymine at position 31. This results in an increase in production of the inflammatory cytokine IL-1 beta. This minor change may predispose individuals to chronic inflammatory conditions by increasing COX2 activity and prostaglandin production. In addition, this SNIP can predispose to hypochlorhydria (low stomach acid production) and H. pylori infection. The good news is that these types of small genetic changes (SNIPS) can often be controlled by appropriate diet and supplementation. If one knew they had this SNIP, it would be important for them to take enzymes, HCl and probiotics and follow the appropriate diet indefinitely.

At this point, I would like to make it clear that I am not saying that IBS will invariably become IBD. I do think, in some susceptible individuals, the data support that this could be a possibility, particularly if the preventive measures mentioned are not employed. In obtaining histories from IBD patients, it is not uncommon for some of them to report that their earlier symptoms were most similar to IBS.

Since there are many similarities in IBS and IBD (Crohn's and ulcerative colitis) that relate to bacteria, inflammation and stress, there are nutritional options that can be incorporated with benefit: higher fiber (more insoluble), omega-3 fish oils, probiotics, digestive enzymes, antioxidants, vitamins and minerals. At the same time, minimizing sugar, simple carbohydrates, known food allergens and stress can be most helpful. It is interesting to note that some of the deficiencies found in IBD, namely zinc, folate, iron and vitamin B12, are the very ones that are poorly absorbed in a low-acid environment. It is well known that stomach acid levels decline with age, acid-blocking drugs and genetic susceptibility.

Another factor is vitamin D deficiency. The best way to supplement would be 30 minutes of sunshine per day. However, after age 60, humans do not tend to make vitamin D through the skin as easily as younger people. Fortunately, supplementation with oral vitamin D works quite well to increase vitamin D3 levels. (See Vitamin D in the Appendix for more information.)

I have had patients who were able to implement much of the above, avoid surgery and continue to be in long-term remission. Unfortunately, with advanced Crohn's or ulcerative colitis, surgery is the only option. Surgery for Crohn's usually involves resection of the severely diseased small bowel, and surgery for ulcerative colitis involves removal of all, or most all, of the colon. If not done correctly, there can be disastrous results. If the surgery is successful, most return to normal lives, but can still have recurrent disease. Surgery does not address the cause of these conditions. This is why, with post-surgical patients, I have stressed optional nutritional approaches and lifestyle changes.

Depending upon their level of awareness, doctors may also advise their IBS patients to eat smaller meals, chew thoroughly, reduce fat intake, increase water consumption, and eliminate gas-forming foods, refined foods and sugar. Some may recommend the use of digestive enzymes with meals, probiotics (to increase friendly bacteria), glutamine (to help heal the bowel wall) and peppermint oil (enteric-coated capsules have been used to help soothe and relax intestinal muscles).[29]

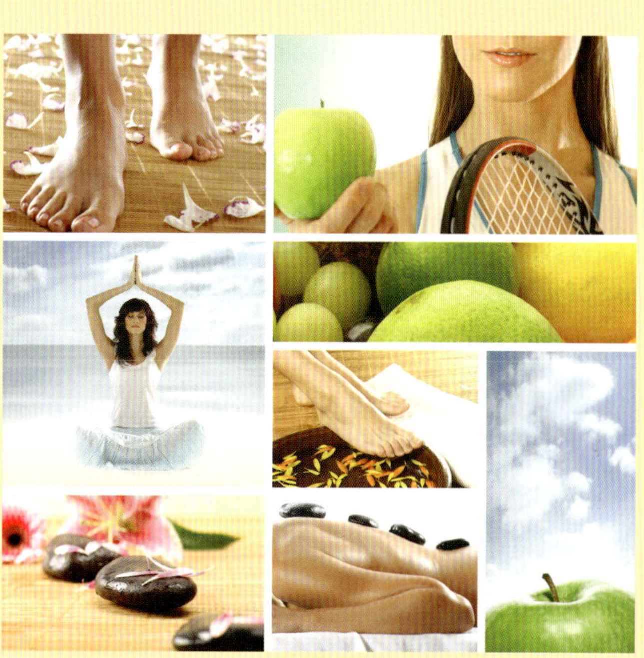

Lactose Intolerance

What Is It?

Lactose intolerance (also known as lactose malabsorption or lactase deficiency) is the name given to the condition in which the body is unable to digest lactose (milk sugar). Put another way, the body cannot break down lactose into its component sugars—glucose and galactose. Normally, this breakdown is performed by the enzyme lactase, which is manufactured in the lining of the small intestine. Lactase, however, is absent or deficient in the intestines of lactose-intolerant people making it difficult for them to handle milk and other dairy products.

It is important to note that lactose intolerance is not the same as a milk allergy, which is an immune response to one or more of the components in the milk, usually a protein. Poor protein digestion is believed to play a role in allergies because the immune response is triggered to react to the presence of unfamiliar undigested proteins in the gut lining or in the bloodstream. The person who is allergic to milk products, however, is not necessarily lactose intolerant since lactose intolerance is a function of poor enzyme activity and not an allergic reaction. (See the Allergies section for more information on food allergies.)

What Causes It?

There are three main types of lactose intolerance, which are summed up well by the Colorado State University:[1]

- Primary lactose intolerance – the most common form in which lactase gene expression turns off in childhood, and the individual is relatively lactase-deficient as a teenager and adult
- Secondary lactose intolerance – a number of diseases affecting the small intestine (inflammatory conditions, bacterial, viral or parasitic infections) can result in temporary lactase deficiency in individuals that are normally lactose tolerant. In most cases, this deficiency resolves in a few weeks.
- Congenital lactase deficiency – rare disorder in which lactase is deficient from birth.

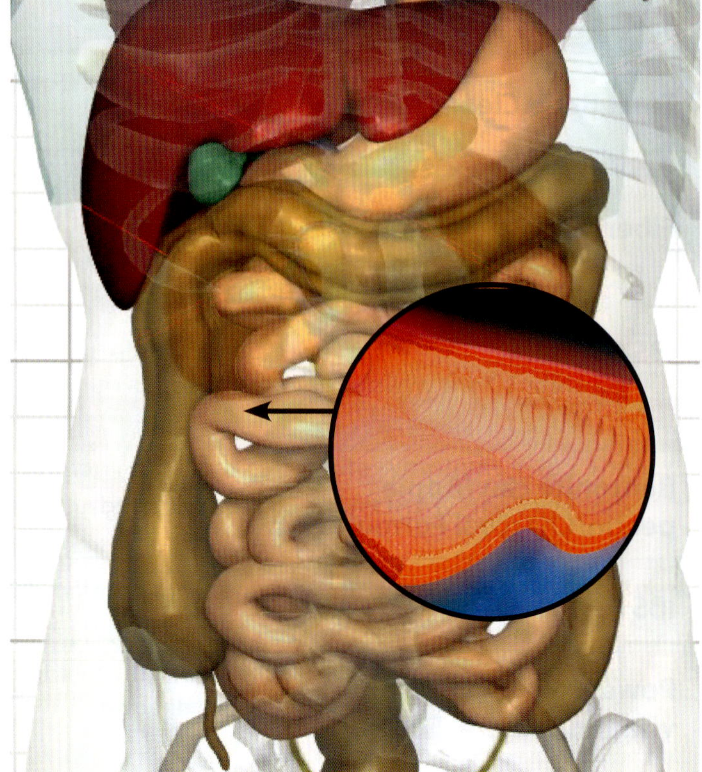

Illustration of an inflamed intestine

Lactose intolerance normally occurs in adults, though it may less frequently affect children. It can occur in infants after a severe bout of gastroenteritis which damages the intestinal lining.[2]

People who are intolerant to the lactose in milk may likewise be sensitive to sugar alcohols such as sorbitol, maltitol and xylitol; and should check labels for the presence of these substances.[3]

When lactose is not thoroughly broken down in the small intestine for any of the reasons discussed, all or some of it enters the colon intact. That portion of unsplit lactose that reaches the large intestine serves as food for bacteria residing there. As these bacteria feed upon the undigested milk sugar, gases and irritating acids are produced giving rise to unpleasant symptoms.

Lactose intolerance affects up to 75 percent of the world's population.[4] It is especially prevalent among people of Asian, African, Native American, Mexican and Mediterranean ancestry, affecting an estimated 70 to 90

Hidden Sources of Dairy Products

- Hot dogs
- Lunch meats (unless Kosher)
- Most non-dairy creamers
- Pancake, biscuit and cookie mixes
- Protein powder drinks
- Salad dressings
- Bread and other baked goods
- Processed breakfast cereals
- Instant potatoes, soups and breakfast drinks
- Margarine
- Candies and other snacks
- Pasta
- Puddings
- Sauces
- Anything that contains:
  - Casein
  - Lactose
  - Caseinate
  - Curds
  - Milk by-products
  - Dry milk solids
  - Non-fat dry milk powder
  - Whey
  - Sodium caseinate

percent of people within these groups.[5] Least affected (10 to 15 percent) are people of Northern or Western European ancestry.[6,7] An estimated 50 million Americans are lactose intolerant.[8]

People with Crohn's disease (an inflammatory bowel disease) and celiac disease (gluten sensitivity) are often lactose intolerant due to damage of the intestinal lining from the disease processes that interfere with lactase production.

What Are the Signs and Symptoms?

Within a short time—usually 30 minutes to two hours—of ingesting milk or dairy products, the lactose intolerant person will develop mild to severe symptoms that may include:

- Abdominal cramps
- Gas and bloating
- Diarrhea
- Nausea
- Headaches
- Acne

The onset of gastrointestinal symptoms may follow the ingestion of even small amounts of lactose, although individual tolerances to the milk sugar vary greatly. Some people are affected by the presence of minute amounts while others are able to tolerate a glass or two of milk. Some people may have a lactase deficiency and yet be without symptoms. They would not be considered lactose intolerant.

Lactose intolerance can be caused by gut inflammation. If symptoms of lactose intolerance become severe, it can cause leaky gut and lead to other problems in the body. Although lactose intolerance is rare in infants, when it occurs the following symptoms may appear: foamy diarrhea with diaper rash, slow weight gain and development, and vomiting.[9]

Some dairy products tend to cause more problems than others. Ice cream is often especially difficult for people with lactose intolerance to handle because some manufacturers add extra lactose to enhance its texture.[10] Hard, aged cheeses such as Parmesan, on the other hand, are relatively low in lactose, and so are generally easier to handle.[11] Fermented dairy products, such as yogurt (with live, active cultures), are usually well tolerated by people with lactose intolerance, as these products have been predigested by bacteria so that most of the lactose is broken down.[12,13]

How Is It Diagnosed?

Anyone suspecting that they may be lactose intolerant can do a simple self-test: Eliminate all sources of dairy products and those products that may contain lactose for at least two weeks to see if symptoms disappear. If they do not, then it is less likely that lactose intolerance is the cause. However, since some people do not have classic symptoms, this approach may not be sufficient. If symptoms do subside, it may be either lactose intolerance or milk allergy. If you are able to tolerate lactose-free or lactose-reduced dairy products, or are able to drink milk when lactase enzyme drops are added (or lactase supplements taken beforehand), the problem can be narrowed down to lactose intolerance. If a milk allergy is

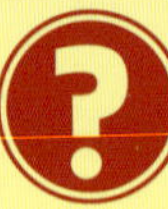

Did You Know

- An estimated 50 million Americans suffer from lactose intolerance, which is an inability to properly digest milk sugar, or lactose.
- This condition, which results in a variety of discomforts such as abdominal cramps and diarrhea, is rarely present at birth, but rather develops over a period of time.
- Lactose can be found in dairy products and in some medications.
- Lactose is the base for more than 20 percent of prescription drugs and about 6 percent of over-the-counter medications.

the cause of the problem, there would be no improvement of symptoms expected with the ingestion of lactase.

It may take some detective work to eliminate all dairy products, as these are often hidden in commonly consumed processed foods. Refer to the chart in this section for a list of known and possible hidden sources of dairy products.

Lactose is also used as a filler in some medications and many types of birth control pills.[14] In fact, it is the base for more than 20 percent of prescription drugs and about six percent of over-the-counter medications.[15]

There are three main diagnostic tools used by the medical profession to identify lactose intolerance: the lactose tolerance test, the hydrogen breath test, and the stool acidity test. The last of these is used for infants and small children who may be prone to dehydration that may result from diarrhea caused by the lactose ingestion required in the first two tests.[16] The test simply measures the amount of acid in the stool which will be elevated in the lactose intolerant person. Undigested lactose, fermented by bacteria in the colon, creates lactic acid and other short-chain fatty acids that can be detected in the stool. Additionally, glucose may be found in the stool sample as a result of unabsorbed lactose in the colon.[17]

The lactose tolerance test is a blood test that measures blood sugar levels. The patient fasts overnight and then drinks a lactose-containing liquid. Blood samples are then taken by a technician to measure blood sugar levels. Blood sugar levels should increase significantly after the ingestion of the lactose if the body is properly digesting it. If the lactose is not completely broken down into glucose, the blood sugar level does not rise significantly, and the diagnosis of lactose intolerance is confirmed, especially if symptoms of the disorder are manifesting.[18]

Another good test for lactose intolerance is checking for the genetic polymorphism 13910 C/T with a genetic analysis of the blood or saliva. If people know they have this they will be more prone to the symptoms of lactose intolerance, and would be wise to minimize lactose in their diet. They might also be more careful to maintain a healthy balance of probiotics and enzymes in their diet as well. If someone has symptoms of lactose intolerance and they know their genetic test is negative for lactose intolerance and the hydrogen/methane breath test is positive, it would indicate secondary lactose intolerance. This occurs when a small intestinal bacterial overgrowth or dysbiosis destroys the lactase enzyme on the mucosal surface in a similar way as with conditions like IBS and IBD.

What Is the Standard Medical Treatment?

There is no known cure for lactose intolerance. However, the symptoms may be controlled or eliminated with diet modifications. For the minority of severe cases and for young children,[19] total and complete elimination of all lactose from the diet may be necessary. In this case, special lactose-free dairy products (often available in supermarkets) or dairy substitutes (such as rice milk, nut milk, seed milk, oat milk or goat's milk) may be used. These dairy substitutes may be made at home or purchased in a health food store or in some supermarkets.

The majority of those suffering from lactose intolerance will be able to include some dairy products in their diet, especially if one or more of the following are used:

- Lactose-reduced dairy products
- Lactase enzyme supplements to be used in conjunction with meals that contain dairy foods
- Fermented dairy products, such as yogurt, kefir, sour cream, acidophilus milk, hard cheeses and buttermilk

Those who need to strictly avoid all dairy products due to lactose intolerance will want to look to other sources of calcium in their diets. Rich sources would include green vegetables (especially leafy and uncooked), sesame seeds (soak them before eating to deactivate enzyme inhibitors), salmon and sardines.

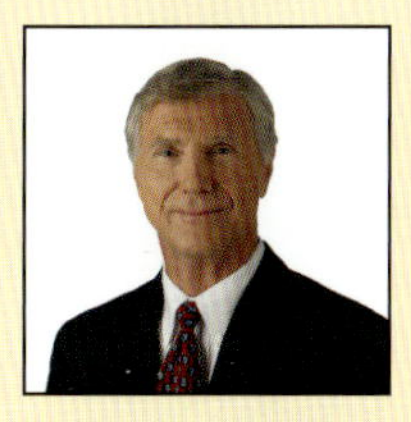

Dr. Smith's Comments

Lactose intolerance increases with age. This may be due to chronic low-grade microbial infection of the small bowel (Candida or bacterial overgrowth). In either case, the brush border enzymes produced by the gut lining will be decreased. Lactase is the enzyme shown to be often the most depleted; it is needed to split the milk sugar lactose. If this does not happen efficiently, symptoms of bloating, diarrhea and malabsorption of calcium may occur.

It is important to note that some patients with osteoporosis may be lactose intolerant. They have increased bone turnover and decreased bone mass, especially in older men and postmenopausal women. Impaired vitamin D status (not enough sunshine) and low calcium absorption have been implicated (AJCN; vol. 22, pp 201-207, 2003). As mentioned previously, low stomach acid, which also occurs with age, may be a significant factor in poor calcium absorption leading to osteoporosis. (See the Osteoporosis section for more information on this condition.)

Lactose intolerance may be an unexpected factor in IBD or IBS, and should routinely be ruled out in these conditions.

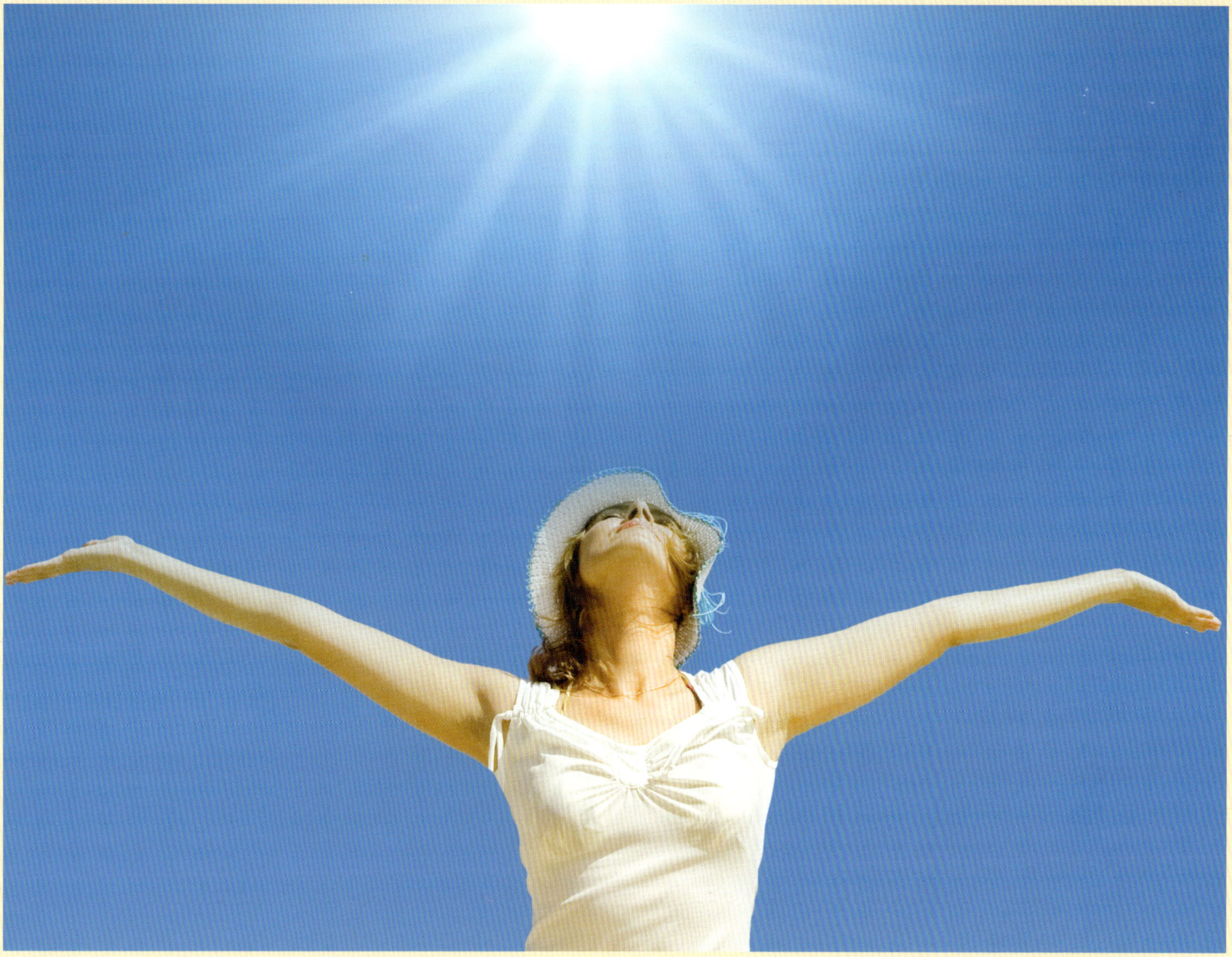

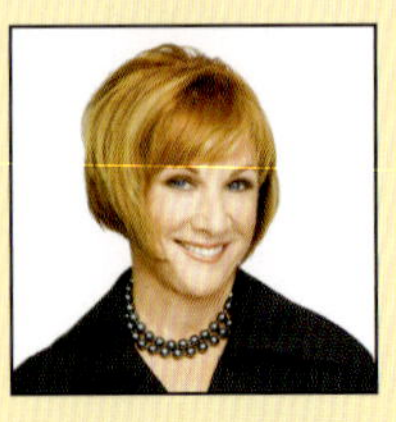

Brenda's Bottom Line

The symptoms of lactose intolerance—gas and bloating, abdominal cramping, loose stools or diarrhea—are also symptoms of a few different digestive conditions. Be sure that your symptoms are not actually the result of one of these conditions. (See the Rule Out list below.)

If you do determine that your symptoms are only the result of eating dairy, then this condition is easy to manage.

There is a spectrum of severity in people with lactose intolerance. Some people react to even the smallest amount of lactose. Other people can eat certain diary products in moderation, but develop symptoms when they overindulge. Determine where on this spectrum you are. From there, you can experiment with taking a lactose-digesting enzyme formula which will help to digest any lactose that you eat. Dosage will vary depending on where you are on the spectrum.

This condition can be easy to manage, but paying attention to your symptoms and making the appropriate changes accordingly is important because, if not controlled, gut imbalance can develop.

Rule Out:

- Food sensitivity (See the Gluten Sensitivity or Allergies section.)
- Candida overgrowth (See the Candidiasis section.)
- Parasitic infection (See the Parasitic Disease section.)
- Irritable bowel syndrome, IBS (See the IBS section.)
- Inflammatory bowel disease, IBD (See the IBD section.)

Diet

- If there is increased inflammation in the digestive tract, a three-day juice fast would be helpful.
- After that, follow the Fiber 35 Eating Plan. (See the Appendix.)
- Some people can tolerate hard cheeses like parmesan, and yogurt because they are relatively low in lactose.
- Eat plenty of foods high in calcium like: black strap molasses, apricots, broccoli, collard greens, kale, spinach, salmon and sardines.

Lifestyle

- Read product labels carefully. In addition to milk and milk solids, you must be aware of the dairy ingredients in processed foods.

Complementary Mind/Body Therapies

- Acupuncture could be helpful during an episode of lactose intolerance.
- Colon hydrotherapy is recommended for lactose intolerance.

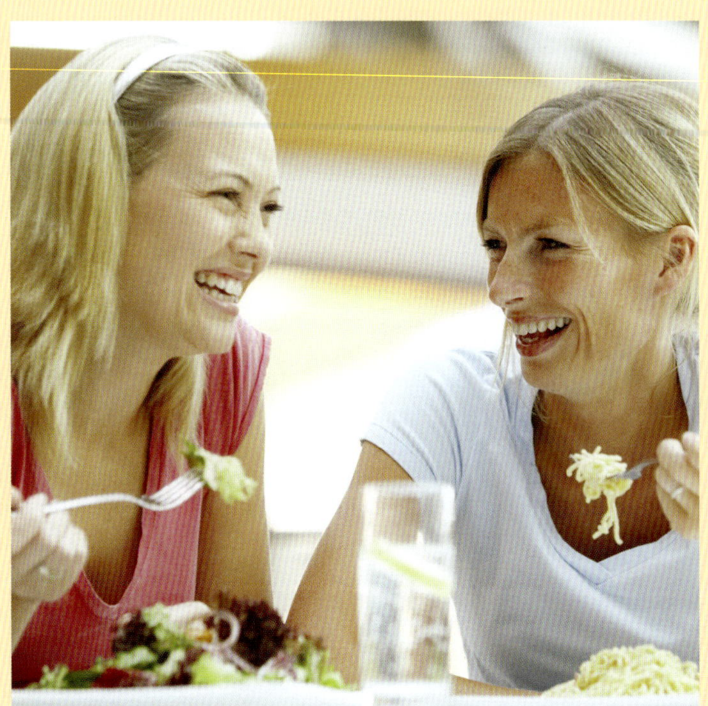

Recommended Nutraceuticals	Dosage	Benefit	Comments
Critical Phase	Daily maintenance recommendations should also be taken during this phase unless otherwise indicated.		
Bentonite clay / Apple pectin / Charcoal Formula	Take as directed for diarrhea	Helps absorb toxins and relieve diarrhea.	Take with plenty of water.
Helpful			
Calcium	1,000 mg daily	Ensures enough calcium is ingested if avoiding dairy.	Take with magnesium to aid absorption.
L-Glutamine Powder with Gamma Oryzanol	5,000-10,000 mg daily in divided doses	Helps repair the intestinal lining reducing permeability and severe reactions to foods.	Take in powder form.
Daily Maintenance			
Digestive Enzymes specific for lactose	Take with lactose containing foods	Helps break down dairy, helps to reduce reactions to undigested lactose.	Look for a formula containing lactase, lipase and papain (protease).
Omega-3 Fatty Acids	At least 2 grams daily of EPA/DHA combination	Helps restore moisture to the intestinal tract. Provides lubrication.	Look for a concentrated, enteric coated fish oil.
Fiber	4-5 grams twice daily	Helps produce healthy bacteria levels and good elimination.	Use in conjunction with high fiber diet to reach 35 g daily.
Probiotics	50-80 billion culture count daily	Replaces beneficial bacteria which can help to digest lactose and maintain intestinal health.	Some people may be sensitive to dairy-derived probiotics. Look for a dairy-free formula.
Vitamin D_3	At least 1,000 iu daily	Helps heal leaky gut, decrease inflammation and increase overall health.	Research is showing many health complications as a result of low vitamin D levels.

See further explanation of supplements in the Appendix

Leaky Gut Syndrome

What Is It?

As food passes through the stomach into the small intestine, nutrient absorption occurs through the semi-permeable mucous lining of the wall of the small intestine. This membrane also shields the bloodstream from unwanted toxins, pathogens and undigested food. In this respect, the gut lining is a vital part of the body's immune system because it limits the volume of potential invaders. Leaky gut syndrome (or increased intestinal permeability) is a condition that develops when the mucous lining of the small intestine becomes too porous, allowing entry of toxins, microorganisms and undigested food particles, as well as pathogens, into the bloodstream. The function of the mucous lining of the small intestine can be compared to that of a window screen which lets air in, but keeps bugs out. It is also like the skin in that it sloughs off a layer of cells naturally every three to five days, and produces new cells to maintain healthy function.

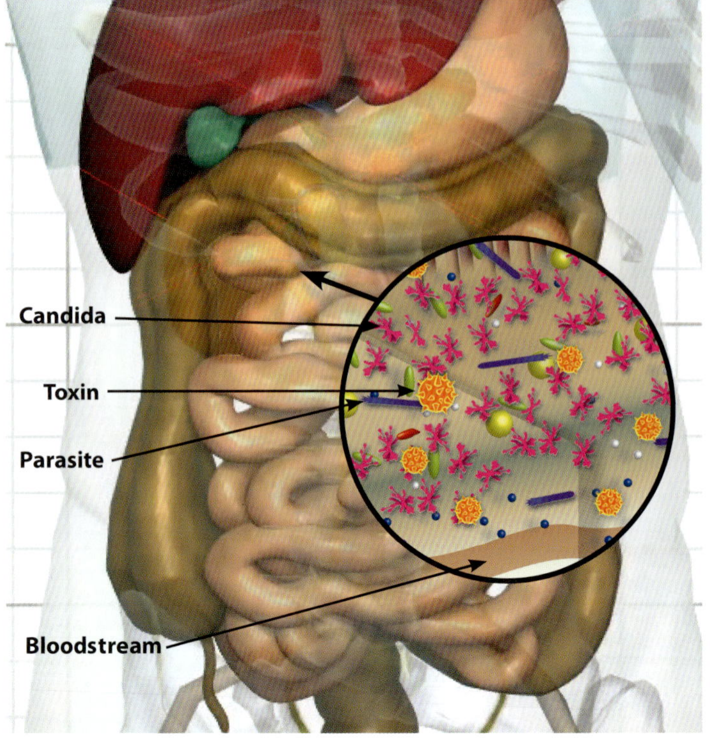

Illustration of leaky gut formation

What Causes It?

When digestion is impaired by such factors as stress, processed food consumption, inadequate chewing, excessive fluid intake with meals, improper food combining, and overeating, it can lead to an excessively permeable (leaky) gut. Here's why: When bacteria present in the intestine act upon undigested food particles, toxic chemicals and gases are produced. These intestinal toxins, known as endotoxins, can damage the mucosal lining resulting in increased intestinal permeability. As a result of repeated attacks by these toxins, the gut lining erodes over time. This is the basic mechanism by which leaky gut comes into being. It can also be caused or aggravated by a number of other factors, including:

- Alcohol (gut irritant)
- Caffeine (gut irritant)
- Parasites (introduced into the body by contaminated food and water)
- Pathogenic bacteria (introduced into the body by contaminated food and water)
- Pathogenic Candida infection (due to overgrowth)
- Food sensitivities
- Chemical food additives (dyes, preservatives, flavorings, etc.)
- Pesticide-laden foods
- Enzyme deficiencies (as found in celiac disease and lactose intolerance)
- Diet of refined carbohydrates ("junk" food)
- Prescription hormones (like birth control pills)
- Mold and fungal mycotoxins (in stored grains, fruit and refined carbohydrates and found in water-damaged buildings)
- Heightened exposure to environmental toxins
- Dental toxins (from restorative materials and invasive procedures)
- Free radicals
- Stress

Perhaps the greatest contributors to leaky gut are the drugs listed below:

- NSAIDs (Nonsteroidal anti-inflammatory drugs, like aspirin and Motrin)
- Antacids

Digestive Care

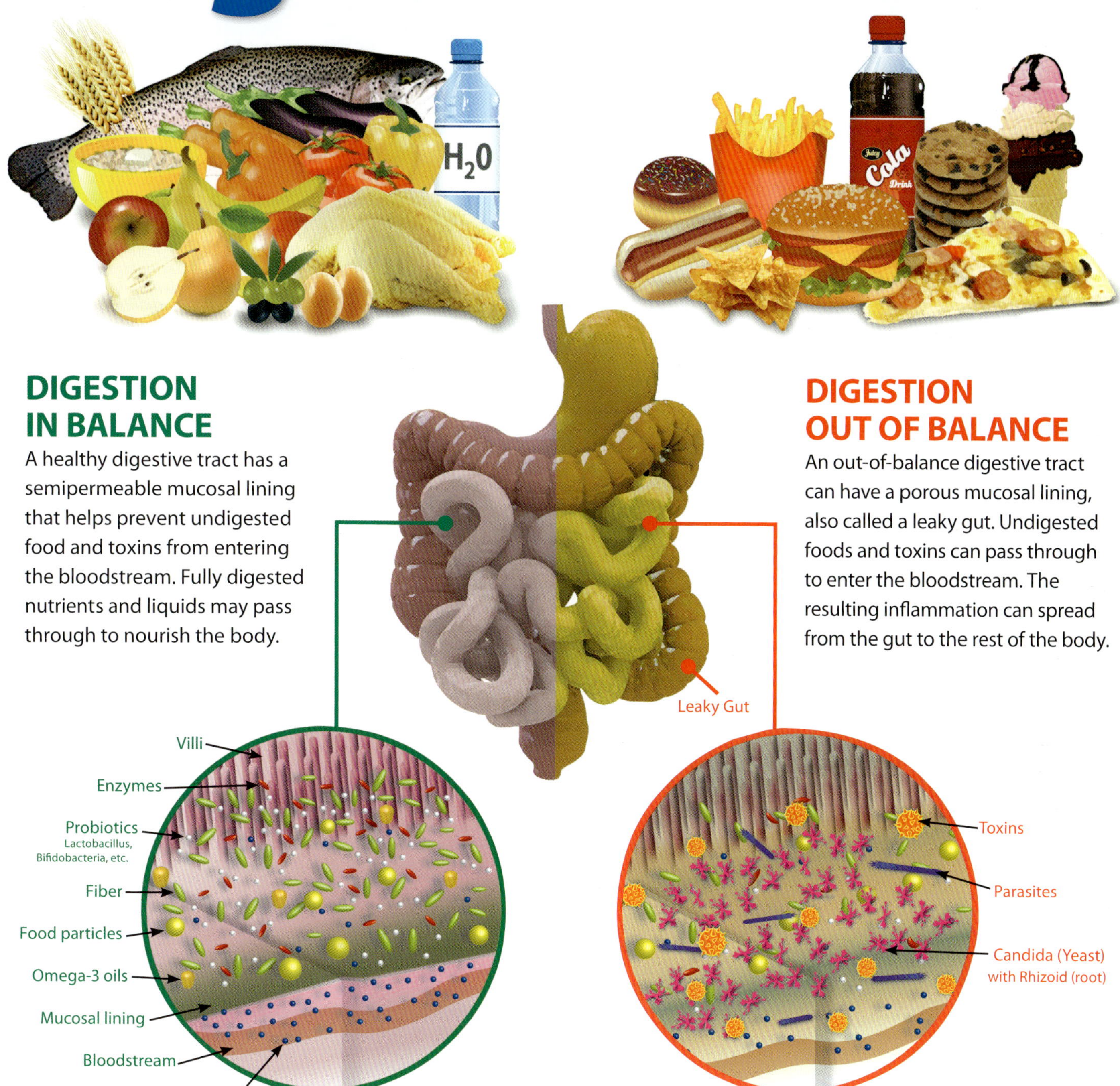

DIGESTION IN BALANCE

A healthy digestive tract has a semipermeable mucosal lining that helps prevent undigested food and toxins from entering the bloodstream. Fully digested nutrients and liquids may pass through to nourish the body.

DIGESTION OUT OF BALANCE

An out-of-balance digestive tract can have a porous mucosal lining, also called a leaky gut. Undigested foods and toxins can pass through to enter the bloodstream. The resulting inflammation can spread from the gut to the rest of the body.

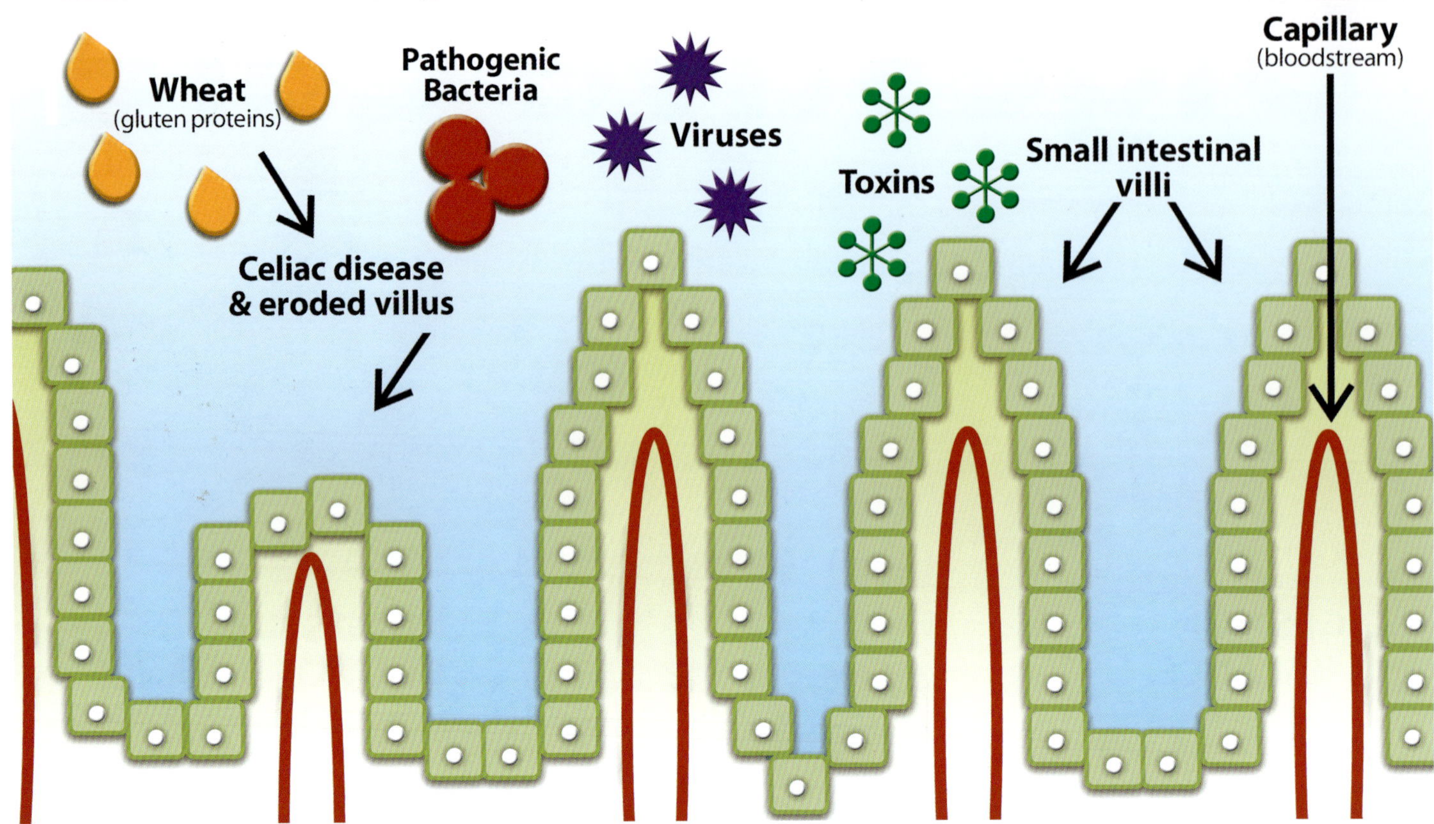

- Steroids (includes prescription corticosteroids such as prednisone and hydrocortisone)
- Antibiotics (which lead to overgrowth of bad bacteria in the GI tract)

Prolonged use of NSAIDs blocks the body's natural ability to repair the intestinal lining.[1] Once endotoxins have eroded this membrane, it becomes permeable rather than semi-permeable. ("The screen on your window gets holes in it.") Now the toxins, pathogens and food particles, which would normally not be permitted to enter the system, literally leak into the bloodstream. The body then attacks these unwanted toxins, developing antibodies to fight the foreign substances.

People of any age can have leaky gut syndrome. Those who regularly take any of the drugs listed previously would very likely suffer from the syndrome whether they've been diagnosed with it or not. People with digestive problems (with or without symptoms) will probably have an underlying leaky gut condition, as will people who routinely use large amounts of alcohol and caffeine, and those who eat a diet that is high in refined carbohydrates and chemical food additives, which is, unfortunately, the Standard American Diet (SAD).

Anyone who has had significant toxic exposure may develop leaky gut. Gut-damaging toxins may come from pathogens such as bacteria, viruses, fungi and parasites, or from chemicals and heavy metals in the environment (or in the mouth in the form of dental restorations). Folks who have autoimmune diseases such as those listed below most likely have an underlying gut permeability problem as well.

What Are the Signs and Symptoms?

The long-term net result of leaky gut syndrome is the likely development of autoimmune disease in which the body attacks its own tissues. There are some 80 recognized autoimmune diseases. These include:

- Lupus
- Alopecia areata
- Rheumatoid arthritis
- Polymyalgia

- Multiple sclerosis rheumatica
- Fibromyalgia
- Chronic fatigue syndrome
- Celiac disease
- Vitiligo syndrome
- Thyroiditis
- Vasculitis
- Crohn's disease
- Ulcerative colitis
- Urticaria (hives)
- Diabetes
- Psoriasis

Physicians are becoming increasingly aware of the importance of the GI tract in the development of autoimmune diseases. In fact, researchers now estimate that more than two-thirds of all immune activity occurs in the gut.[2] Allergies can develop when the body produces antibodies to the undigested proteins derived from previously harmless foods. These antibodies can get into any tissue and trigger an inflammatory reaction when that food is eaten. Depending on where this inflammation occurs in the body—in the joints, brain, lungs, blood vessels or gut—a variety of chronic illnesses can develop as a result.[3]

Other disorders associated with leaky gut include eczema, psoriasis, pancreatic insufficiency, candidiasis, non-alcoholic fatty liver disease (NAFLD), multiple chemical sensitivities and even heart disease. Leaky gut can aggravate existing conditions as well, for it can give rise to such symptoms as:[4]

- Fatigue
- Joint pain
- Muscle pain

Did You Know

Digestive disorders, including indigestion, nausea and vomiting, currently drive almost 38 million Americans into their doctor's offices each year.

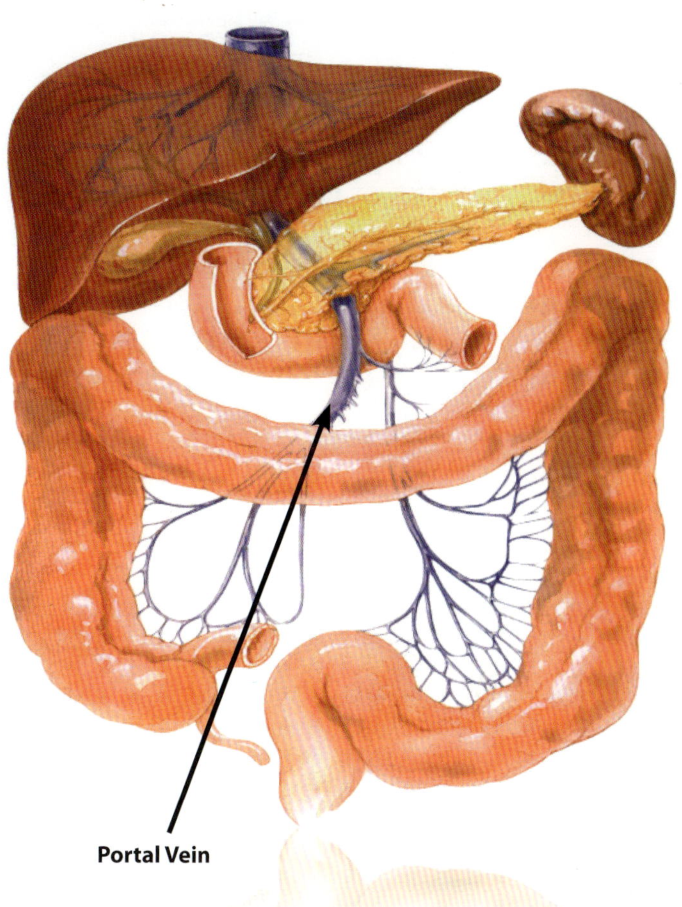

Toxins from a leaky gut flow directly to the liver, via the portal vein, increasing liver toxicity.

- Fever
- Abdominal discomfort
- Diarrhea
- Skin rashes
- Memory deficit
- Shortness of breath

Leaky gut syndrome can also cause malabsorption, and thus, deficiencies of many important nutrients—vitamins, minerals and amino acids—due to inflammation and the presence of potent toxins. This malabsorption can also cause gas, bloating and cramps, and can eventually lead to such complaints as fatigue, headaches, memory loss, poor concentration and irritability. The set of symptoms known collectively as irritable bowel syndrome (IBS)—bloating and gas after eating and alternating constipation and diarrhea—has also been linked to leaky gut syndrome, as has the more serious inflammatory bowel disease.

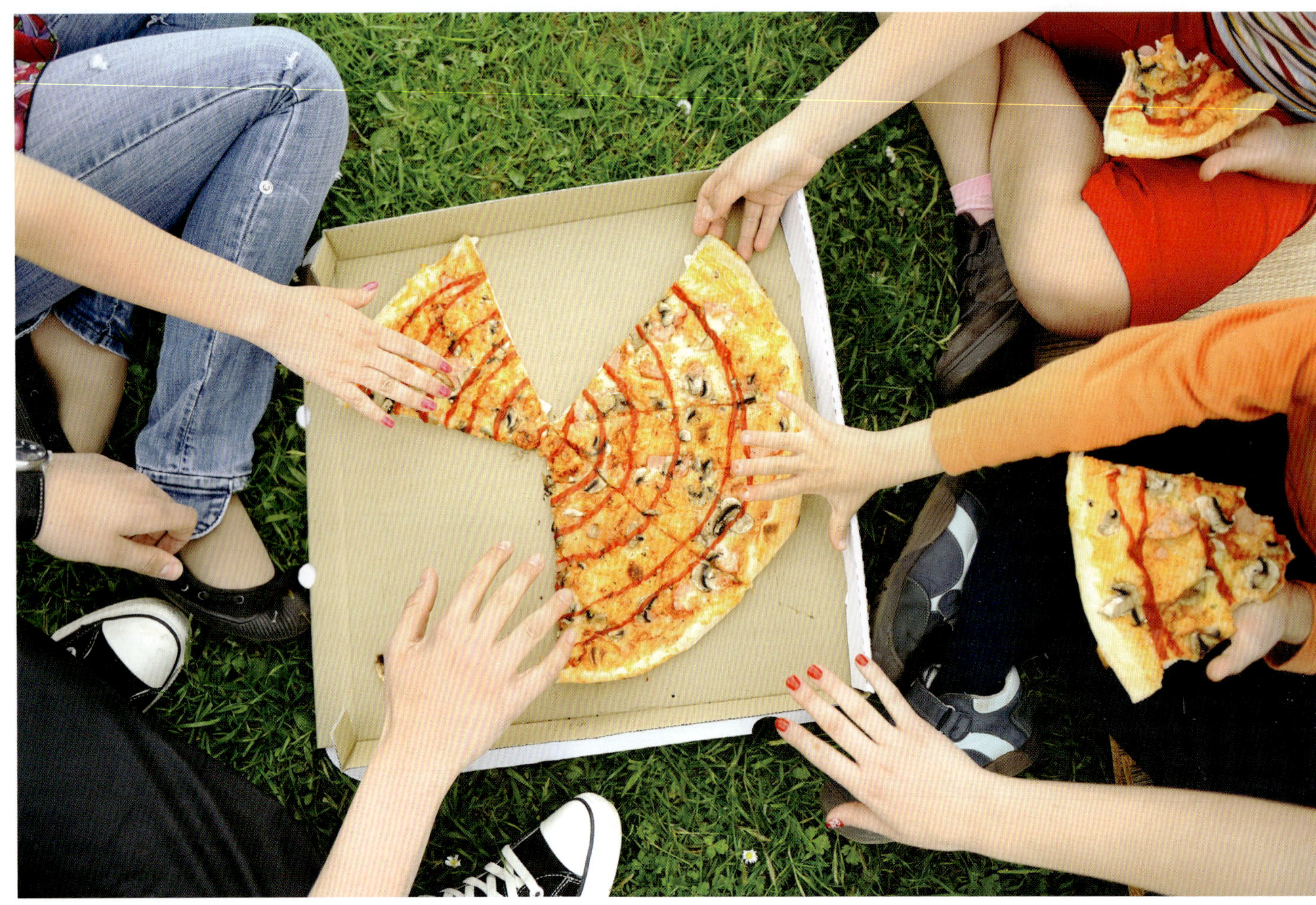

Leaky gut has been associated with such cognitive dysfunctions as autism in children. It has been found that some autistic children seem to react to the MMR (measles, mumps, rubella) vaccine with inflammation in the gut lining.[5] It is this inflammation that causes the gut to leak, allowing proteins such as gluten (from most grains) and casein (from milk) to enter the bloodstream, causing an allergic reaction to foods containing those proteins. (See the Autism section for more information.)

Once toxins enter the bloodstream through the leaky gut, their first stop is the liver. When the liver is called upon to work overtime due to toxic overload, toxins either re-circulate or are deposited in the liver or other places in the body. When they re-circulate to the intestines, they further irritate the lining, increasing its permeability. The recirculation of toxins can occur through the body's normal mechanism of entero-hepatic recirculation in which toxins go from liver to bile to intestines to the bloodstream and then back to the liver to start over. The food allergies and sensitivities that result from leaky gut create inflammation that causes the gut to leak even more. So, once leaky gut develops, it tends to become progressively worse if measures aren't taken to correct it.

How Is It Diagnosed?

The intestinal permeability assessment, which measures the absorption of mannitol and lactulose (two non-metabolized sugars), is described in the Appendix.

What Is the Standard Medical Treatment?

Since leaky gut syndrome is not a focus of conventional medicine, there really is no standard medical treatment. The conventional medical doctor will focus upon treating conditions that arise from leaky gut syndrome—and that treatment will likely be through use of drugs and/or surgery. Those nutritionally oriented physicians familiar with leaky gut will take a different approach, described, at least in part, at the end of this section.

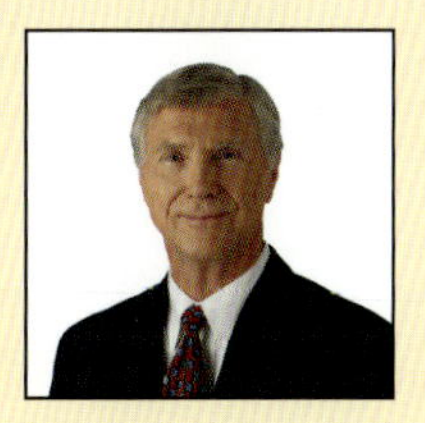

Dr. Smith's Comments

Increased intestinal permeability, whether it is intermittent or chronic, may be a major contributing factor to most diseases. It has been well established that there are at least four factors that can lead to increased permeability:

1) food allergies and sensitivities
2) malnutrition
3) dysbiosis (abnormal immune response to flora of low virulence or even normal flora)
4) hepatic stress

(Please go to www.mdheal.org by Leo Galland, MD, for further details.)

From birth throughout life, maintaining a well-nourished intestinal lining and overlying mucus with beneficial bacteria is of paramount importance in controlling intestinal permeability. There is an excellent review article about this in the American Journal of Clinical Nutrition (Oct 2003, pages 675-683). This is a hallmark description of how mucus is made by the intestinal lining, how it is the gel layer of the mucus that allows for bacterial adhesion, how there is crosstalk between the bacteria and intestinal lining, and how these vibratory signals profoundly affect what type of immune response is elicited by the intestinal immune system. Suffice it to say that a balance of soluble and insoluble fiber, the right ratio of essential fatty acids, beneficial bacteria, digestive enzymes, and supplements for building and maintaining the gut lining would be a very wise dietary choice for everyone to make on a regular basis.

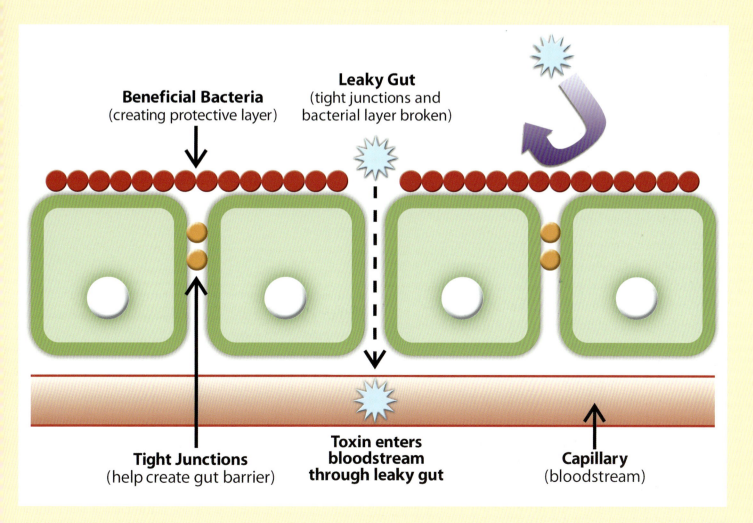

Beneficial Bacteria
(creating protective layer)

Leaky Gut
(tight junctions and bacterial layer broken)

Tight Junctions
(help create gut barrier)

Toxin enters bloodstream through leaky gut

Capillary
(bloodstream)

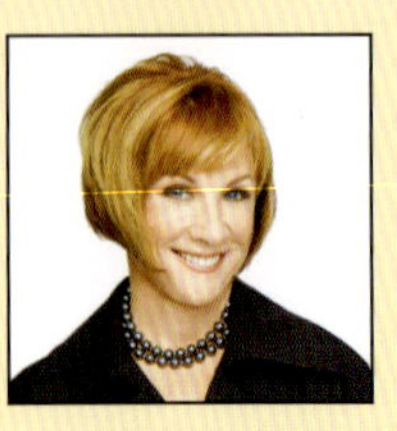

Brenda's Bottom Line

Leaky gut syndrome is the crux of all the conditions in this book. When the gut is imbalanced and inflamed, the integrity of the intestinal lining breaks down. This allows toxins, pathogens and undigested food particles to enter into the bloodstream which triggers an immune response involving yet more inflammation and a dysregulation of the immune system. All these factors contribute to the development of many different chronic diseases.

"Leaky gut syndrome is a major part of the gut connection to so many health conditions that affect the rest of the body."

Leaky gut syndrome is a major part of the gut connection to so many health conditions that affect the rest of the body. I cannot stress enough the importance of rebuilding the gut lining. The gut lining needs to be intact so that the beneficial bacteria can adhere to it properly, creating the proper defense against invading pathogens and toxins, and being able to communicate with the immune system, which is connected to the gut lining. If this gut protection system is not in place, chronic and recurrent health conditions will develop.

Reducing toxic exposure is of prime importance in preventing and reversing leaky gut syndrome. Both exotoxins (from the outside environment) and endotoxins (produced inside the body by bacteria and poor digestive conditions) can contribute to leaky gut. Eliminating these toxins, maintaining regular elimination, and healing the intestinal lining are key steps in healing a leaky gut.

Rule Out:

- Candida overgrowth (See the Candidiasis section.)
- Parasitic infection (See the Parasitic Disease section.)
- Food sensitivity (See the Gluten Sensitivity and Allergies section.)
- Lactose intolerance (See the Lactose Intolerance section.)

Recommended Testing

- Comprehensive stool analysis (CSA) (See the Appendix.)
- Food sensitivity test (See the Appendix.)
- Intestinal permeability test (See the Appendix.)

Diet

- If Candida is an underlying condition, follow the Candida Diet. (See the Appendix.)
- For maintenance, follow the Fiber 35 Eating Plan. (See the Appendix.)

Lifestyle

- Avoid or minimize the use of NSAIDs (aspirin, ibuprofen, etc.) and antibiotics.
- Avoid use of antacids.
- Reduce toxic exposure to chemicals. Clean up your environment, and eat organic food as much as possible.

Complementary Mind/Body Therapies

- Stress can be a major component of this disease, so find ways to reduce it with therapies such as meditation, yoga, deep breathing, massage, biofeedback, or music therapy.
- Acupuncture may be helpful as it targets the meridians associated with the digestive system, and it is also a stress reducer.
- Colon hydrotherapy may be beneficial to improve digestion and intestinal balance.

Recommended Nutraceuticals	Dosage	Benefit	Comments
Critical Phase Daily maintenance recommendations should also be taken during this phase unless otherwise indicated.			
L-Glutamine Powder with Gamma Oryzanol	10,000 mg daily in divided doses	Helps repair the intestinal lining, reducing permeability and severe reactions to foods.	Best taken in powder form.
Helpful			
Total Body Cleanse	See Appendix	Encourages elimination and detoxification.	Herbal formula should support the seven channels of elimination.
Liver Detox	This should follow the Total Body Cleanse. See Appendix	Encourages detoxification involving the liver.	Should contain milk thistle seed extract containing silymarin, phosphatidylcholine, selenium and herbs.
Antioxidant Supplement	Use as directed	Protects tissue from damage.	You can purchase a high-potency antioxidant formulation from most health food stores.
High Potency Multi-vitamin/mineral	Use as directed	Provides needed nutrients that can be deficient with those with a leaky gut.	Powder or liquid formulation helpful due to easier assimilation and absorption.
Daily Maintenance			
L-Glutamine Powder with Gamma Oryzanol	5,000 mg daily in divided doses after critical phase	Helps repair the intestinal lining, reducing permeability and reducing severe reactions to foods.	Best taken in powder form.
Digestive Enzymes	Take with meals	Helps digest and absorb nutrients from food.	If low stomach acid is found find a formula that contains hydrochloric acid.
Probiotics	50 to 200 billion culture count daily	Numerous benefits to intestinal health, helps reduce permeability and inflammation.	Look for high amount of bifidobacteria, the main beneficial bacteria in colon.
Omega-3 Fatty Acids	At least 2 grams daily of EPA/DHA combination	Helps restore moisture to the intestinal tract and reduces inflammation.	Look for a concentrated, enteric coated fish oil.
Fiber	4-5 grams twice daily	Helps produce healthy bacteria levels and good elimination.	Use in conjunction with high fiber diet to reach 35 g daily.
Vitamin D_3	At least 1,000 iu daily	Helps heal leaky gut, decrease inflammation, increase overall health.	Research is showing many health complications as a result of low vitamin D levels.

See further explanation of supplements in the Appendix

Parasitic Disease

What Is It?

A parasite is an organism that lives off another organism. Parasites living inside the human body will feed off cells, energy, digested food and supplements. Technically, parasites would include bacteria, viruses and fungi, as well as worms and protozoa (single-celled microscopic organisms). For the purposes of this book, however, only worms and protozoa will be considered under the category of parasites. There are more than 3,000 varieties of parasite,[1] and they all fall within one of four categories:[2]

- **Tapeworms** (Cestoda) – These large parasites generally reside in the intestinal tract, and can grow up to 12 meters in length. The most common varieties are beef and pork tapeworms.
- **Roundworms** (Nematoda) – Also known as threadworms, these parasites range from 0.2 centimeters to 35 centimeters in length. They may reside in the intestinal tract or migrate into lymphatic vessels, the pancreas, heart, lungs, liver or body cavities.
- **Protozoa** – These microscopic single-celled parasites migrate through the bloodstream to all parts of the body.
- **Flukes** (Trematoda) – These parasites range in length from one to two and a half centimeters. They generally travel through the tissues to the liver, kidneys, lungs or intestinal tract.

Some human intestinal parasites include:

- Enterobius sp.
- Giardia lamblia
- Cryptosporidium
- Blastocystis hominis
- Necator americanus
- Entamoeba histolytica
- Dientamoeba fragilis
- Ascaris sp.
- Strongyloides stercoralis
- Dipylidium caninum
- Toxocara sp.
- Trichinella sp.
- Trichuris sp.

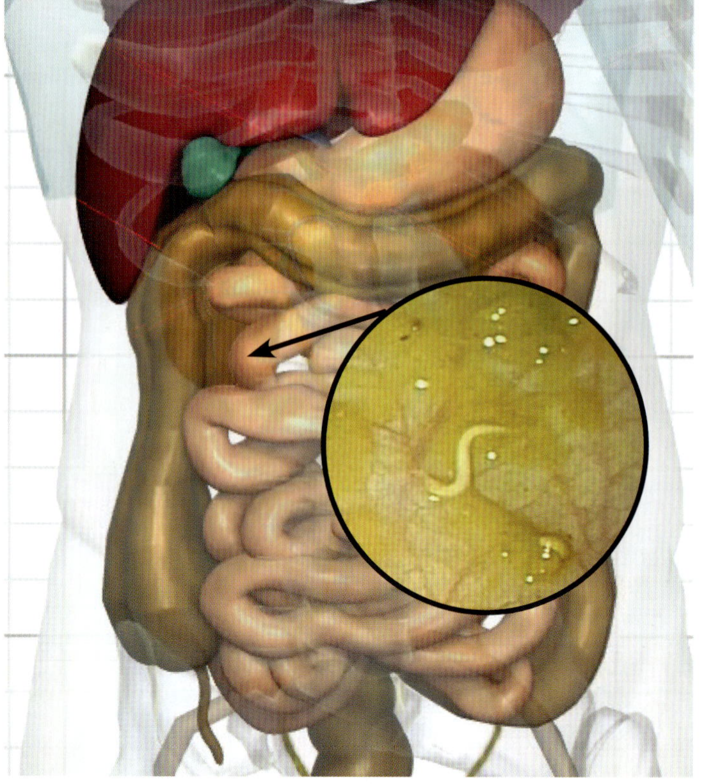

Endoscopic view of roundworm (yellow) in the small intestines

Parasites that affect other areas of the body include:

- Babesiosis
- Leishmaniasis
- Toxoplasmosis
- Trichomoniasis
- Trypanosoma (chagas and sleeping sickness)
- Plasmodium falciparum (malaria)

What Causes It?

Parasites are ubiquitous, which is to say they are everywhere. While precautions can be taken to avoid them, some degree of exposure is probable even when extreme care is taken to prevent parasitic infection. While everyone is exposed to parasites to some degree, not everyone will suffer equally from their ill effects.

What determines whether parasites will set up housekeeping in the body or pass harmlessly through it? While there are many factors at work, the most important is the degree of resistance or the strength of the body's immune system. This, in turn, depends heavily upon exposure to toxins. Some of the damaging chemicals to which people are regularly exposed include pesticides, personal care products, household cleaners, industrial wastes, solvents, drugs, etc. The threat of heavy metals, especially those used extensively in dentistry, such as mercury and nickel, represents another hidden, yet dangerous exposure to toxins. When the body is heavily burdened with these toxins, the table is set for the arrival of the uninvited guest—the parasite. If the body is further weakened through poor diet, infection, other disease processes, or stress in any form, its resistance to parasitic infestation will be lowered further.

Nutritional deficiency appears to contribute to parasite infestations. The effect of nutrition on the internal environment of the body plays a key role in determining whether parasites will pass through harmlessly, or begin to proliferate.

Decreased output of enzymes by the pancreas and deficiency of hydrochloric acid (HCl) in the stomach are two factors that can predispose the body to parasitic infection.[3] Stomach acid is one of the body's first defenses against parasites, for in its presence, parasites are destroyed due to the extremely high acidity.

Parasites can enter the body through the mouth, the nose, and the skin, including through the bottom of the feet. They can also be transmitted via vectors, or insect carriers. Common sources of parasites include:

- Contaminated soil
- Contaminated fruits and vegetables
- Raw or rare meat
- Pets
- Mosquitoes
- Contact with feces (such as through day-care centers)
- Polluted water/tap water
- Contact with someone who has parasites

Another factor that has contributed significantly to the growing parasite epidemic is the widespread use of drugs that suppress immunity. Many of the drugs in common use today are immunosuppressive and therefore increase our susceptibility to parasitic infestation.

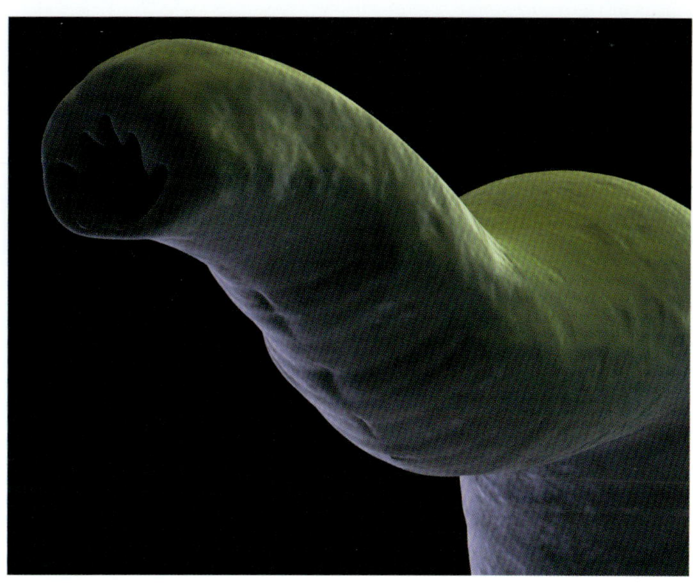

A hookworm illustration

Although many external factors contribute to the parasite problem, by far the biggest factor is an internal one: a toxic colon. Colon toxicity is largely the result of an unwholesome lifestyle and resulting bacterial imbalance in the colon. Once the ideal ratio of good to bad bacteria in the colon is disrupted, the resulting imbalance creates an environment conducive to parasite infestation. Factors that contribute to this imbalance include:

- Antibiotics
- Refined carbohydrates
- Steroid drugs
- Birth control pills
- X-rays/radiation therapy
- Chlorinated water
- Stress
- Low-fiber diet
- Pollution
- Poor digestion and elimination
- Mercury toxicity (often from mercury and nickel dental fillings)

These factors can also set the stage for overgrowth of the yeast Candida albicans. For this reason, Candida and parasites tend to appear together.

It's not just third-world countries, nor foregin travelers, that experience parasite problems as many people believe. No one is immune from parasite infestation. It is a growing problem in industrialized nations, as recent studies show. Dr. Omar M. Amin, of the Parasitology Center in

Scottsdale, Arizona, completed a large parasite study in 2000. His study involved analysis of two fecal specimens from each of 2,896 patients throughout the United States. Dr. Amin found that one-third (32 percent) of the patients tested positive for parasites with one or more of 18 identified species.[4]

While the parasite problem is widespread and growing, it often goes unrecognized. Because parasitic infestation has generally been considered a disease of the tropics, the typical MD is not likely to consider it when making a diagnosis, especially since parasitology is seldom presented in mainstream medical journals or medical schools. There are presently only five nationally reportable parasitic diseases:[5] Cryptosporidiosis, cyclosporiasis, giardiasis, malaria and trichinosis. Apart from the records kept by the Center for Disease Control (CDC) in the United States, there is little tracking for parasites in this country. With lack of information and little training, doctors aren't likely to look for parasites as an underlying cause of illness, which, in fact, they often are. That being the case, accurate statistics are not widely available with regard to parasitic infestation. Nonetheless, a growing number of holistic practitioners are concluding, based on their own clinical observations, that the parasite problem is epidemic in proportions in developed and developing nations.

Cryptosporidium outbreaks from contaminated public water sources continue to be of concern due to the organism's ability to survive chlorination. In 1993, it was estimated that 403,000 people were infected with Cryptosporidium due to poor water quality.[6] Even as recent as 2007, a Cryptosporidium outbreak that affected recreational waters was reported.[7] This indicates that there is still a problem with the organism reaching public water supply.

What Are the Signs and Symptoms?

It is important to bear in mind that parasites can mimic other disorders and/or produce no noticeable symptoms. When they do cause symptoms, a wide range can be displayed. These can include:

- Diarrhea or constipation
- Digestive complaints (gas, bloating, cramps)

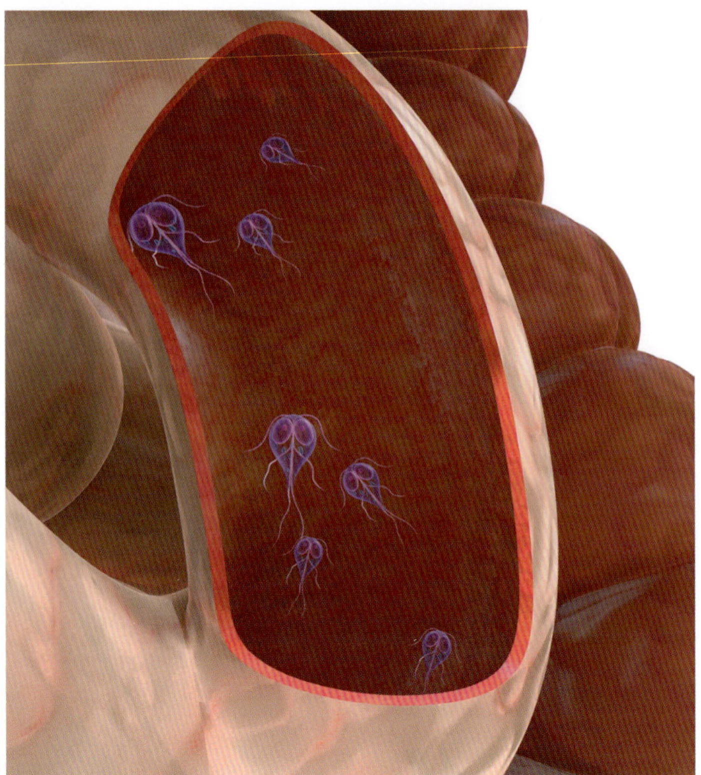

An illustration of Giardia parasite in the intestine

- Irritability/nervousness
- Persistent skin problems
- Granulomas (tumor-like masses that encase destroyed larva or parasites)
- Overall fatigue
- Disturbed sleep
- Muscle cramps
- Joint pain
- Post nasal drip
- Swollen glands
- Teeth grinding
- Prostatitis
- Sugar cravings
- Ravenous appetite (or loss of appetite)
- Weight loss (or gain)
- Headaches/neckaches/backaches
- Itchy anus or ears
- Dark circles under the eyes
- Light sensitivity
- Elevated eosinophils (white blood cells)
- Low-grade fever
- Nose picking
- Nail biting
- Brain fog
- Pain in the umbilicus
- Bedwetting

- Mucus in stools
- Foul-smelling stools
- Coughing
- Food and environmental sensitivities
- Depressed secretory IgA (an antibody)

Parasites can affect tissue anywhere in the body. Some of the disorders that have been associated with them include arthritis, appendicitis, recurrent yeast infections, allergies, asthma, bronchitis, anemia, irritable bowel syndrome, frequent colds and infections, lactase deficiency, fibromyalgia, gallbladder problems, malnutrition, urinary tract infections, prostatitis, and colitis.[8] Over time, a parasite infection can depress immunity and cause leaky gut syndrome (see the Leaky Gut Syndrome section), which leads to nutritional absorption problems and has been associated with allergies and other autoimmune diseases.

Because they can get into the blood and travel to any organ, parasites can cause problems that are often not recognized as parasite-related. This can result in an incorrect or incomplete diagnosis. For example, chronic infection with Giardia lamblia (giardiasis), considered the most common parasite to affect humans in the US, can be an undetected element or missing diagnosis in chronic fatigue syndrome. Giardial or Blastocystis hominis infection can both be mistaken for irritable bowel syndrome (IBS)[9] or duodenal ulcer.[10] Symptoms of the amoeba Entamoeba histolytica can mimic ulcerative colitis or IBS.[11]

Most people don't realize it, but it is not only parasites that can cause damage to the body but also the waste they give off. Giardia lamblia, for example, invades the upper intestine and gives off toxins that damage enzymes (causing lactose intolerance when the lactase enzyme is damaged). Giardia is often found in mountain streams and in some city water systems, as it is not killed by chlorine. Cryptosporidium is another protozoan that has contaminated some city water supplies. It was the second most prevalent parasite found by Dr. Amin in his 2000 study. The first was Blastocystis hominis.

Interestingly, one-third of B. hominis infections were not associated with any symptoms in Dr. Amin's study.[12] Until recently, this disease-causing organism was considered to be a harmless yeast. In 1967, it was reclassified as a protozoan and deemed a pathogen.[13] It is not unusual for parasites that were once considered harmless to be reclassified as pathogens. Dr. Amin found, in fact, that some protozoa considered as non-pathogenic unexpectedly caused symptoms in 73 to 100 percent of the cases studied.[14] This points to a continuing need to reassess the pathogenic potential of parasites.

The waste products from parasites poison the body and force the organs of elimination to work overtime stressing the liver. As the detoxification mechanisms become overwhelmed, nutritional reserves are depleted, and the immune system weakens. The net result is disease development.

How Is It Diagnosed?

A stool analysis is usually used to detect parasites. However, parasites can be difficult to detect since they tend to hide in the lining of the intestine, and can live in other organs. If parasites are in the heart or lungs, they will not show up in stool regardless of how well it's analyzed.

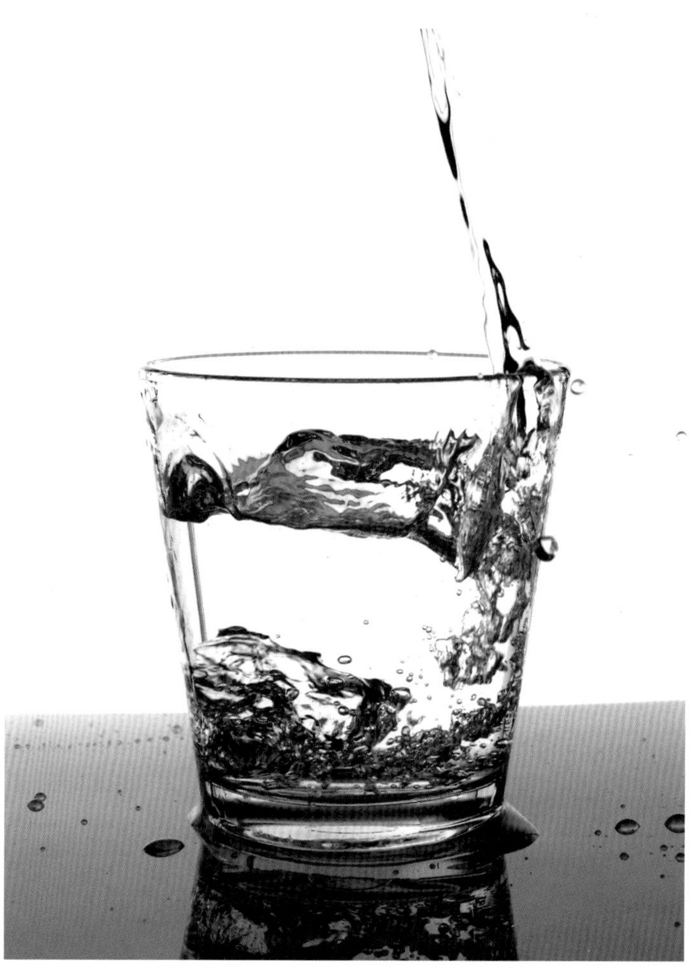

Did You Know

- Over time, parasites can be a contributing cause to chronic diseases such as arthritis, multiple sclerosis, asthma, edema, appendicitis and cancer.
- Mainstream medicine tends to overlook parasites as a possible primary cause for many well-known diseases costing patients many frustrating hours, and costing the health care systems many millions of dollars in unnecessary diagnostic tests and ineffective pharmaceutical treatments.

In fact, a single random solid stool sample, analyzed in the traditional manner, is unlikely to even reveal the presence of intestinal parasites. Specialized testing (see the Appendix for laboratory information) is often needed to detect parasites that can be difficult to spot as they go through different stages of their life cycles. Some doctors use purged stool analysis; the patient is given a laxative beforehand to liquefy the stool and loosen embedded parasites. Multiple stool samples are then submitted for analysis. Another approach is the rectal swab test, designed to detect those parasites that live in the mucous membranes that line the intestinal tract.

Another approach, though an invasive one, is to obtain a tissue specimen through a biopsy taken with an endoscope. This lighted, flexible tube is passed into the intestine where a tissue sample is removed through the rectum. Pinworms can be detected in a much more low-tech manner: a piece of tape attached to the anus can pick up these worms or their eggs, which can be detected with microscopic analysis. Blood tests can be used to reveal an elevated eosinophil count, a general indicator for an infection by parasites—except for giardia and amoeba, which rarely cause eosinophilia.[15] IgG and IgM antibody testing can be done for giardia and Entamoeba histolytica.[16] Other types of blood tests, sputum tests, urine tests and even radiologic tests can be used to detect various types of parasites with varying degrees of success. Analysis of aspirated fluids and the growth of tissue cultures may also be used.[17]

Parasites have a complex life cycle. Three of the most prevalent parasites found in the United States and worldwide shed at irregular intervals. This means that the parasite might be in the stool two to four days a week but not the rest of the week. If the person is tested for the parasite on a day it is not present, there will be a negative test result. The person would then go untreated. Therefore, it is best for repeat stool samples (at least two to three) to be taken on non-consecutive days.

It is best to have parasite testing done by a laboratory, such as Dr. Amin's, that specializes in parasitology. While testing technique is constantly being modified and improved, false negatives still occur. Therefore, parasites cannot be positively ruled out based on even the best lab results. When positive lab results are found, they can be very helpful in designing an effective treatment protocol.

What Is the Standard Medical Treatment?

When parasites are detected, they are most often treated with drugs, usually Flagyl (metronidazole), despite its many adverse side effects and the fact that many parasites have become Flagyl-resistant.

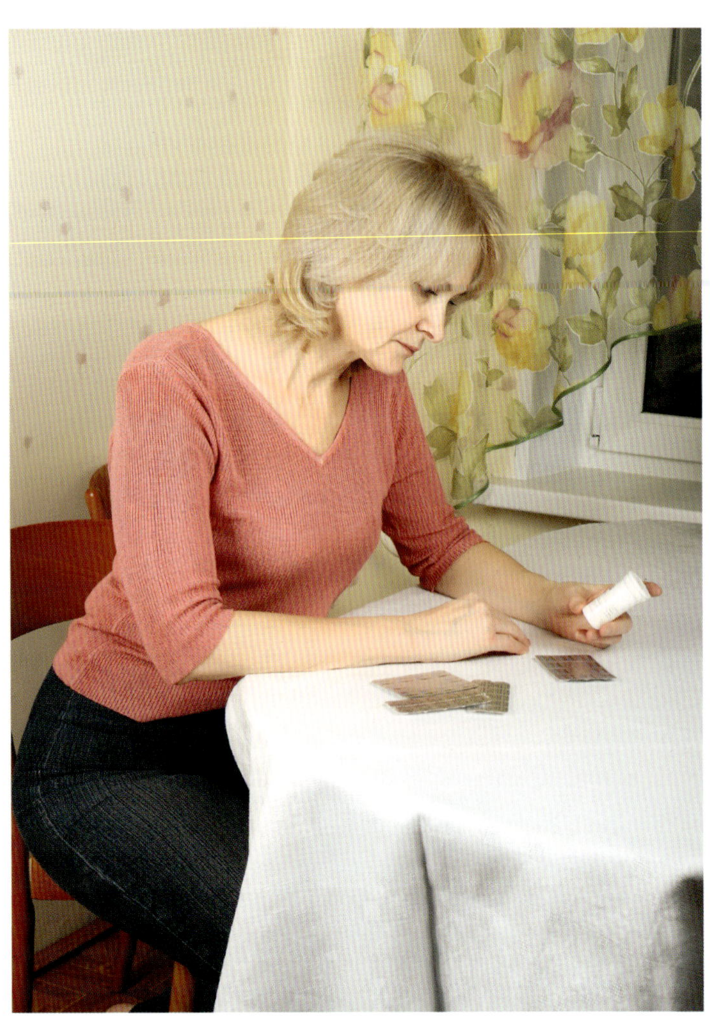

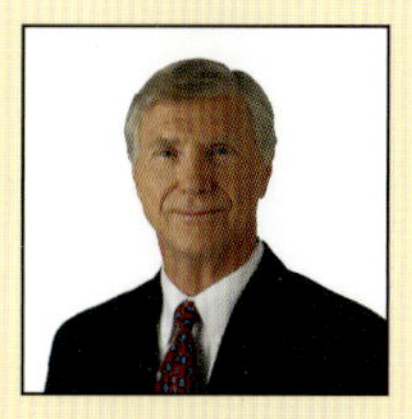

Dr. Smith's Comments

Interestingly, certain parasites may actually be useful in some situations involving human health. Dr. Joel Weinstock and others have shown that an intentional creation of a low-grade infestation with a parasite known as Trichuris suis (pig whipworm) in humans lowers the inflammatory response in patients with inflammatory bowel disease (IBD), namely Crohn's and ulcerative colitis.

Experiments done with humans involved drinking a suspension of Gatorade and 2500 eggs from pig whipworm several times over 4 to 6 months. This did not bother the humans in any way. It turns out the pig whipworm is not a human pathogen, and does not stay in the human more than a few months. However, during this time, it reprograms the gut lining to be more tolerant not only the worms but also to gut microflora. IBD often involves an exaggerated hyperimmune response to normal flora which causes profound inflammation. It appears that the interaction between this parasite and the immune system in the gut lining and gut wall produce immune tolerance. This immune balancing occurs due to an increase in gut levels of what is known as T regulatory lymphocytes.

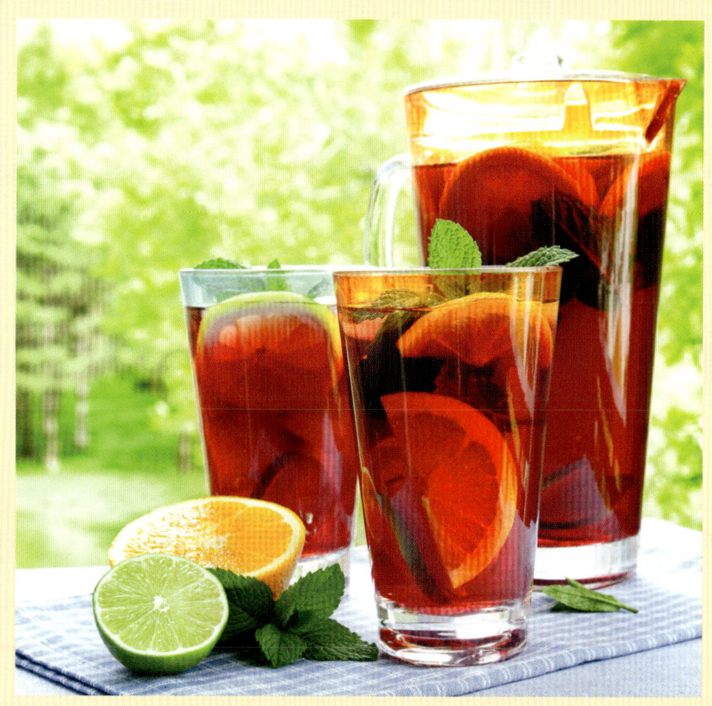

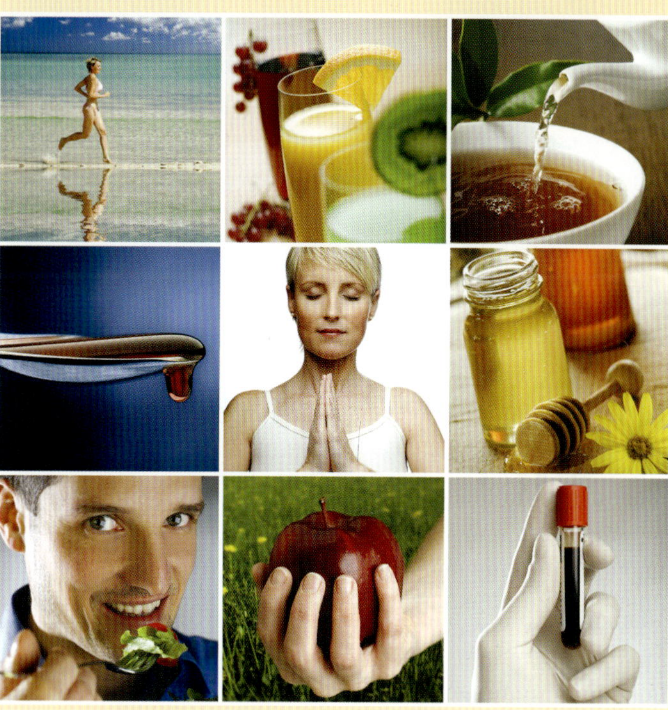

Many of the patients have stayed in remission even after stopping the whipworm therapy.

There have also been some reported benefits using this treatment in autistic children who also often have inflammatory gut issues that closely resemble Crohn's Disease. I believe we will continue to see more beneficial uses of not only probiotics but pro-parasitics as well, both of which can reprogram how our intestines react to the microbes they encounter.

Helminths seemed to stimulate regulatory T cells, an increasingly studied class of immune cells that work to dampen and control immune responses, including both the Th1 and Th2 variety. Science, 2005;305 v9.

However, the immune system may have evolved to operate optimally in the regulated environment of infection, and, in our more hygienic environment, we are prone to overzealous reactions to innocuous targets generating the rapidly increasing levels of allergy and autoimmunity being experienced in the developed world.

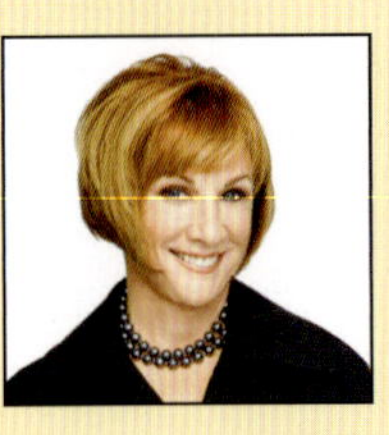

Brenda's Bottom Line

Because it will not always be possible to identify the type of parasite you have or even to know with certainty that you do have parasites (given the limitations of the testing procedures), it is highly advisable to make a parasite cleanse a regular part of your natural detoxification program.

Often the onset of a parasitic infection involves flu-like symptoms which, like the flu, resolve after a week or so. This is because the parasite has gone into a dormant stage. A month or two later, the flu-like symptoms return. In more severe cases, a prescription drug may be necessary in conjunction with the cleansing program. The medication will probably have to be taken more than once due to the cyclic nature of the parasitic life cycle.

A chronic parasitic infection can lead to more serious health conditions. A comprehensive stool analysis (CSA), (see the Appendix) that specifically looks for parasites can be helpful. An interesting note about parasitic infections is that symptoms often increase during the full-moon.

The following program can have fewer side effects than prescription medications, though prescription medication may be needed. It is a good idea to have a health care practitioner's supervision when following the protocol below. This protocol can also be helpful for people who consume sushi frequently, who travel overseas, and for people who swim in lakes and rivers.

Recommended Testing

- Comprehensive stool analysis (CSA) (See the Appendix.) specific for parasites

Diet

- Because Candida and parasites tend to travel together, it is wise to treat for both simultaneously. This will require strict adherence to an anti-Candida diet. (See the Appendix.) You'll want to adhere to this diet for the duration of your parasite cleanse, generally one to three months.
- After that, follow the Fiber 35 Eating Plan for daily maintenance.

Lifestyle

- Do not drink untreated water (filter or purify before drinking).
- Have separate cutting boards for meats/fish and fruits/vegetables.
- Have pets tested/treated for parasites.
- Keep pets away from food preparation areas.
- Don't allow pets to eat out of your dishes.
- Wear gloves when changing cat litter and wash hands afterward. If immune-compromised or pregnant, have someone else do the chore if possible.
- Wash hands before eating.
- Wash hands after gardening.
- Make sure meat is thoroughly cooked (no pink showing).
- Wash hands after handling raw meat.
- Don't eat raw meat or fish.
- Wash vegetables and fruits in a diluted hydrogen peroxide/vinegar bath.
- Freeze fish for 48 hours (beef and pork for 24 hours) before preparing. This will kill any parasite larvae.[18]
- Wash hands after using the toilet.
- Wash hands after changing a baby's diaper.
- Keep your immune system in good shape.
- Do a parasitic cleanse once or twice yearly.

Complementary Mind/Body Therapies

- Stress can be a major component of this disease, so find ways to reduce it with therapies such as meditation, yoga, deep breathing, massage, biofeedback, or music therapy.
- Colon hydrotherapy is excellent for removing waste from the colon and can be helpful during a parasite program.

Recommended Nutraceuticals	Dosage	Benefit	Comments
Critical Phase	Daily maintenance recommendations should also be taken during this phase unless otherwise indicated.		
Total Body Cleanse	See Appendix	Encourages elimination and detoxification.	Herbal formula should support the seven channels of elimination.
Parasite Cleanse	See Appendix	Helps to eliminate parasites and encourage a healthy intestinal microbial balance.	This should follow the above Total Body Cleanse.
Parasitic Digestive Enzyme	Take on empty stomach several times daily	Taken without food can be beneficial in maintaining a healthy intestinal tract.	Make sure formula also contains HCl and L-glutamine.
Bentonite clay / Apple pectin / Charcoal Formula	Use as directed	Absorbs toxins from possible "die off" reaction and improves regularity.	Take with plenty of water.
Helpful			
High Potency Multi-vitamin/mineral	Follow directions on label	Provides needed nutrients that can be deficient in those with parasites.	Powder or liquid formulation would be helpful as it is easier assimilated and absorbed.
Saccharomyces boulardii	10 billion cultures, twice daily	Helps protect against traveler's diarrhea, sometimes innduced by parasites.	Look for formula with other immune enhancing ingredients.
Daily Maintenance			
L-Glutamine Powder with Gamma Oryzanol	5,000-10,000 mg daily in divided doses	Helps repair the intestinal lining reducing permeability.	Best taken in powder form.
Digestive Enzymes	Take with meals	Helps digest and absorb nutrients from food.	If low stomach acid is found find a formula that contains hydrochloric acid.
Probiotics	50 to 200 billion culture count daily	Helps reduce intestinal permeability and inflammation and maintain balance of intestinal microbes.	Look for high amount of bifidobacteria, the main beneficial bacteria in the colon.
Omega-3 Fatty Acids	At least 2 grams daily of EPA/DHA combination	Helps restore moisture to the intestinal tract and reduces inflammation.	Look for a concentrated, enteric coated fish oil.
Fiber	4-5 grams twice daily	Helps produce healthy bacteria levels and good elimination.	Use in conjunction with high fiber diet to reach 35 g daily.
Vitamin D_3	At least 1,000 to 2,000 iu daily	Helps heal leaky gut, decrease inflammation, increase overall health.	Research is showing many health complications as a result of low vitamin D levels.

See further explanation of supplements in the Appendix

Cirrhosis

Liver, Pancreas and Gallbladder

What Is It?

Cirrhosis is a degenerative inflammatory disease in which fatty deposits and dense connective tissue build up in the liver causing hardening, drying and scarring of the organ, as well as a reduction of blood supply to it. Cirrhosis is considered to be a permanent and irreversible condition.

What Causes It?

For years, alcohol abuse was the most common cause of cirrhosis in the United States. Recently though, hepatitis C (a viral disease) surpassed alcoholism as the major cause of this end-stage liver disease. Hepatitis B and D (also viral) can also lead to cirrhosis. Cirrhosis may result from other chronic diseases such as congestive heart failure, advanced syphilis, parasitic flatworm infections,[1] cystic fibrosis and the genetic disorders hemochromatosis (excessive iron accumulation) and Wilson's disease (excessive accumulation of copper in the liver).

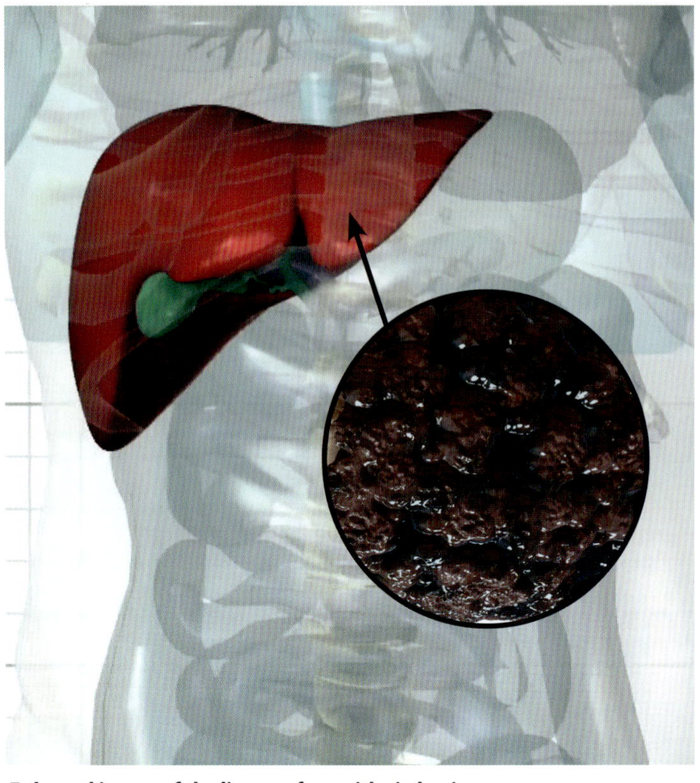

Enlarged image of the liver surface with cirrhosis

Other inherited diseases that can lead to cirrhosis are alpha-1 antitrypsin deficiency (absence of a serum proteinase inhibitor), galactosemia (galactose metabolism disorder due to an enzyme deficiency) and glycogen storage disease.[2] Toxic overload due to drug abuse (street, over-the-counter or prescription) and environmental chemicals (particularly solvents such as formaldehyde, toluene and trichloroethylene)[3] and ongoing exposure to heavy metals, particularly lead and nickel, can pave the way for cirrhosis.[4] Finally, cirrhosis may be the net result of physical injury to the liver, bile duct obstruction, chronic inflammation or malnutrition.

Did You Know

Non-alcoholic fatty liver disease (NAFLD) is a condition involving the accumulation of fat in the liver as a result of pro-inflammatory diet, stress and other factors which lead to insulin resistance. This condition can be completely asymptomatic. People with NAFLD generally are well on their way to metabolic syndrome which includes: insulin resistance, high blood pressure and dyslipidemia (high triglycerides, high total cholesterol, high LDL cholesterol and low HDL cholesterol). Elevated insulin (from insulin resistance) causes storage of fat in and around the liver cells. Metabolic syndrome occurs due to poor diet, lack of exercise, stress, and probably toxicity from heavy metals, bacterial dysbiosis, and fat soluble toxins (like BPA and phthalates).

If NAFLD worsens, it progresses to non-alcoholic steatohepatitis (NASH) which involves inflammation of the fatty liver. There are approximately 30 million people with NAFLD in the U.S. More than 14 million of these have progressed to NASH. These conditions are becoming a significant health concern in the U.S. The complications of NASH include cirrhosis leading to portal hypertension and liver failure which may result in liver transplant or death. NAFLD goes hand in hand with the increase in abdominal obesity; all of which are at epidemic proportions. The good news, however, is that it is reversible with diet, exercise and proper dietary supplementation. (See the NAFLD section for more information on this condition.)

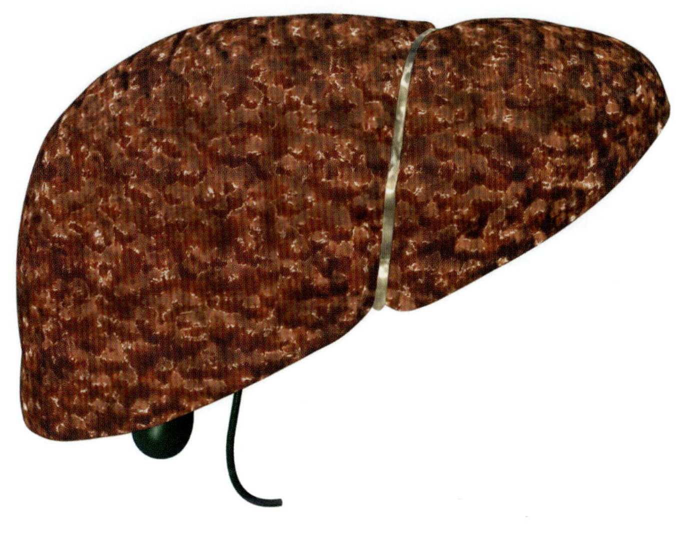

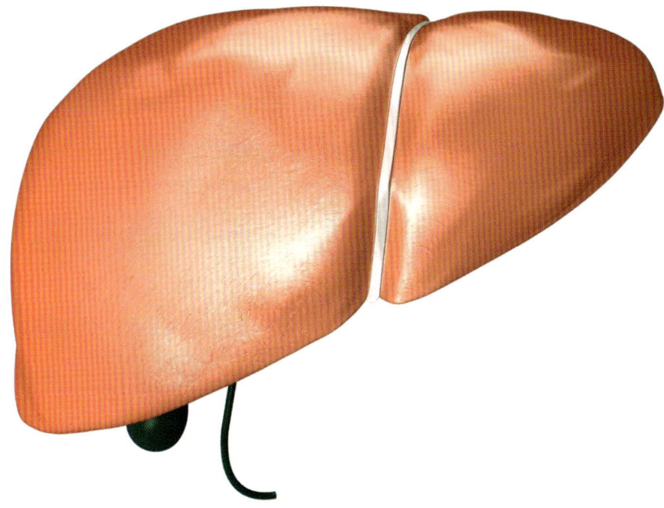

A healthy liver below, cirrhotic liver above

Drugs that can be particularly damaging to the liver include anti-convulsants, antihypertensive methyldopa, chlorpromazine, drugs used to treat tuberculosis and large amounts of acetaminophen (not toxic if taken as prescribed). These drugs are particularly dangerous if combined with alcohol.[5] Synthetic vitamins A and niacin can also damage the liver if taken in excessive amounts over a prolonged period of time.

A precursor to cirrhosis, steatosis (fatty liver), characterized by a buildup of fat in the liver cells without accompanying symptoms, also occurs in association with toxic exposure and alcohol abuse. Diabetes and obesity may additionally contribute to fatty liver that, in turn, leads to inflammation, cell death and fibrosis (formation of fibrous tissue).

An interesting gut-liver connection has been found involving bacterial overgrowth in the small intestine. One study found that almost half of the patients suffering from cirrhosis also had an overgrowth of bacteria in the small intestine.[6] In patients with more severe cases of cirrhosis, the bacteria overgrowth was also more severe.

Cirrhosis and liver disease are the seventh leading causes of death in the United States.[7] Also at high risk for developing cirrhosis would be people whose exposure to heavy metals and environmental chemicals is high and constant. Those who have an occupational or other chronic exposure to solvents may be at particular risk for developing cirrhosis, especially if they are also heavy drinkers, because alcohol is also a solvent.

While cirrhosis commonly affects adults, often becoming a life-threatening problem in the fifth or sixth decades of life, in rare cases, infants may develop it as a result of biliary atresia, a condition in which the bile ducts are absent or injured.[8] Children can also be affected as a result of cystic fibrosis or other inherited disorders.

What Are the Signs and Symptoms?

As serious as cirrhosis is, the early symptoms may be vague and mild. In fact, a full one-third of people with the disease have no clinical symptoms.[9] The diagnosis of cirrhosis is often made during the course of testing for other conditions or during surgery. Sometimes it's not discovered until an autopsy is done. As the disease

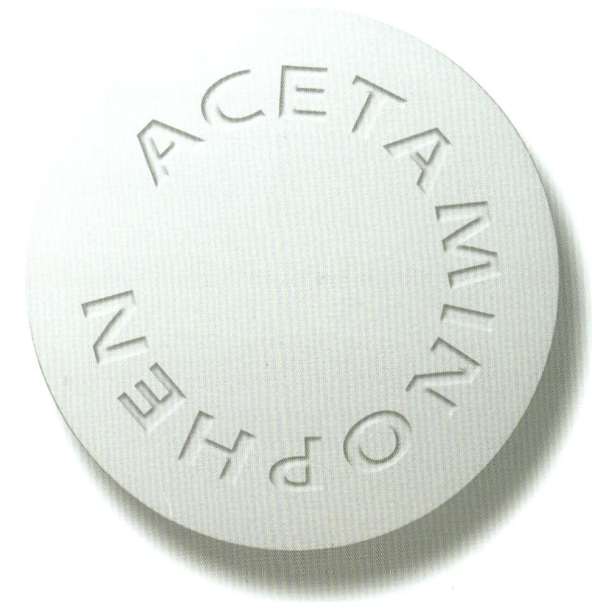

progresses, symptoms become more severe. The list below, so lengthy due to the 500 plus functions of the liver, starts off with early signs and symptoms progressing to those found in late stages of cirrhosis:

- Fatigue
- Loss of appetite
- Nausea or vomiting
- Abdominal swelling
- Upset stomach
- Weakness
- Exhaustion
- Constipation or diarrhea
- Edema (build up of fluid in the legs resulting from the extra load placed on kidneys)
- Light-colored stools
- Indigestion
- Flatulence
- Extreme skin dryness
- Decreased libido

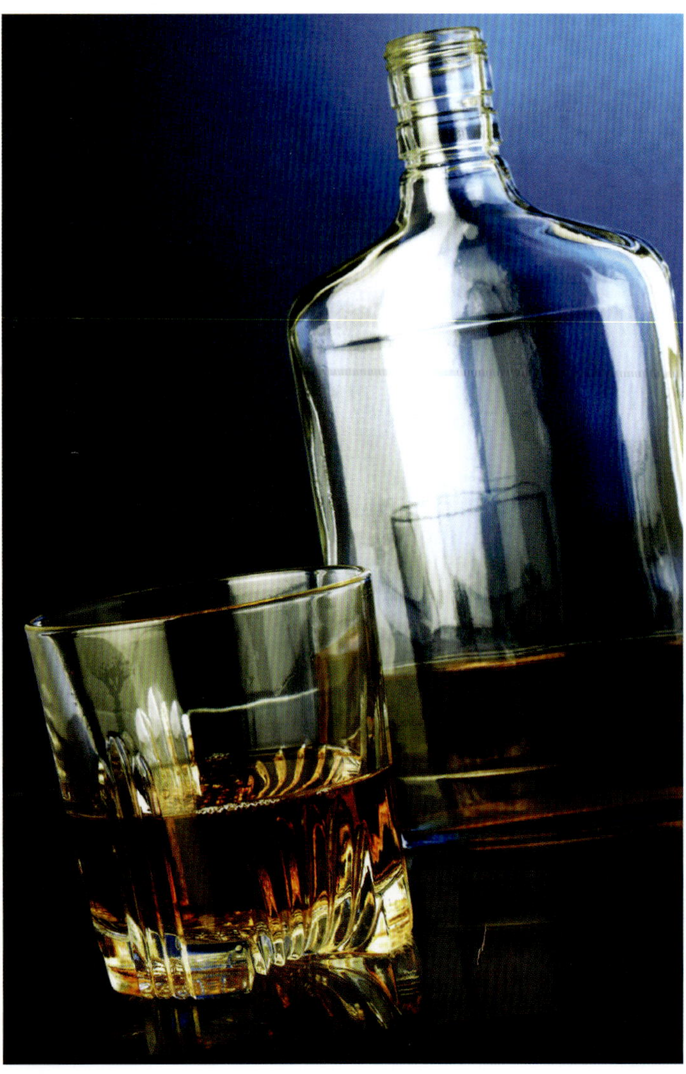

"Serious disorders associated with cirrhosis include insulin resistance, diabetes mellitus, kidney dysfunction, congestive heart failure, osteomalacia and osteoporosis."

- Ascites (fluid accumulation in the peritoneal cavity)
- Red palms
- Enlarged liver
- Generalized itching (due to bile pigments that are deposited under the skin)
- Bruising (due to bleeding under the skin)
- Abnormal bleeding (due to vitamin K deficiency)
- Decreased albumin (blood protein) levels
- Spider angiomas (raised red dots from which small blood vessels radiate)
- Lowered platelet count
- Varicosities (in stomach, rectum, and esophagus)
- Jaundice (yellowed skin resulting from elevation of bilirubin—the yellow pigment the liver produces when it recycles worn-out blood cells)
- Bright yellow or brown urine
- Anemia
- Gallstones (due to alterations in the bile from the primary condition causing cirrhosis)
- Varices (new blood vessels) in stomach and esophagus (formed when blood from intestines tries to find a way around the blocked liver
- Fever
- Testicular atrophy
- Gynecomastia (enlargement of the male breast)
- Loss of chest and armpit hair
- Psychotic mental changes (such as extreme paranoia) resulting from build up of toxins in the blood that reach the brain without being detoxified by the damaged liver
- Facial veins
- Decreased absorption of glucose and vitamins
- Altered hormone production
- Portal hypertension (high blood pressure in the veins connecting the liver with the intestine, stomach and esophagus)

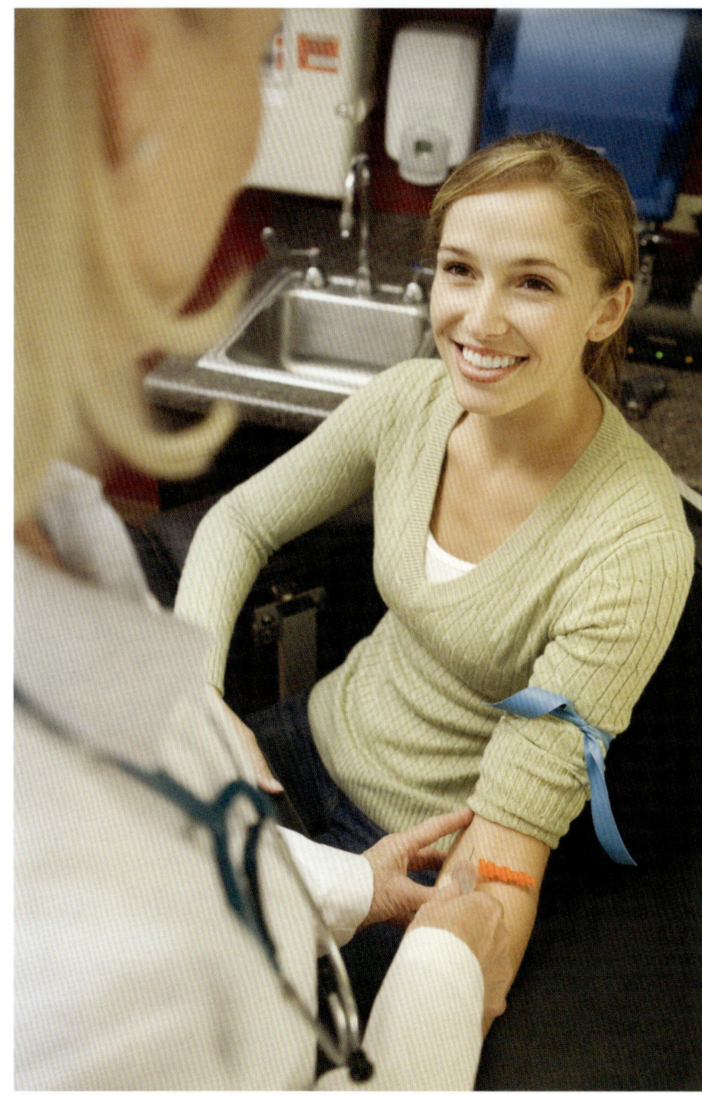

If left untreated, cirrhosis can lead to such severe complications as gastrointestinal hemorrhage, ammonia toxicity, kidney failure, liver failure, hepatic coma and, ultimately, death.

Serious disorders associated with cirrhosis include insulin resistance, diabetes mellitus, kidney dysfunction, congestive heart failure, osteomalacia and osteoporosis. Those with cirrhosis have a higher incidence of liver and other cancers than those in the general population, and are at risk for developing malnutrition, kidney disorders, stomach ulcers, diabetes mellitus and severe drug reactions.

Although cirrhosis is initially a silent disease (no symptoms), eventually symptoms do develop as a result of the loss of functioning liver cells and distortion of the liver by scarring. This scar tissue blocks the flow of blood through the liver. The loss of normal liver tissue slows the processing of nutrients, hormones, drugs and toxins, as well as the production of proteins and other substances by the liver.[10]

As liver cells die, production of the blood protein albumin decreases leading to edema (water retention in cells or tissues) and ascites (fluid accumulation in the lining of the abdominal cavity), as well as a tendency to bruise and bleed easily (proteins are needed for blood clotting). Cirrhosis can also lead to the creation of varices. Varices are dilated veins that form in the stomach and esophagus when blood from the intestines tries to find a way around the blocked liver. These varices can burst creating a life-threatening situation.

How Is It Diagnosed?

The diagnosis of cirrhosis will entail the use of several diagnostic tests in addition to a complete physical examination and thorough medical history. Diagnostic work-ups may include such blood tests as a complete blood count, liver enzymes, blood proteins, electrolytes and hepatitis B screening. Radiologic procedures could include computerized axial tomography (CT scan), an ultrasound of the liver, gallbladder and bile ducts, and an isotope vein injection study known as a liver/spleen scan. A more invasive study would be vascular imaging of the liver. A laproscopic exam, which involves inserting devices through tiny incisions in the abdomen, may also be done to obtain videos and biopsies of the liver.

What Is the Standard Medical Treatment?

There is no cure for cirrhosis. Medical treatment is aimed at delaying or stopping progression of the disease, minimizing damage to liver cells and reducing complications. Where the cause of the cirrhosis is a

Did You Know

More than 27,000 Americans die from cirrhosis annually making it the country's third leading cause of death for people between the ages of 25 and 59, and the seventh leading cause of death overall.

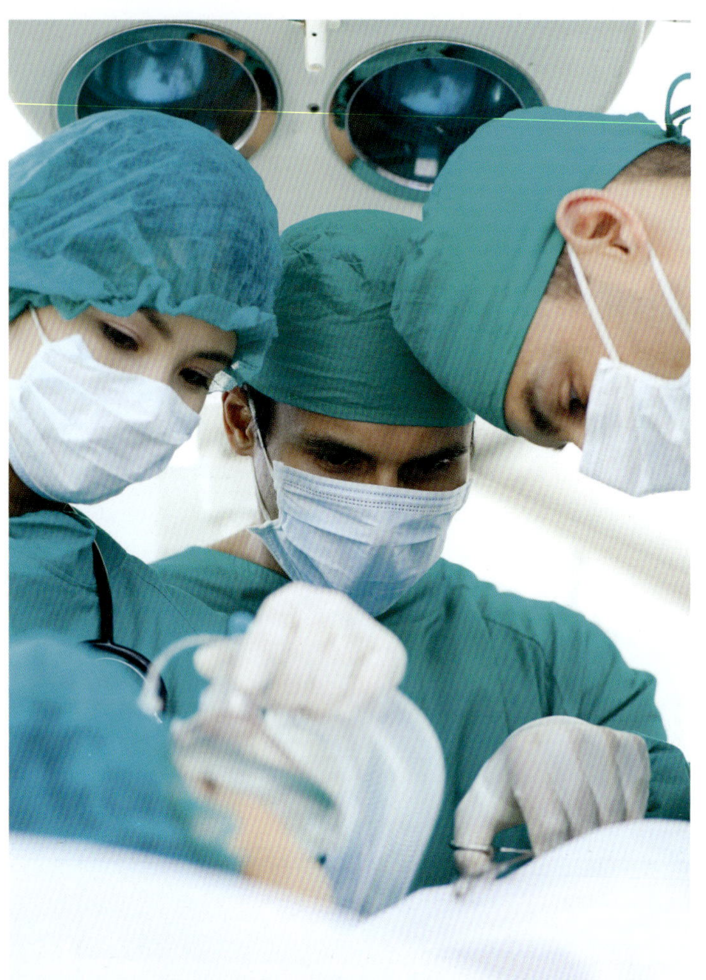

Elevated blood ammonia can be a serious complication resulting in coma. Lactulose, a synthetic sugar that is not absorbed by the body, has been used in some cirrhosis cases to assist in removal of ammonia from the blood.[11] Neomycin and other antibiotics have been used to decrease intestinal bacteria that produce ammonia.[12] Finally, a restriction of dietary protein may be used to decrease ammonia levels. Such a restriction will result in less toxin formation in the digestive tract. Where infections, such as spontaneous bacterial peritonitis, develop, antibiotics are used. Immunosuppressive drugs, such as cyclosporine and methotrexate, have been used with cirrhosis patients in an effort to facilitate survival, but at a cost, as these drugs have serious side effects.

"Where the cause of cirrhosis is a known toxin, removal of that toxin can usually stop progression of the disease."

known toxin, such as alcohol, removal of that toxin can usually stop progression of the disease, and, in time, some degree of liver function may be restored.

Where hepatitis is the underlying cause of the cirrhosis, the patient may be treated with steroids or antiviral drugs to reduce injury to liver cells. Medications are also typically used to treat such symptoms as itching and water retention (edema and ascites) resulting from portal hypertension. To address the later problem, a salt-restricted diet may be imposed. If unsuccessful, diuretic drugs may be employed. As a last resort, a shunt (using the patient's own veins, cadaver veins, or prosthetic grafts) may be surgically implanted to divert blood flow from the portal vein to another blood vessel in an effort to take some of the pressure off the portal venous system and prevent variceal bleeding.

Other treatment modalities—beta-blocking blood pressure medications and sclerotherapy (injection of a scarring chemical into the vein) or even endoscopic stapling of varices may also be used.

A generic drug called colchicine, used to treat gout, has also been used to improve liver function and survival in cirrhosis patients since it inhibits collagen (a protein in the body that makes up scar tissue).[13] This drug, however, carries with it serious gastrointestinal side effects. Ursodiol, a gallstone-dissolving drug with fewer side effects, has been used to improve symptoms of cirrhosis, is

It is imperative that drugs metabolized in the liver (most are) be used with extreme caution in the cirrhosis patient since detoxification of these drugs is extremely problematic. When the liver stops working, the only treatment option is liver transplant. The encouraging news here is that 80 percent of patients receiving liver transplants are still alive five years after the transplant.[14]

Because no wonder drugs have been developed to treat cirrhosis, and because all drugs can have devastating side effects, all viable natural alternatives should be considered in treatment of the cirrhosis patient, with an emphasis on nutritional supplementation.

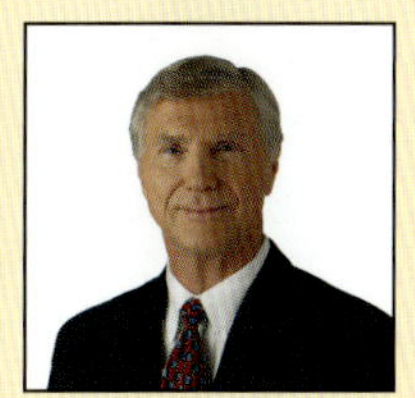

Dr. Smith's Comments

Cirrhosis is a process of ongoing deposition of collagen in the liver with resultant fibrosis or hardening of the liver. The serious clinical problems of cirrhosis are:

Seriously compromised liver function leading to liver failure and the need for liver transplant.

Creation of portal hypertension, which occurs when the fibrous scarring of the liver obstructs the flow of blood to and from the liver. When this happens, the inflowing blood to the liver from the abdominal organs must go through alternative venous routes around the liver in order to get back to the heart. These alternate veins can become dilated and actually rupture. This can be a serious cause of upper gastrointestinal bleeding. These veins are called varices, and they are usually located in the esophagus, stomach and duodenum. To stop the bleeding often requires endoscopy, or, at times, surgery. Surgery either involves ligating (tying off) the bleeding veins, or doing some type of shunt, which is a venous detour around the liver blockage. With advanced cirrhosis, it is unlikely that nutrition can reverse the situation, but it might slow it down.

Ascites due to cirrhosis result from the accumulation of a clear fluid in the abdomen that can cause massive abdominal swelling. Such swelling pushes on the diaphragm, and can compromise respiration and even affect blood flow through the kidneys. It is thought to be due to a portion of plasma exuding out of the veins as a result of the backpressure from the cirrhotic liver. It can be controlled sometimes with diuretics, but, when severe, it is necessary to drain it with a needle or to surgically shunt it into a neck vein to return blood flow to the heart.

It is thought that cirrhosis is a chronic inflammatory process. This inflammation can be due to ongoing viral infection, toxic exposure (often alcohol) and absorption of toxins from the gut, which can also lead to autoimmune liver disease. Whatever the cause, the inflammation creates an oxidative stress environment (excess free radical exposure). The oxidative process is thought to be one of the factors that promotes the deposition of collagen, which is one of the early steps leading to cirrhosis of the liver. Supporting evidence comes from Gastroenterology [1997; 113: 1069-73]. This article showed in a small group of hepatitis C patients that vitamin E (d-alpha tocopherol), 1200 I.U. daily, prevented stellate cell activation and hepatic collagen production, both of which are important steps in the development of hepatic fibrosis or cirrhosis. A wide variety of supplements may be helpful, including alpha lipoic acid, glutathione, silymarin, N-acetyl-cysteine, glycine, glutamine, selenium, B vitamins and vitamin C.

"The inflammation of cirrhosis can be due to ongoing viral infection, toxic exposure (often alcohol) and absorption of toxins from the gut."

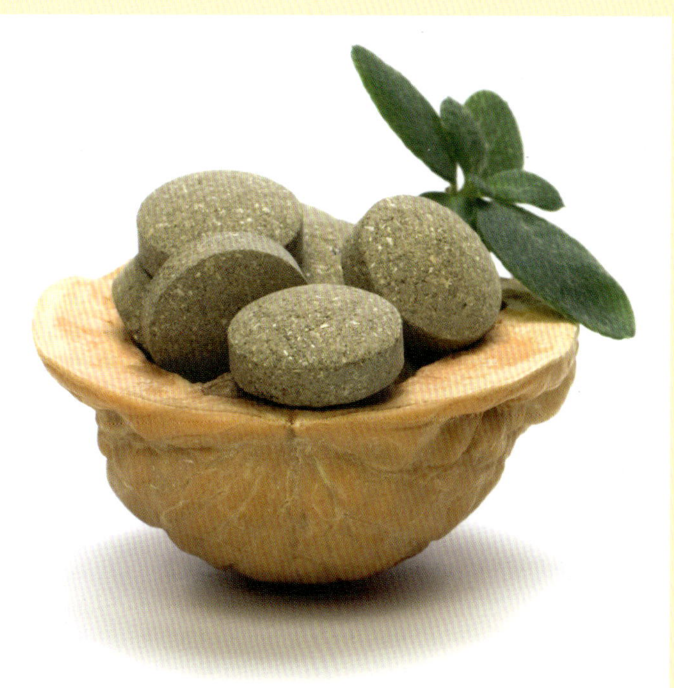

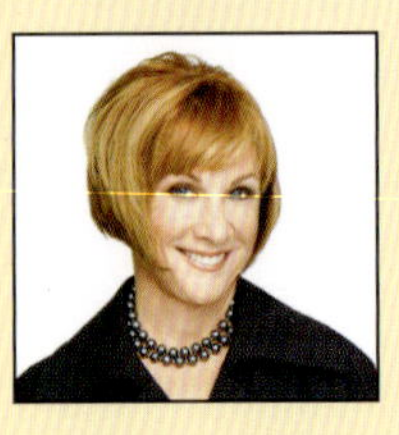

Brenda's Bottom Line

Cirrhosis is a progressive liver condition that can be fatal. But the liver regenerates at a rapid rate, so healing is possible with the proper changes. My friend's mother had severe cirrhosis, and was told by doctors that she would die within two weeks. Her cirrhosis was largely due to alcohol use, so she quit drinking immediately, and she is still alive today.

Removing any toxin exposure is an important part of healing the liver. Healthy digestive function plays a big role in supporting liver function as well, because any toxins in the gut are transported directly to the liver. If gut imbalance exists, it can overburden the liver leading to the inflammation and scarring of cirrhosis.

Follow the protocol below and on the next page to help support healthy gut and liver function. For the cleansing recommendations, if you are experiencing diarrhea, skip the Total Body Cleanse and begin the Candida Cleanse instead.

Diet

- Follow the Fiber 35 Eating Plan found in the Appendix of this book. Include plenty of raw fruits and vegetables.
- You may need to watch protein (especially from animal sources) if ammonia levels are high.
- If you do eat animal protein, limit it to small quantities of poultry and fish.
- Watch fats, especially fried foods, saturated and trans fats. If the liver is too damaged, it may not be able to handle fat-soluble vitamins like A, D, E and K, except in small amounts.
- Keep refined carbohydrates (sugar, white bread, white pasta, white rice, etc.) out of your diet. Carbohydrate consumption should be in the form of vegetables and whole grains.
- Do not overeat. Eat small meals more frequently.
- Do not consume alcohol (most important!).

Lifestyle

- Medications can be stressful for the liver. Take with caution.
- Do not become constipated. Use the LifeStep (see the Appendix) for proper elimination posture.
- Do not smoke, and avoid second-hand smoke.
- Clean up your environment, as all chemicals and toxins can affect liver function.

Complementary Mind/Body Therapies

- Stress can be a major component of this disease, so find ways to reduce it with therapies such as meditation, yoga, deep breathing, massage, biofeedback, or music therapy.
- Colon hydrotherapy is beneficial to remove toxins.

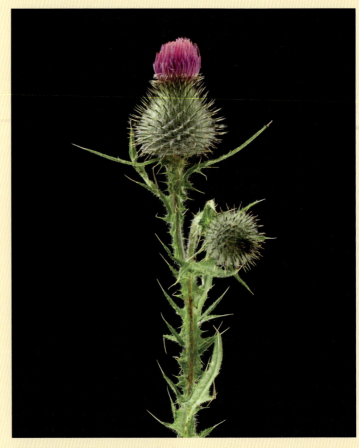

Milk thistle is liver-supporting herb

Recommended Nutraceuticals	Dosage	Benefit	Comments
Critical Phase	Daily maintenance recommendations should also be taken during this phase unless otherwise indicated.		
Total Body Cleanse	See Appendix	Encourages elimination and detoxification.	Herbal formula should support the seven channels of elimination.
Liver Detox	This should follow the Total Body Cleanse. See Appendix	Encourages detoxification involving the liver.	Should contain milk thistle seed extract containing silymarin, phosphatidylcholine, selenium and herbs.
Helpful			
SAMe	180 mg daily	Helps improve liver function.	Do not use if you have bipolar disorder or are taking antidepressants.
L-Glutamine Powder with Gamma Oryzanol	5 grams twice daily	Helps maintain the health and integrity of the intestinal lining.	Added gamma oryzanol may help relieve pain associated with gastrointestinal complaints.
High Potency Multi-vitamin/mineral	Follow directions on label	Provides needed nutrients that can be deficient in those with cirrhosis.	Powder or liquid formulation would be helpful as it is easier assimilated and absorbed.
Antioxidant Supplement	Use as directed	Protects tissue from damage.	You can purchase a high-potency antioxidant formulation from most health food stores.
Daily Maintenance			
Critical Liver Support Formula	Use as directed	Enhances liver detoxification.	Should include milk thistle seed extract containing silymarin, N-acetyl-cysteine, alpha lipoic acid L-glutathione.
Fiber	4-5 grams twice daily	Helps produce healthy bacteria levels and good elimination.	Use in conjunction with high-fiber diet to reach 35g daily.
Digestive Enzymes	Take with meals	Helps digest and absorb nutrients from food to reduce liver stress.	If low stomach acid is found find a formula that contains hydrochloric acid.
Omega-3 Fatty Acids	At least 2 grams daily of EPA/DHA combination	Reduces inflammation.	Look for a concentrated, enteric coated fish oil.
Probiotics	30 - 80 billion culture count twice daily	Restores bacterial balance and pH of colon and promotes regularity.	Look for high amount of bifidobacteria, the main beneficial bacteria in colon.

See further explanation of supplements in the Appendix

GALLSTONES

What Is It?

Gallstones are the most common digestive problem associated with the gallbladder. Gallstones can be solid, semi-solid or soft masses that are composed of one or more of the following: cholesterol, bile pigment (bilirubin), bile salts, inorganic minerals (usually calcium) and the phospholipid lecithin. Gallstones can range in size from as small as a grain of sand to as large as a golf ball. Very often they are the size of small pebbles. A person can have a single stone, dozens, or even hundreds of stones.

When bile production, circulation, or quality is compromised, gallstones can occur. The liver produces bile (a yellowish-brown or green fluid), excretes toxins into it and then sends it to the gallbladder. It is the job of the gallbladder to hold that bile in storage until food enters the small intestine. At that time, the gallbladder should contract, sending bile through the cystic and bile ducts into the duodenum (upper portion of the small intestine). To break down and emulsify fat from food. Bile also helps increase peristalsis and retard putrefaction.

There are two major types of gallstones: cholesterol stones and pigment stones. Cholesterol gallstones make up 80 percent of gallstone cases in the U.S., while pigment gallstones make up the remaining 20 percent of cases.[1] Cholesterol stones contain more than 70 percent cholesterol; some are pure cholesterol.[2] Pigment stones are made up of calcium and bilirubin with a mucous protein core.[3]

What Causes It?

A number of factors appear to contribute to gallstone formation. Primary among them are:

- Inherited body chemistry
- Body weight
- Gallbladder motility (movement)
- Diet
- Pregnancy
- Birth control use

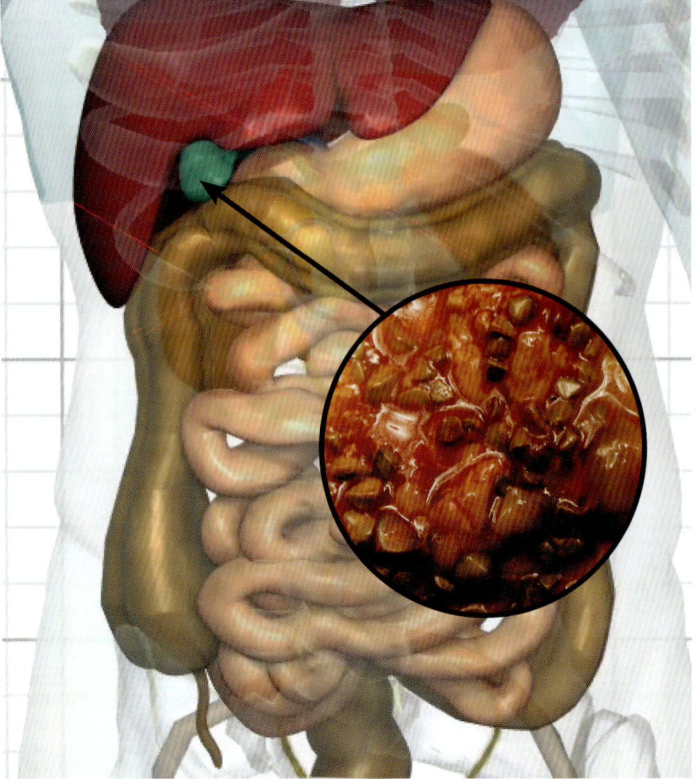

Endocopic image of gallstones in the gallbladder

- Hormone replacement
- Toxin exposure
- Parasitic infection
- Constipation
- Food allergy
- Lack of exercise
- Low stomach acid

During the normal course of digestion, about 98 percent of the bile acids that are secreted from the liver and released by the gallbladder are reabsorbed in the ileum (lower portion of the small intestine). When the ileum is impaired in its ability to reabsorb these bile acids, the bile acid pool is reduced, as is the rate of bile secretion. The net result is an increased risk of developing gallstones.

When the liver produces too much cholesterol or an insufficient quantity of bile salts, then cholesterol crystals can precipitate out of solution and form cholesterol stones.[4] Excess cholesterol in the bile can result from obesity or pregnancy, while a deficiency of bile salts can result from the use of bile salt binding drugs used to treat high cholesterol. A bile-salt deficiency is also found in Crohn's disease, a serious gastrointestinal disorder usually affecting the ileum.

The risk of developing gallstones during pregnancy is elevated not just because of the added body weight, but also due to increased estrogen levels. Women on birth control pills or hormone replacement therapy are therefore also at greater risk of developing gallstones than women not on these therapies. Increased estrogen levels may increase cholesterol levels in the bile and decrease gallbladder movement.[5] Additionally, exposure to some environmental chemicals, such as pesticides and plastics, affects the body in the same way as excessive estrogen,[6] and so could conceivably play a role in gallstone formation.

Cholesterol stone formation is accelerated if gallbladder contractions are sluggish, as they tend to be when there is too much cholesterol in the bile. This can happen after a person has undergone prolonged fasting or followed a very low-calorie diet. Some cholesterol-lowering drugs can also slow gallbladder contractions causing incomplete emptying of bile.[7] Delayed emptying of the gallbladder gives cholesterol more opportunity to crystallize into stones.

The hormone largely responsible for the contraction of the gallbladder is cholecystokinin, or CCK. CCK also triggers the pancreas to release enzymes. When fatty food enters the duodenum, CCK is released and travels to the gallbladder causing it to contract. Secretin, to a lesser extent, also triggers this contraction.

What's more, it has been shown that in patients using proton pump inhibitors, 26 percent had impaired biliary function.[8] This could be due to a decreased amount of secretin, which is triggered by the presence of stomach acid.

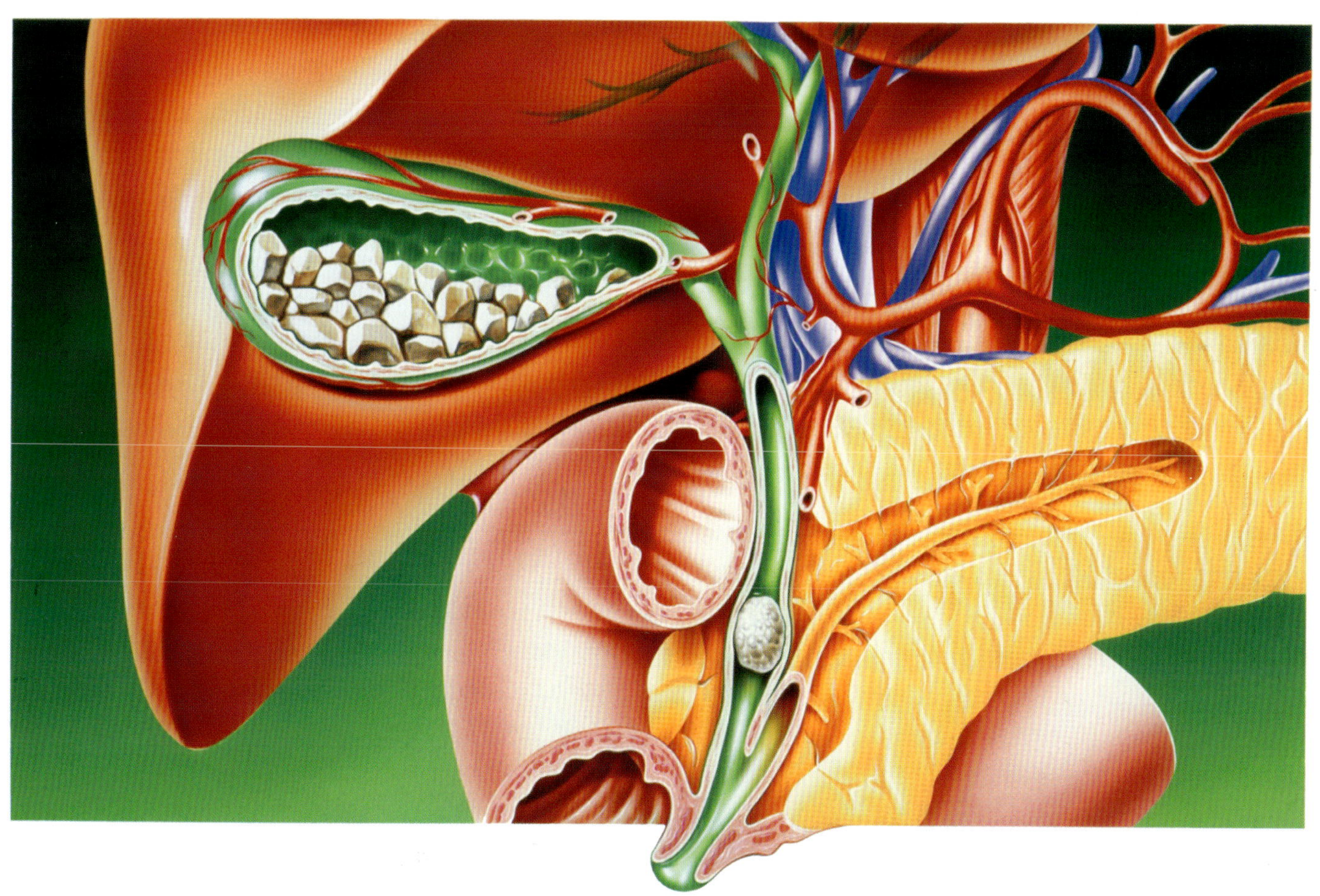

Illustration of gallstones in the gallbladder (green) and common bile duct. Gallstones are hard deposits of salts or cholesterol that form in the gallbladder when the chemical composition of bile is upset. They are most common in women, the elderly and the obese, and usually cause no symptoms unless one becomes stuck in the bile duct, which can lead to acute pain, jaundice, infection, and the formation of a liver abscess. If necessary the gallbladder may be surgically removed.

The bilirubin found in pigment stones is created as part of the body's normal functioning, resulting from the following steps:

- The spleen removes worn out red blood cells from the bloodstream.
- These red blood cells release hemoglobin, a red pigment.
- Hemoglobin is converted to the yellow pigmented bilirubin.
- Bilirubin is picked up by the liver and released into the bile.

Pigment stones can form when the body destroys too many red blood cells, a condition called hemolysis, present in hereditary blood disorders such as sickle cell anemia. Pigment stones can also result from alcoholic cirrhosis of the liver. The risk of developing pigment stones is also increased in the patient who has had intestinal surgery.

Diet is less of an influence in the development of pigment stones than in cholesterol stones. It is believed that low-fiber, high-cholesterol diets (those high in animal fats) and diets high in starchy foods contribute to the formation of cholesterol stones.[9] Over-consumption of fatty and fried foods and refined sugar, as well as inadequate intake of foods containing the vitamins E, B and C, are also factors thought to contribute to gallstone formation.[10]

There appears to be a genetic component to gallstones, for they tend to run in families and are more common in some races than others. Parasitic infection can also play a role, for such infection can lead to a build up of calcium-based stones. Constipation is another condition that can set the stage for development of gallstones. Food allergies also appear to play a role, for allergenic foods may cause swelling of the bile ducts resulting in impaired bile flow from the gallbladder.[11] Lack of exercise can also contribute to stone formation. In fact, physical activity can reduce the risk of stone formation by 20 to 40 percent.[12] Dehydration is another contributing factor. Adequate water intake is necessary to dilute toxins in the body.

The amount of stomach acid produced by the body seems to also play a role in gallstone formation, for stomach acid and fat stimulate the hormones that make the gallbladder contract. A deficiency in hydrochloric acid may impair gallbladder contraction and result in back up of bile.[13]

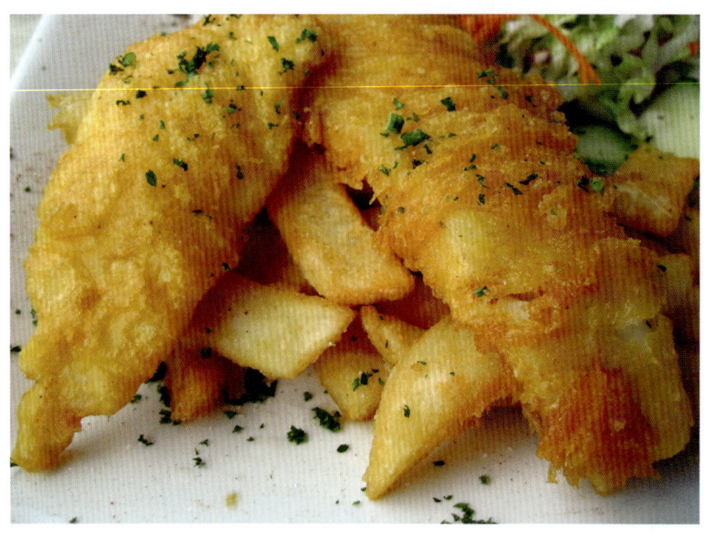

Once gallstones have formed, they can block the flow of bile from the liver and gallbladder. At times, they can obstruct the pancreas and intestine, as well, creating medical emergencies.

Those most prone to biliary problems (problems related to bile and associated structures through which it flows, including gallstones) are people who can be described by the five F's: fair, fat, female, fertile, and 40. Women are decidedly more prone to gallbladder formation (two to four times more likely to be affected than men),[14] especially when pregnant, taking birth control pills or on hormone replacement therapy.

While gallstones can affect people of any age, the risk for developing them increases with age, especially as middle age approaches. It is believed that the majority of adults over 60 have gallstones,[15] though most will be unaware of it due to lack of symptoms. While more than 20 million Americans have gallstones, about 80 percent are asymptomatic (without symptoms).[16]

While increased levels of cholesterol in the bile can cause formation of cholesterol gallstones, it is important to know that the level of cholesterol in the bile does not correlate with the total cholesterol in the blood. There does, however, appear to be an association between increased serum triglyceride levels and less-soluble bile.[17]

What Are the Signs and Symptoms?

Most people who have gallstones never have symptoms.[18] Early symptoms are characterized by incomplete fat digestion. When fat is not completely digested, bacteria in the colon act upon undigested portions of it, resulting in:

- Gas
- Fatty stools that float
- Foul-smelling stools
- Abdominal distention and bloating
- Chronic belching

Once the stone begins to form, its radius increases at an average rate of 2.6 mm per year, eventually reaching a size of a few millimeters to more than a centimeter. Symptoms occur an average of eight years after formation of the stone begins.[19] The presence of stones creates the possibility that inflammation of the gallbladder (cholecystitis) may develop as a result of stones lodging in the cystic duct (connecting the gallbladder to the common bile duct which empties into the duodenum causing a backflow of bile). Serious symptoms may occur when stones become large enough to obstruct bile ducts. These may include:

- Pain in the upper right abdomen (may radiate to the right shoulder, to the back or to the area under the sternum and mimic a heart attack), especially after a fried or fatty meal

Did You Know

- Gallstones are very common. Over one million people are diagnosed each year. They occur in one out of five women by age 60, and they are half as common in men.
- Gallstones occur more commonly in older people and in people who are overweight or who lose weight suddenly.
- They also occur more frequently in women who have been exposed to higher amounts of the hormone estrogen over their lifetime by having multiple pregnancies, by taking birth-control pills or by taking hormone replacement after menopause.
- More than 80 percent of people with gallstones have no symptoms, and do not require treatment.
- Even when gallstone attacks subside on their own, 50 percent of the time the symptoms will return within a year.

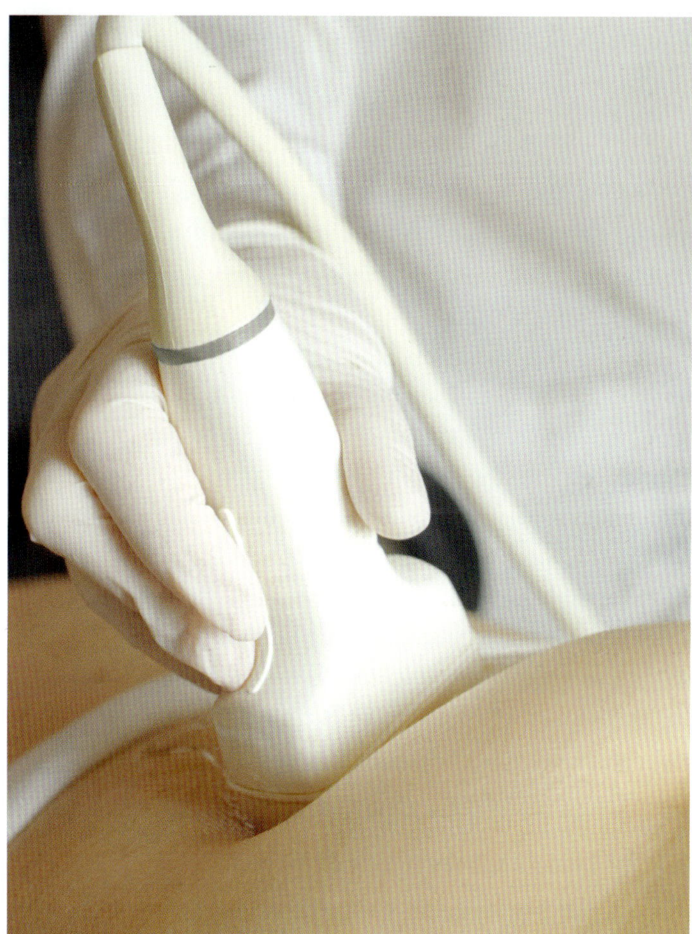

Ultrasound procedure to detect gallstones

- Nausea and vomiting
- Malaise (feeling bad all over)
- Loss of appetite
- Constant itching (the result of bile salts entering the bloodstream)
- Chills, fever (due to infection)
- Jaundice (yellow coloration of skin and whites of the eyes)
- Brown or bright yellow urine
- Light or clay-colored stools
- Shaking
- Food intolerances
- Fatigue
- Headaches
- Anxiety, irritability

Attacks of gallbladder pain can last anywhere from 20 minutes to several hours. Pain that occurs when a gallstone blocks the flow of bile from the gallbladder is referred to as biliary colic. Prolonged blockage of bile ducts can cause severe damage to the gallbladder, liver or pancreas and may even be fatal.[20]

How Is It Diagnosed?

Those called "silent" gallstones (those causing no symptoms) are often detected during a diagnostic work up that is done for unrelated reasons. Gallstones may appear on an abdominal X-ray, CT scan, MRI scan or abdominal ultrasound. Ultrasound is the diagnostic tool most frequently used to rule out gallstones when they are suspected. Ultrasound (or pulse-echo sonography) is a non-invasive, painless procedure that involves passing a probe externally over the abdomen. Sound waves are introduced into the body through this probe. If gallstones are present, the waves will bounce off them, revealing their location via an image that appears on a monitor. Other benefits of ultrasound are that it can show gallbladder distension (swelling) and thickness of the gallbladder wall as well as inflammation. Ultrasound will also help detect liver cysts, tumor blockage of bile ducts and pancreatic tumors and cysts.

"Most conventional doctors are unaware of the role that food allergies or sensitivities can play in gallstone formation."

Endoscopic ultrasound, where an ultrasound probe is built into the tip of an endoscope (a flexible lighted tube inserted into GI tract), can be used to find small stones in the gallbladder and common bile duct that cannot be detected by conventional ultrasound.[21]

A hepatobiliary (liver-bile duct) scan with an intravenous isotope (radioactive for an element), which is concentrated in the liver and excreted into the bile to be stored in the gallbladder, is an important functional test that can differentiate asymptomatic stones from those stones blocking the ducts. If the test is positive, the gallbladder will not be seen on the imaging screen, as the isotope will not be able to enter the gallbladder due to cystic duct blockage. This is usually an indication for gallbladder removal surgery. With a negative test, the gallbladder and bile ducts are well visualized, and the patient's gallstones may not be causing their problem. However, if the gallbladder is not contracting properly, the gallstones may still be a concern. A more complex and difficult test is

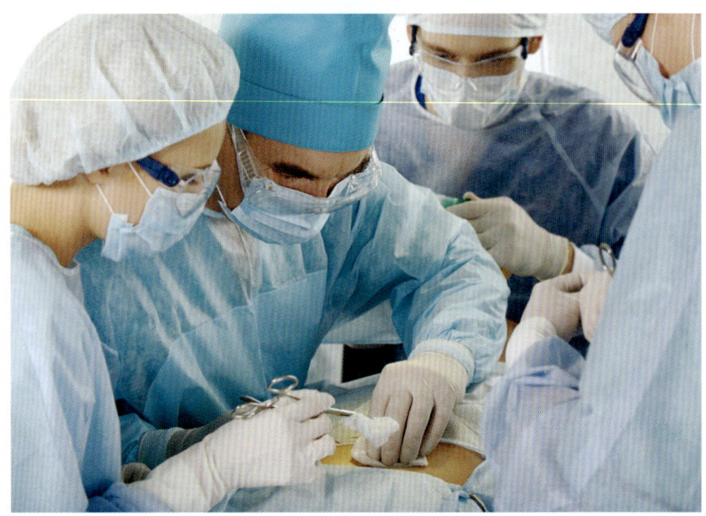

endoscopic retrograde cholangiopancreatography (ERCP). This is generally reserved for more complex and hard to diagnose cases. ERCP is useful for showing strictures or scar tissue of bile ducts or of the sphincter of Oddi.[22]

Gallstones cannot be diagnosed strictly on the basis of symptoms, for there are other conditions that can cause the same type of abdominal pain or intolerance to fatty food. These conditions include irritable bowel syndrome (IBS), gastroesophageal reflux disease (GERD), sphincter of Oddi dysfunction (dysfunction of a tight valve at the junction between the common bile duct and the duodenum),[23] ulcers (usually duodenal), antral gastritis and parasitic disease.[24] When gallbladder disease is suspected, the following should be ruled out: pancreatitis, duodenitis, gastritis and esophagitis[25]—all conditions involving inflammation. In addition, a cardiac evaluation with an ECG and cardiac enzymes may be indicated since heart problems can present as gallbladder disease.

Most conventional doctors are unaware of the role that food allergies or sensitivities can play in gallstone formation. Those who are aware of this relationship may order a food sensitivity test (see the Appendix) to detect these.

Those physicians who are aware of the role that low HCl levels may play in gallstone formation may order a Heidelburg test (see the Appendix) to measure levels of stomach acid.

Additionally, physicians usually order a liver function profile since elevation of liver enzymes is commonly an indicator of gallbladder problems.

What Is the Standard Medical Treatment?

When gallstones are silent (causing no symptoms), no treatment is generally recommended, and, unfortunately, all too often no lifestyle modifications are recommended to prevent future problems. Those problems can take the form of a gallbladder infection, which invariably will be treated with antibiotics. If the patient does not respond to antibiotic treatment and/or if the bile duct is blocked by gallstones, surgical removal of the gallbladder will most likely be the treatment of choice due to the drawbacks inherent in other conventional treatments including: stone removal, widening of the sphincter between the end of the common bile duct and the intestine to allow easier passage of stones, and use of drugs and other techniques to break up stones.[26]

Non-surgical approaches to gallstones are generally used for those patients who are unable to tolerate surgery. One such approach involves oral dissolution therapy using bile salts (chenodeoxycholic acid and ursodeoxycholic acid). Here medication that alters the composition of the bile is taken by mouth. The bile salts used in this approach promote increased cholesterol solubility. While this is a desirable effect, there are drawbacks to oral bile-salt therapy: it works only on cholesterol stones; it can have undesirable side effects, including mild diarrhea and possible liver damage; it is extremely slow-working, taking six months or more to dissolve stones; complete disappearance of stones happens only in a minority of cases; there is a tendency of stones to recur after dissolution; and full-dose therapy must be continued indefinitely, or stones may re-form when the drug is discontinued.[27]

Contact dissolution is another non-surgical approach in the treatment of gallstones. Here, a chemical, methyl-tert-butyl ether (MTBE), is injected directly into the gallbladder through a catheter passed through the abdominal wall. The downside of this therapy is that the MTBE has an extremely unpleasant odor; it causes pain in the upper abdomen; it may cause nausea and vomiting; it may cause damage to the kidneys if it escapes from the gallbladder; and recurrence of stones is possible.[28]

Extracorporeal shock-wave lithotripsy (ESWL) is another non-surgical treatment for gallstones. This is a non-invasive but expensive procedure involving the use of

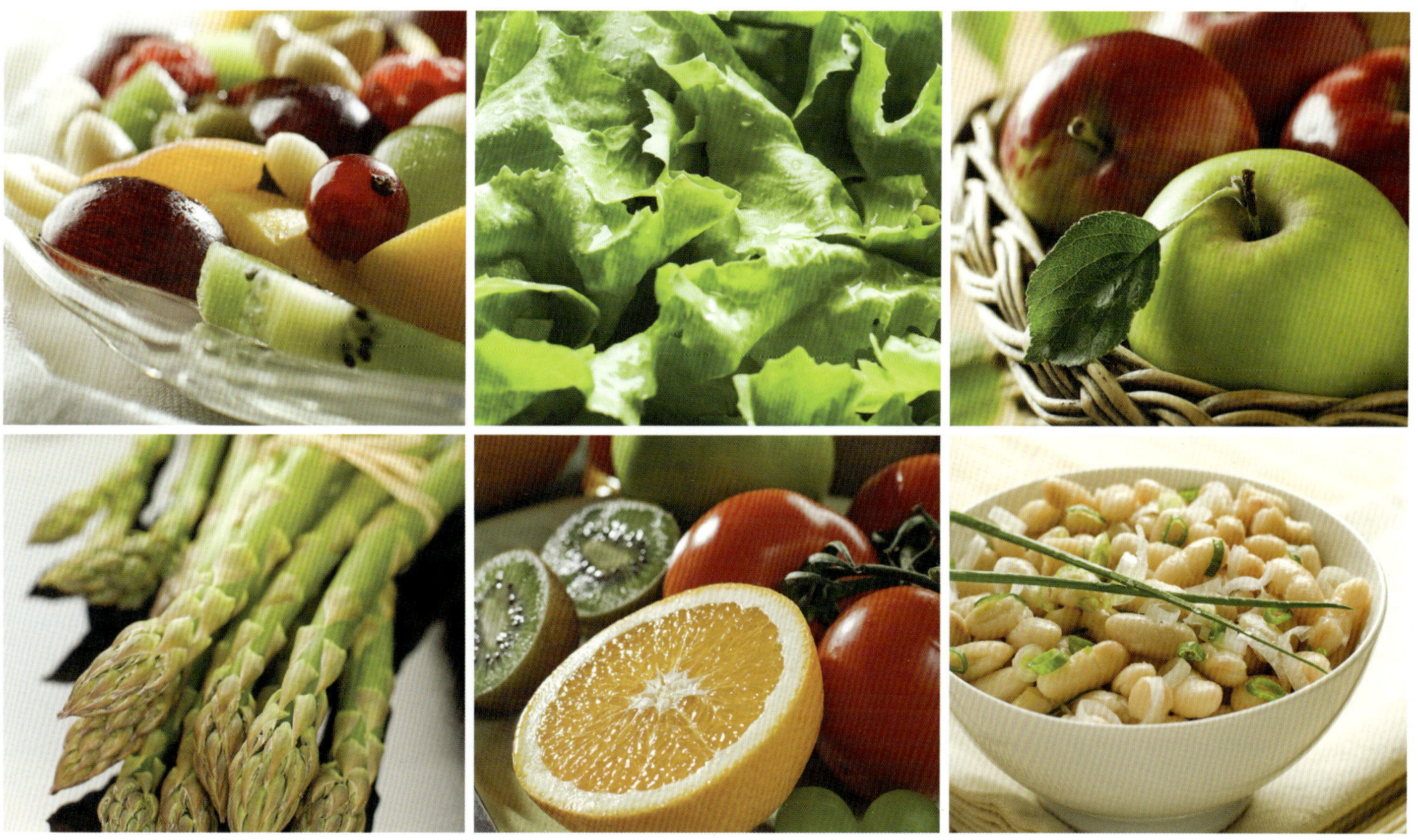

"Conventional medicine views the gallbladder as a dispensable organ."

sound waves to break up stones. It only works for small cholesterol stones that are not calcified (less than 10 percent of the typical gallbladder cases seen in the U.S.), and no more than three stones can be treated at a time. Although this procedure has worked well in combination with bile-salt therapy, there have been some associated side effects (biliary pain and some bleeding into the kidney).[29]

The non-surgical approaches described above are, according to the "Merck Manual" (the physician's guide to diagnosis and treatment), " … now largely unavailable owing to greater patient acceptance of laparoscopic cholecystectomy."[30] Translation: Patients prefer to have their gallbladders removed. In fact, gallbladder removal is one of the most commonly performed surgical procedures.[31]

Removal of the entire gallbladder to cure the gallstone problem may seem extreme, but the thinking is this: Simply removing the stones does no good; the abnormal bile would re-form them.[32] In addition, the damaged lining of the gallbladder tends to allow for recurrent stone formation. Medicine views the gallbladder as a dispensable organ. After all, certain animals (rats, horses, pigeons) get along without a gallbladder as can most humans. A common temporary side effect can be diarrhea. This usually clears in one to two months as the liver and the intestines begin to compensate for having no gallbladder. About one percent of patients may have chronic diarrhea.

The type of cholecystectomy (gallbladder removal) most commonly done today is the laparoscopic variety introduced in 1988. Known as "keyhole surgery," it involves entering the abdomen through the navel, with three additional small incisions made for the insertion of instruments and a small video camera. The video camera is attached to an external monitor used to guide the surgeon's movements. There are several advantages of laparoscopic over conventional (open) cholecystectomy, which involves a 5- to 8-inch incision and one week of hospitalization.

These advantages include:
- Less pain
- Quicker healing
- Improved cosmetic results
- Fewer complications

In addition to gallstones in the gallbladder, it is possible to have stones retained in the cystic duct or common bile duct at the time of gallbladder removal. This can be prevented by taking an X-ray at the time of surgery. There are also cases where stones are formed in the liver ducts due to sluggish bile flow and infection. In all these cases, common bile-duct exploration would be needed. Laparoscopic exploration is one such method. For smaller gallstones, endoscopic retrograde cholangiopancreatography (ERCP) is used with sphincterotomy to remove the gallstones through the sphincter of Oddi, located at the end of the common bile duct leading into the duodenum.

Open surgery is still used today for complex cases and when complications are encountered in the laparoscopic approach. With either surgery, complications are possible. These include:

- Injury to the common bile duct – This is the most common complication; it can cause leakage of bile and/or infection, and may necessitate corrective surgery. Scarring of any part of the duct may lead to obstruction causing repeated complex operations. Severe disability and even death can result if the problem is not completely corrected.
- Adhesions – These are unnatural connections of body tissues.
- Leftover stones in the bile duct – This usually can be handled with endoscopic removal of the stones via the ampulla of Vater (opening of the bile duct into the duodenum).
- Bile leakage from the gallbladder bed in the liver. This can cause subhepatic abscess formation requiring either radiologic or surgical drainage.
- A portion of the cystic duct left behind – When this happens, retained stones can enter the common bile duct and cause problems.

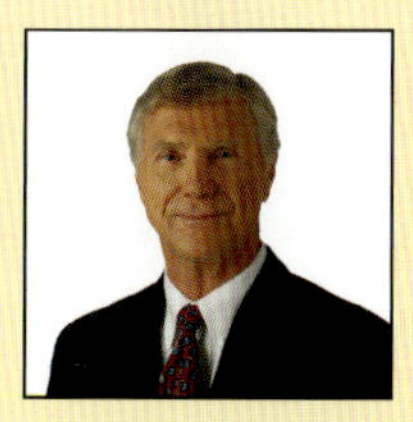

Dr. Smith's Comments

I have seen many patients present with classical signs and symptoms of acute cholecystitis; namely right upper-abdominal pain, with radiating pain under the right scapula (shoulder blade); nausea and vomiting, especially after a fatty meal; and yes, commonly with the five Fs: female, fair, fat, fertile, and 40; with gallstones on ultrasound.

However, I would like to point out that there are many other possible presentations ranging from the signs and symptoms of a heart attack, to heartburn, indigestion, ulcers or even small bowel obstruction. In fact, gallstone ileus is a condition whereby a large gallstone migrates through the wall of an inflamed gallbladder right through the wall of a piece of intestine adherent to the gallbladder. The large stone now in the intestine can cause a bowel obstruction, which often requires surgery unless it is small enough to pass.

Some patients have no symptoms, and do not even have gallstones, but can be acutely and deathly ill from what is known as acalculus cholecystitis (without stones and an inflamed gallbladder). This is an extreme example of toxic or infected bile, which can be due to increased intestinal permeability (leaky gut).

Many hospitalized patients are not eating for various reasons, and are on many medications, including antibiotics. This sets the stage for serious malnutrition of the intestinal lining. Most people are not aware that the intestinal lining feeds itself before any food is absorbed into the bloodstream. From the bloodstream and lymphatics, food is then taken to the liver for processing and detoxification if necessary.

In the presence of malnutrition, overgrowth of yeast and/or pathogenic bacteria (often as a result of antibiotics) and stress, there can be a pathologic increase in intestinal permeability. Viral and bacterial particles and toxins, and poorly digested food remnants (especially in the colon) that have been sitting there for

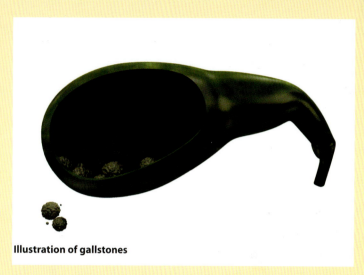

Illustration of gallstones

days can now go to the liver via the circulation. When the liver is overwhelmed, some substances are detoxified but others get by untouched. In addition, if there is a shortage of sulfur-containing amino acids, the liver itself will take some toxins and convert them into new compounds that are even more toxic.

Thus, there can be highly toxic and/or infected bile that literally burns the liver, bile ducts and gallbladder. When the gallbladder stores this infected toxic material, it then starts destroying the wall of the gallbladder and is absorbed into the blood creating a true surgical emergency. If the patient is too sick to be operated upon, radiology can place a drain in the gallbladder as a temporary treatment.

To make matters worse, the infected toxic bile enters the duodenum and begins a destructive path of inflammatory damage to the duodenum, pancreas and small intestine. This greatly exacerbates the original problem; the inflamed pancreas will not deliver needed enzymes, and the inflamed small intestine will be more damaged allowing more toxins to leak through and creating a dangerous vicious cycle for the body.

The above example is indicative of how the intestine, liver, gallbladder and pancreas are all interconnected, not only in health, but in disease as well.

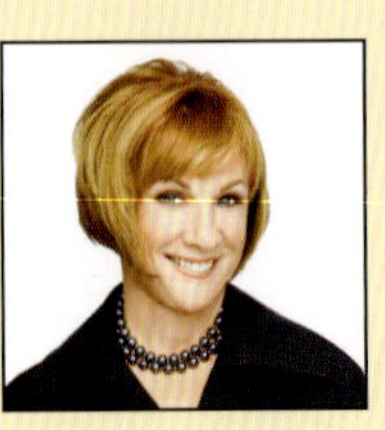

Brenda's Bottom Line

Clearly, at times, there may be no alternative to gallbladder removal, depending on the individual case. In many instances, however, diet and lifestyle modification can play a key role in halting the growth of gallstones and reducing the frequency and severity of gallbladder attacks. Most nutritionally-oriented physicians are aware that a high-fiber diet featuring whole grains, fruits and vegetables can reduce the amount of cholesterol in bile and the tendency to form stones. Reduced fat intake (namely, less meat and dairy products) means less cholesterol in the bile which may prevent further stone formation. Such doctors would also advocate a low-sugar diet based on the fact that several studies have indicated that people who eat a lot of sweets are more likely to develop gallstones.[33] This may be due to the fact that increased sugar entering the liver activates its conversion into triglycerides and then into cholesterol. The liver is the first line of defense against elevated blood sugar from the diet.

In dealing with gallstones, the stimulation of bile flow is essential. Gallstones often form due to stagnation in the flow of bile, which can be likened to a constipation of the gallbladder. In the liver, bile flows through tributary-like ducts that merge into a larger duct that flows into the gallbladder. Stimulating this flow is essential, and can be done with natural ingredients found in liver support formulas.

If the gallbladder has already been removed, for a period of about six months, bile flow through the digestive system is not regulated. To soak up excess bile, you need to increase your daily intake of soluble fiber. The easiest way to do this is with a soluble fiber supplement. (See the chart on the next page.)

Rule Out:

- Foods sensitivities (See the Gluten Sensitivity and Allergies sections.)
- Parasites (See the Parasitic Disease section.)
- Low HCl in the stomach – Heidelberg test. (See the Appendix.) A simple test of low stomach acid is to take a hydrochloric acid capsule (500 mg to 650 mg) before a meal. Then, with each subsequent meal, add another capsule until you feel a burning sensation. Then back off to the previous dose.

Recommended Testing

- Foods sensitivity test (See the Appendix)
- Heidelberg pH test (See the Appendix)

Diet

- Follow the Fiber 35 Eating Plan in the Appendix of this book. A two- to three-day juice fast would be beneficial especially in cases of gallbladder inflammation.
- Decrease coffee intake (coffee intake increases dehydration)
- Reduce intake of sugar and refined carbohydrates as this has been associated with gallstones.
- Don't skip breakfast (fasting longer than 14 hours elevates gallstone risk).
- Drink plenty of water (about half the body weight in ounces), necessary to dilute bile.
- Avoid spicy and fried foods.

Lifestyle

- If overweight, lose weight slowly; no crash dieting.
- Avoid synthetic hormones.
- Chew food well for best digestion.
- Exercise daily to reduce risk of gallstones.

Complementary Mind/Body Therapies

- Colon hydrotherapy could be helpful in cases of constipation and will assist in liver detoxification. Try it with the Steps of Cleansing program or Liver Detox program. (See the Appendix.)
- Acupuncture can be beneficial for gallbladder problems.

Recommended Nutraceuticals	Dosage	Benefit	Comments
Critical Phase	Daily maintenance recommendations should also be taken during this phase unless otherwise indicated.		
Total Body Cleanse	See Appendix	Encourages elimination and detoxification.	Herbal formula should support the seven channels of elimination.
Liver Detox	This should follow the Total Body Cleanse. See Appendix	Encourages detoxification involving the liver and gallbladder.	Should contain milk thistle seed extract containing silymarin, phosphatidylcholine, selenium and herbs.
Helpful			
High Potency Multi-vitamin/mineral	Use as directed	Provides needed nutrients that may be deficient.	Powder or liquid formulation would be helpful as it is easier assimilated and absorbed.
Vitamin D_3	At least 1,000 to 2,000 iu daily	Vitamin D may not be absorbed well with gallbladder dysfunction.	Research is showing many health complications as a result of low vitamin D levels.
Peppermint oil	0.2 -0.4 ml 3 times daily	May help to dissolve gallstones.	Be sure to use enteric coated peppermint oil.
Daily Maintenance			
Lecithin	1200 mg lecithin with meals	Emulsifies fat, helping with its digestion.	May use phosphatidylcholine instead, 500 mg daily.
Critical Liver Support Formula	Use as directed	Enhances liver and glallbladder function.	Should include milk thistle seed extract containing silymarin, N-acetyl-cysteine, alpha lipoic acid L-glutathione.
Digestive Enzymes	Take with meals	Helps digest and absorb nutrients from food to reduce liver and gallbladder stress.	Formula containing betain HCl may be helpful for those with low stomach acid.
Omega-3 Fatty Acids	At least 2 grams daily of EPA/DHA combination	Reduces inflammation.	Look for a concentrated, enteric coated fish oil.
Fiber	4-5 grams twice daily	Promotes regular bowel movement and absorbs excess bile.	Look for a soluble/insoluble fiber blend. Use in conjunction with high fiber diet to reach 35 g daily.
Probiotics	30 - 80 billion culture count twice daily	Restores bacterial balance and pH of colon and promotes regularity.	Look for high amount of bifidobacteria, the main beneficial bacteria in colon.

See further explanation of supplements in the Appendix

HEPATITIS

What Is It?

Hepatitis involves inflammation of the liver. There are many different types of hepatitis, each identified by what causes it. Viral hepatitis is the most prevalent type. Hepatitis can also be defined in terms of the severity of the case, with three separate categories: acute (inflammation lasting less than six months), chronic (inflammation lasting more than six months) and fulminant—a particularly serious form of acute hepatitis associated with jaundice, coagulopathy (blood clotting dysfunction) and encephalopathy (brain dysfunction).[1]

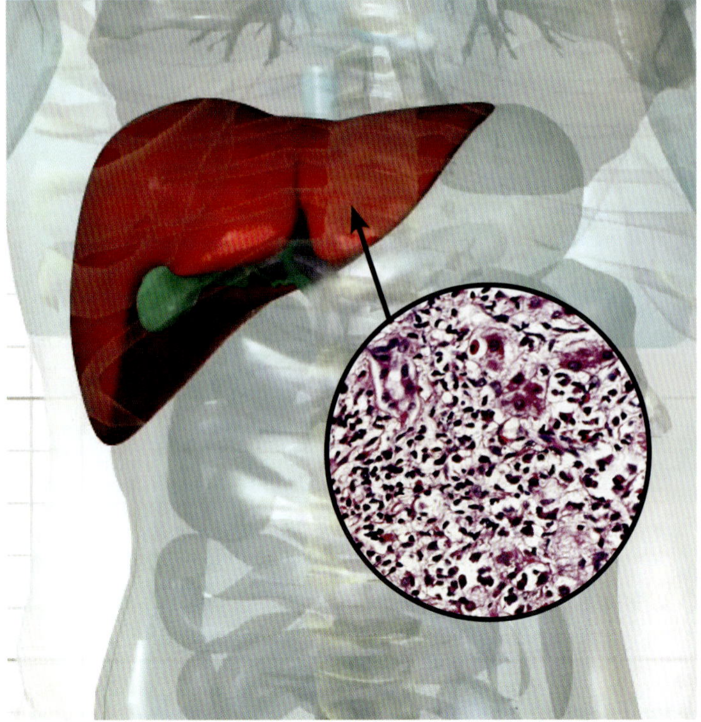

Microscopic chronic hepatitis

What Causes It?

Although most cases of hepatitis are thought to be caused by viruses, other factors may also be involved. These include excessive use of alcohol, street drugs, some medications (both prescription and over-the-counter), injury to the liver, and exposure to environmental toxins. Even environmental toxins absorbed through the skin can damage the liver. Chlorinated hydrocarbons and arsenic are examples of agents that are severely toxic to the liver. Obesity may also be a causative factor in hepatitis, for excess weight means excess fat deposited in the liver causing inflammation known as fatty liver hepatitis, or non-alcoholic steatohepatitis (NASH).[2]

NASH begins as another condition, non-alcoholic fatty liver disease (NAFLD), which involves fat buildup in the liver without much inflammation. NAFLD and NASH are associated with insulin resistance,[3] found in metabolic syndrome and type 2 diabetes. People with abdominal fat are prone to these conditions that can largely be controlled and/or reversed through lifestyle changes involving diet and exercise. (See the NAFLD section for more information on this condition.)

One or more of seven specific viruses (listed alphabetically as hepatitis A through G), may attack the liver causing hepatitis. Two other viruses, the transfusion-transmitted virus (TTV) and SEN-V (named for the person from whom it was first isolated), may also cause the disease. Indeed, other viruses that primarily target organs other than the liver may also attack the liver causing inflammation. These include such viruses as Epstein-Barr, cytomegalovirus and herpes simplex.

Hepatitis D is a virus that only affects people who have hepatitis B. It is the least common, but most serious of the hepatitis viruses. Hepatitis E, rarely found in the U.S., is similar to hepatitis A. Evidence for the existence of hepatitis F is at present only anecdotal. The last hepatitis virus to be discovered (in 1995) was hepatitis G. It does not appear to be a significant cause of acute or chronic hepatitis.[4]

Yet another variety of the disease is autoimmune hepatitis. Celiac disease, or gluten sensitivity, has been shown to be highly prevalent in those people with autoimmune hepatitis.[5] For this reason, early screening for gluten sensitivity is recommended.

The three most common types of viral hepatitis are hepatitis A, B and C (HAV, HBV, HCV). These will be the focus of discussion.

There are more than 1,000 drugs and chemicals that can injure the liver causing drug-induced hepatitis. Some of the major ones are cimetidine, clindamycin, warfarin, diazepam, ibuprofen, metronidazole, phenytoin, and salicylates (aspirin).[6] Street drugs can also damage the liver causing inflammation. Both cocaine and the amphetamine known as ecstasy can cause acute hepatitis.[7] Use of intravenous and intranasal drugs has long been associated with the transmission of HBV and HCV. Cigarette smoking, while not a direct cause of hepatitis, can increase susceptibility to the liver-toxic effects of some drugs, such as those listed above. Smoking also decreases the liver's detoxification ability.

Interestingly, low levels of stomach acid (hydrochloric acid, or HCl) have been associated with chronic hepatitis.

Although hepatitis B has a high rate of transmission through sexual contact, both hepatitis C and A can also be transmitted sexually to a lesser extent. How the three major hepatitis viruses can be spread:

Hepatitis A
HAV is found in the stool of HAV-infected persons. HAV is usually spread from person to person by putting something in the mouth (even though it may appear to be clean) that has been contaminated with the stool of a person with hepatitis A. This can happen when people don't wash their hands after using the toilet, and then touch other people's food. HAV may also be spread from mother to baby during childbirth.

Hepatitis B
HBV is found in blood and certain body fluids. It is spread when blood or body fluid from an infected person enters the body of a person who is not immune to the virus. HBV is spread through unprotected sex with an infected person, needle sharing when injecting drugs, exposure to needle sticks or sharps (sharp medical tools) on the job, or from an infected mother to her baby during childbirth. Exposure to blood in ANY situation can be a risk for transmission.

Hepatitis C
HCV is found in blood and certain body fluids. It is spread when blood or body fluids from an infected person enters another person's body. HCV is spread through sharing

Risk Factors Associated with the Three Major Hepatitis Viruses[10]

Hepatitis A

- Children in cities and states where routine hepatitis A vaccination is recommended
- Household contacts of infected persons
- Sex partners of infected persons
- Persons traveling to countries where HAV is common (everywhere except Canada, Western Europe, Japan, Australia and New Zealand)
- Injecting and non-injecting drug users
- People eating food or drinking water that is infected with the virus
- Persons with chronic liver disease

Hepatitis B

- Persons with multiple sex partners
- Persons diagnosed with a sexually transmitted disease
- Sex partners of infected persons
- Injecting drug users
- Household contacts of infected persons
- Infants born to infected mothers
- Infants/children of immigrants from areas with high HBV rates
- Health care and public safety workers who are exposed to blood
- Persons with severe kidney disease (including predialysis/dialysis)
- Persons traveling to and from areas where HBV is common

Hepatitis C

- Injecting drug users
- Recipients of clotting factors made before 1987
- Hemodialysis patients
- Recipients of blood/solid organs before 1992
- People with undiagnosed abnormal liver test results
- Infants born to infected mothers
- People having sex with an infected partner (possibly)

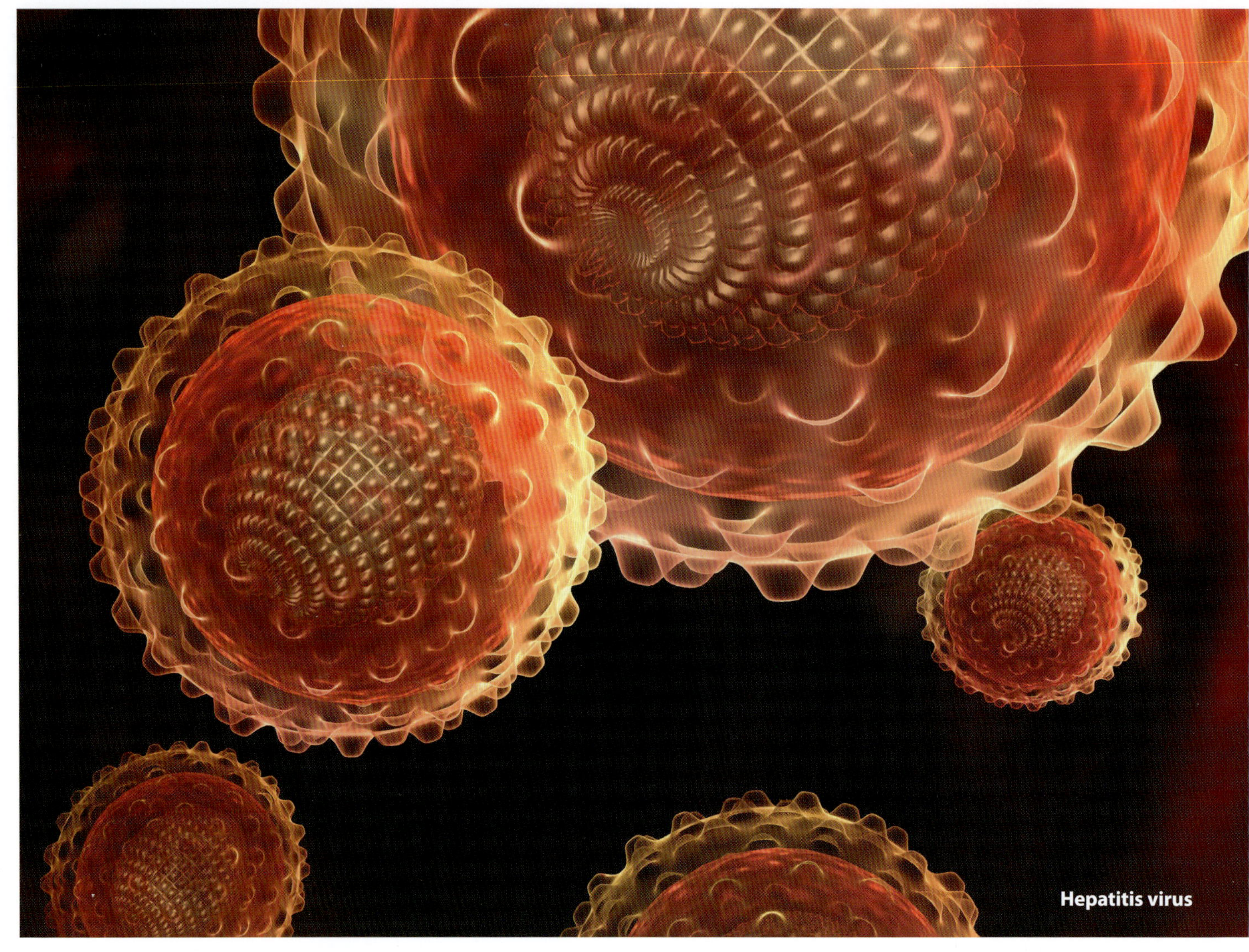

Hepatitis virus

needles, through exposure to needle sticks or sharps on the job, or sometimes from an infected mother to her baby during birth.

Both HCV and HBV (also known as serum hepatitis) can be transmitted via transfusion of contaminated blood, though improved screening of donated blood has decreased the incidence of this kind of transmission. HAV (infectious hepatitis), in addition to being transmitted through fecal contamination of food or water, can infect a person who has eaten raw shellfish from polluted waters.[8] Of the three major types of viral hepatitis, HCV is the most serious, since 85 percent of infections with this slowly progressive, but ultimately devastating virus lead to chronic liver disease.[9]

While HBV and HCV can lead to chronic (long-term) hepatitis, with HAV, there is no chronic infection, and it can only be contracted once.

People of any age may develop hepatitis. The most common age of onset for HBV is between 15 and 24 years, while the HCV virus is generally activated after age 40.

Generally speaking, those at greatest risk for developing any type of hepatitis would be those with a weak immune system and heavy body burden of toxins from any source. Additionally, those with lowered levels of stomach acid would be at increased risk for developing chronic hepatitis. Since HCl levels tend to decline as we age, risk for developing the chronic form of the disease would tend to increase with age as well. There may well be other, as yet unidentified, risk factors involved for each of the hepatitis viruses.

Vaccines are presently available for HAV and HBV, but not for HCV. There is some controversy regarding the safety and efficacy of these vaccines, especially HBV[10] and HAV, which are now a routine part of the recommended infant

Did You Know

- Up to 85 percent of those with hepatitis C, and a smaller number of those with hepatitis B, develop long-lasting (chronic) hepatitis. Some people with hepatitis B become lifelong carriers of the illness, and can spread the hepatitis infection to others. Patients with chronic hepatitis C also are infectious, and can spread the virus through blood-to-blood contact.
- About five percent of adults who get hepatitis B will develop a long-lasting form of the disease. The rate is much higher for babies and young children. A small percentage of these patients eventually develop cirrhosis or liver cancer.
- Up to 80 percent of people infected with hepatitis C will develop chronic infection, and about 20 percent to 30 percent of these patients will develop cirrhosis or liver cancer.
- Since the early 1990s, improved techniques for screening donated blood have greatly reduced the risk of catching hepatitis B or C from blood transfusions. According to the U.S. National Institutes of Health, the current risk of catching Hepatitis B or C is one in 205,000 units of transfused blood.
- In the United States today, most infectious cases of hepatitis are caused by an infection with one of the hepatitis viruses (A, B, C, D or E).

immunization program. The argument prevails that very few infants in the 0 to 1 age group are at risk for these diseases, and yet, there are reports of adverse reactions to these vaccines in that age group.

What Are the Signs and Symptoms?

While some people with viral hepatitis have no symptoms, those who do, regardless of virus type, may experience any or all of the following:

- Fever
- Weakness
- Nausea/vomiting
- Headache
- Muscle aches
- Fatigue
- Dark urine
- Light stools
- Jaundice (yellow pigment to the skin and whites of the eyes)
- Low levels of stomach acid (HCl)
- Abdominal discomfort
- Elevated bilirubin (bile pigment) in the blood
- Flu-like symptoms (mild to severe)
- Joint aches/inflammation
- Diarrhea
- Itchy skin lesions
- Personality changes

Unlike HBV and HCV, the onset of HAV symptoms is sudden. Acute forms of HBV and HCV may develop into chronic forms increasing the risk for liver failure and death from cirrhosis and liver cancer.

It is important to know that hepatitis causes some degree of liver damage, even in the absence of symptoms.

How Is It Diagnosed?

Diagnosis of viral hepatitis may be made on the basis of symptoms, and confirmed with blood tests that show an elevation of liver enzymes, such as SGPT, GGPT, SGOT and alkaline phosphatase, which leaks out into the blood when liver cells are damaged.[11] Another type of blood test is also used, one which shows the presence of viral antigens (compounds that are foreign to the body resulting in the formation of antibodies against them) or antibodies (chemical bullets) that bind antigens. Viral type (A, B, C, etc.) is identified on the basis of types of viral antigens or specific antibodies in the blood.

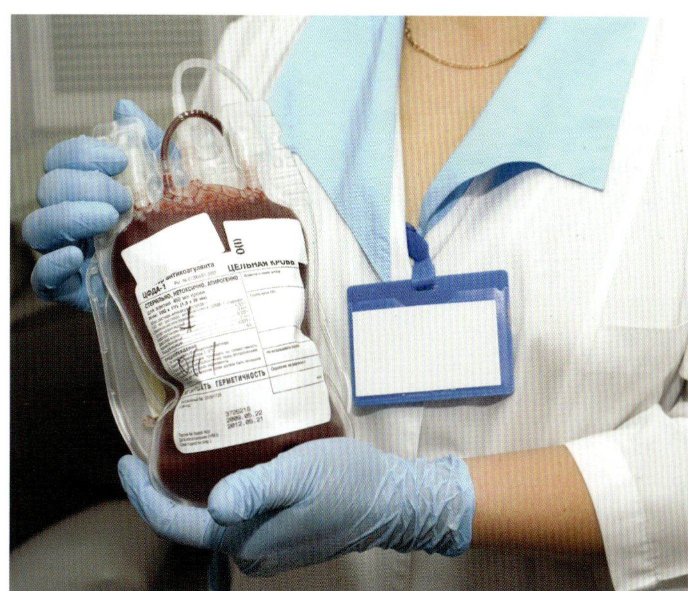

Healing HOPE Testimonial

"I recently did the Liver Detox, due to liver anomolies, high enzymes and upper quadrant discomfort that baffled doctors for some time. I did the detox two times, with about a month between each one. My liver enzymes were retested, and they dropped to normal readings from almost triple the numbers two months earlier. The detox, along with the diet and lifestyle recommendations, helped me to heal."
– Keith

In addition to liver enzymes, hepatitis is monitored by counting viral particles. This is done by measuring the RNA of viral particles by a technique known as polymerase chain reaction. In the case of hepatitis C, the higher the level of HCV-RNA, the more aggressive the chronic infection.[12] As patients respond to treatment, their viral particle count, measured by PCR, drops lower, ideally to zero. A liver biopsy (a piece of liver tissue obtained with a needle) can be performed to confirm the diagnosis and identify the type and degree of damage.

What Is the Standard Medical Treatment?

There is no cure for hepatitis. Treatment is aimed at protecting the liver and preventing further damage to it.

There is no treatment for hepatitis A beyond rest and fluid replacement and a nourishing diet as recovery progresses. Basically, the disease is left to run its course, giving the body supportive therapies only. Drugs would only tax the liver. Drug therapy is, however, used in treatment of both HBV and HCV in their chronic phase. Alphainterferon and lamivudine are the two drugs licensed for the treatment of chronic hepatitis B, while interferon, pegylated interferon and ribavirin are licensed for the treatment of chronic hepatitis C. Often drug combinations are used for treatment of HCV. Acute HBV and HCV are treated in the same manner as HAV with rest and fluid replacement. All hepatitis patients are advised to avoid alcohol. Strenuous exercise should also be avoided, as should liver-toxic drugs and chemicals. Additionally, special care should be taken with hygiene during the contagious phase of the disease (two to three weeks prior to onset of symptoms up through three weeks after onset of symptoms). Contact with others should be avoided during this time. It is especially important not to share personal care items (such as razors, toothbrushes and washcloths) that may have blood on them.

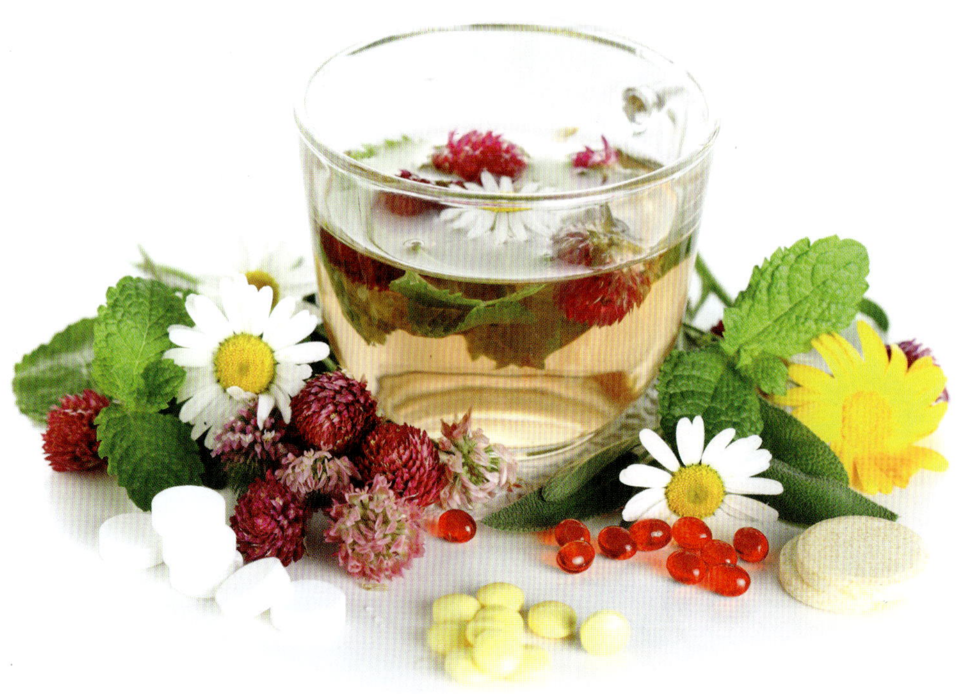

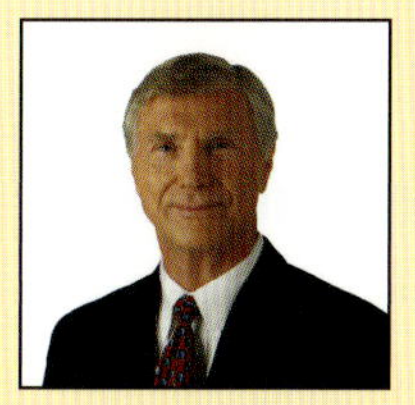

Dr. Smith's Comments

As mentioned in the text, hepatitis is inflammation of the liver that can come from many sources. The major causes of hepatitis are chemical toxicity, alcohol and viral illnesses. Nutritional supplements can be helpful in all of these areas.

I would like to share an example that relates to glutathione levels in white blood cells in hepatitis. There is an article entitled: "Antioxidant status and glutathione metabolism in peripheral blood mononuclear cells from patients with chronic hepatitis C." The investigators wanted to see what role oxidative stress could play in the pathogenesis of hepatitis C virus infection. They investigated the oxidant/antioxidant status in peripheral blood mononuclear cells from patients with chronic hepatitis C and controls.

Lipid peroxidation products and superoxide dismutase activity in peripheral blood mononuclear cells were higher in chronic hepatitis C patients than in healthy subjects, while glutathione S-transferase activity was reduced in patients as compared to controls. S-transferase is a selenium-dependent enzyme. In addition, 35 percent of patients with chronic hepatitis C showed lower levels of reduced glutathione and higher levels of oxidized glutathione than normal controls.

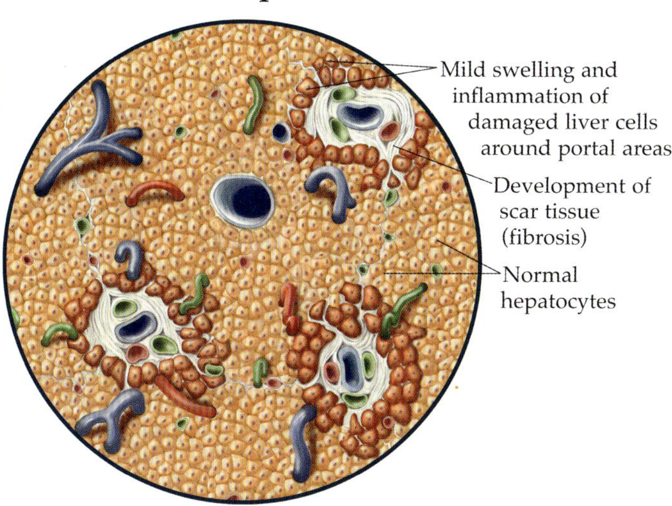

Microscopic liver cross section

Conclusions: Oxidative stress is observed in peripheral blood mononuclear cells from chronic hepatitis C patients. This process might alter lymphocyte function and facilitate the chronicity of the infection [Journal of Hepatology, Vol. 31 (5) (1999) pp. 808-814].

The above examples support the need for nutritional support in patients with chronic hepatitis B or C. As one can see, looking at the last example, the oxidative stress and resulting glutathione depletion affects not only the liver but also the immune blood cells.

I think a complete nutritional and supplemental program, as outlined in the following section, would certainly benefit patients while they are receiving anti-viral therapy (Interferon and Ribavirin). Continued support after the viral count is down may help prevent relapse of the infection.

Two good tests to monitor would be the liver detoxification test and a comprehensive stool analysis (CSA). The liver detox test demonstrates the liver's ability to detoxify caffeine, Tylenol and aspirin, (good indicator of overall detoxification capacity), and gives an idea of what nutrients may be needed. The stool analysis is a good indicator of any digestive problems showing up in the stool. This is important since whatever happens in the stool may indicate what is in store for the liver. Many people may not be aware that the liver takes the full burden of whatever is happening in the intestinal tract. Therefore, minimizing toxicity in the intestinal tract will help to restore and maintain liver function. This is clearly seen in primary sclerosing cholangitis where up to 70 percent of the patients with this disorder have had IBD. The IBD is usually ulcerative colitis, but if it is Crohn's, it always involves the colon. This is compelling evidence of the colon and liver connection.

NAFLD / NASH

What Is It?

Non-alcoholic fatty liver disease (NAFLD) describes a spectrum of chronic liver disease in people who drink little to no alcohol. The first stage of this disease involves a buildup of fat in the liver, also known as fatty liver, or steatosis. In some people, this fat accumulation causes inflammation and scarring, or fibrosis, at which point the condition is considered non-alcoholic steatohepatitis (NASH). This inflammation can lead to severe scarring of the liver—yet another condition known as cirrhosis—if enough tissue is damaged. (See the Cirrhosis section for more information.) If enough of the liver is damaged from scarring, liver failure could occur. This entire spectrum of liver disease is known as NAFLD.

It has recently been recognized that NAFLD may lead to the development of cardiovascular disease (CVD).[3] This occurs for a couple of reasons. It has been suggested that NAFLD may directly cause atherosclerosis and vice versa, in addition to the ability of many of the individual risk factors of NAFLD, themselves, to lead to CVD.

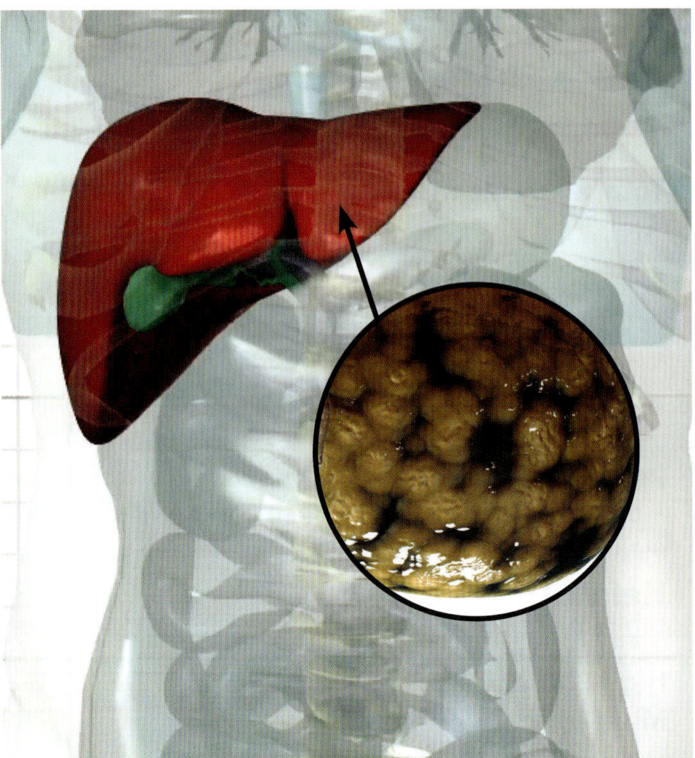

Enlarged image of a fatty liver

What Causes It?

In NAFLD the liver has trouble breaking down fats resulting in a buildup of fat in the liver. There are many different factors contributing to the development or worsening of NAFLD. These include:[4,5]

- Obesity
- Metabolic syndrome
- Insulin resistance
- Type 2 diabetes
- High triglycerides
- High cholesterol
- Oxidative stress
- Dysbiosis
- Leaky gut
- Inflammation
- Candida overgrowth
- Gluten sensitivity / celiac disease
- Milk (casein) allergy
- Poor diet
- Toxins
- Certain medications
- Family history and genetics

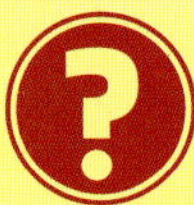

Did You Know

A cause for concern with NAFLD comes from the evidence that NASH can progress to liver cancer.[1] In 100 percent of NASH patients, a particular marker that detects liver cell proliferation (which is what occurs in liver cancer) was found.[2]

Obesity is a major risk factor in the development of NAFLD. In fact, 90 percent of obese people may develop chronic liver injury.[6] It is thought that obesity is the most common cause of NAFLD.[7] Since the obesity rate in the U.S. has increased so drastically in the past few decades, and is projected to continue increasing, NAFLD is becoming more common, and will likely continue this trend. Abdominal fat is an especially important factor in NAFLD, even in people who are not overweight.[8]

Obesity, Insulin resistance ▷ **Fatty Liver + dysbiosis** ▷ **Oxidative stress + inflammation** ▷ **NAFLD spectrum**

It is thought that insulin resistance and oxidative stress are two of the main processes of NAFLD.[13] Dysbiosis contributes to this process by inducing inflammation.[14]

NAFLD is closely related to the components of the metabolic syndrome, most notably insulin resistance, another risk factor for NAFLD, which leads to type 2 diabetes. Some consider NAFLD to be part of the metabolic syndrome.[9] Others view it as a consequence of the metabolic syndrome.[10] Some of the individual components of the metabolic syndrome can lead to NAFLD. These include: insulin resistance, abdominal fat, high triglycerides and bad cholesterol (LDL and VLDL). Insulin resistance causes an increase in the amount of glucose in the liver, which is converted into fat and accumulates. High insulin levels, which coincide with insulin resistance, also decrease the burning of fat because, when insulin levels are high, the body incorrectly thinks that it does not have enough energy (in the form of glucose), so fat storage is increased as a back-up storage source.[11]

A main feature of NAFLD is oxidative stress, being a direct result of the excess fat accumulated in the liver. It is thought that oxidative stress is largely responsible for the advancement of fatty liver to NASH and cirrhosis.[12] Oxidative stress causes inflammation which damages the liver. Another contributor is a lack of antioxidants, which counteract oxidative stress.

Dysbiosis, or an imbalance in the intestinal microbes (bacteria, fungi, parasites), plays an important role in the development of NAFLD. The gut-liver connection is illustrated in a number of ways. One major way in which intestinal dysbiosis leads to NAFLD is when microbial endotoxins (toxins produced by bacteria), such as lipopolysaccharide (LPS), trigger an inflammatory reaction in the liver.[15,16] Small intestinal bacterial overgrowth (SIBO), another term for dysbiosis, has been found in 50 percent of NASH patients.[17] The dysbiosis itself leads to a condition known as increased intestinal permeability, or leaky gut syndrome, promoting the ability of partially undigested food particles and toxins (both microbial and otherwise) to enter through the compromised intestine and into the blood supply, which flows first to the liver. Leaky gut and dysbiosis are both associated with NAFLD.[18] (See the Leaky Gut Syndrome section for more information on this condition.) Maintaining a healthy balance of intestinal bacteria is an important step in protecting the liver from damage.

Inflammation is a major component of NAFLD. Inflammation can occur for a number of reasons. The fat itself, which accumulates in the liver, can cause inflammation. But inflammation can also come from an imbalance, or dysbiosis that begins in the gut. The most prominent inflammatory chemical associated with NALFD is tumor necrosis factor alpha (TNF-alpha).[19] TNF-alpha is involved in all stages of NAFLD. Interestingly, TNF-alpha is produced in large amounts in response to endotoxins, like LPS, produced by bacteria. This further supports the gut-liver connection.

Overgrowth of the intestinal yeast Candida may also be at the basis of liver damage, via leaky gut. Candida overgrowth is a form of dysbiosis, largely caused by one organism, the yeast Candida albicans. An interesting connection to NAFLD occurs when Candida organisms ferment simple sugars in the gut into alcohol. This is also known as "auto-brewery" syndrome.[20] Other pathogenic bacteria are also able to produce alcohol in the gut. The alcohol can contribute to oxidative stress in the liver.[21] In addition, the alcohol can further oxidize to acetaldehyde at toxic levels, contributing to the development of leaky gut[22] and further liver toxicity. Indeed, obese women with

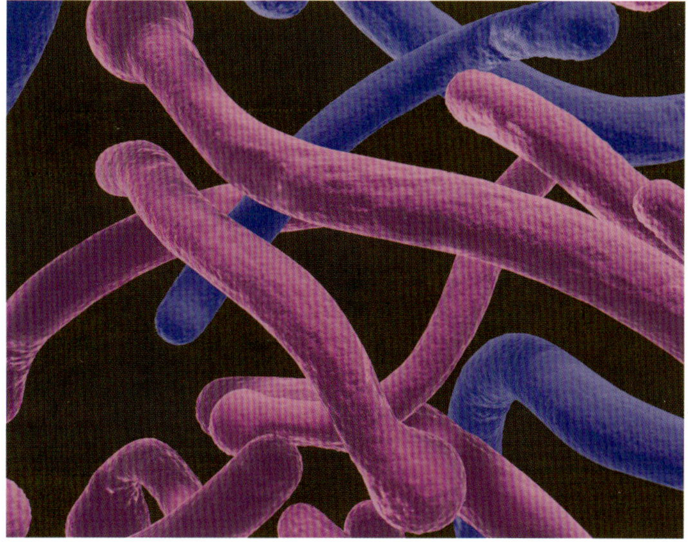

Illustration of Candida albicans

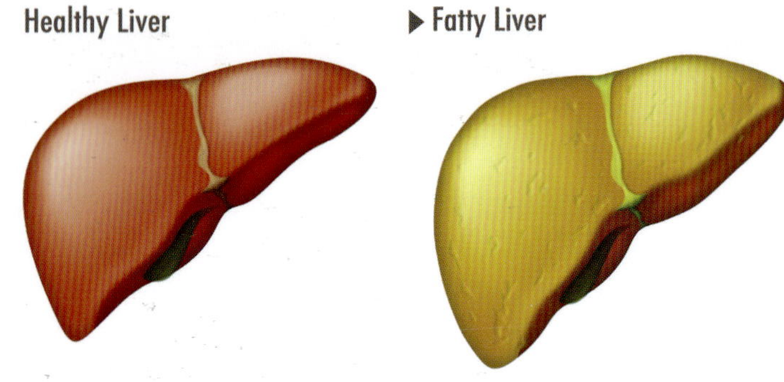

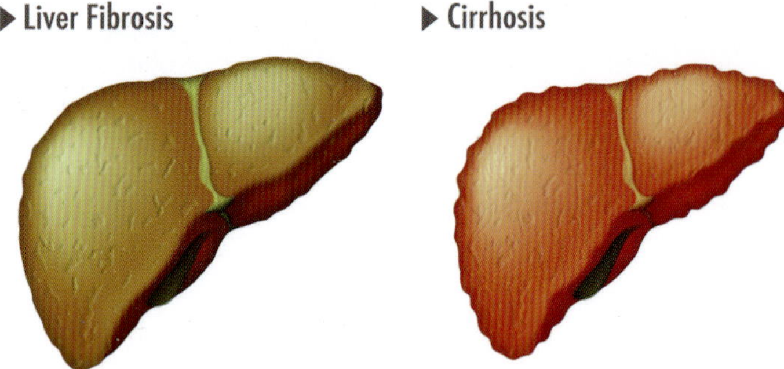

NASH have been found to have increased breath-alcohol levels without having consumed alcohol.[23] This is said to be due to intestinal bacterial overgrowth. Given the fact that alcoholic fatty liver disease involves the same disease process as non-alcoholic fatty liver disease (NAFLD), it is not surprising that an internal production of alcohol by dysbiotic microorganisms is involved in NAFLD.

Gluten sensitivity, or the more advanced celiac disease, may also contribute to the development of NAFLD, again by way of leaky gut syndrome, in a similar way as dysbiosis. Gluten sensitivity involves the inability of the body to completely digest gluten. The body becomes sensitive to the gliadin protein, a component of gluten. This sensitivity involves an immune response against the gliadin, resulting in inflammation inside the intestine. This inflammation destroys the lining of the intestine, creating a leaky gut. The partially digested gluten can then enter the bloodstream through the leaky gut, and the inflammatory immune response continues in the bloodstream and into the liver where liver damage occurs as a result of inflammation.[24]

Liver abnormalities are common in people with celiac disease—over 40 percent have increased blood levels of the liver enzyme transaminase.[25] This is a common finding in NAFLD and other liver diseases. In patients with celiac disease who follow a gluten-free diet, these enzyme levels return to normal. Within a year of following a gluten-free diet, 75 to 95 percent of patients with celiac disease were found with normalized liver enzyme levels.[26] Even in severe liver disease, a gluten-free diet has been shown to prevent liver failure.[27]

In addition, milk allergy can also cause liver damage by way of a leaky gut.[28] It may be that the most important part of these processes is the leaky gut, since it allows the entrance of excess toxins into the liver. Maintaining a healthy intestinal lining is a critical part of supporting liver health.

Poor diet is also involved in the development of NAFLD. This is illustrated by the fact that obesity and insulin resistance, both largely due to poor diet, are main factors contributing to NAFLD. But poor diet may be a factor even if obesity or insulin resistance are not taken into account. For example, a diet which included a high intake of meat and soft drinks and a low intake of omega-3 fats was found in NAFLD patients, even with normal body mass index (BMI).[29]

Like the endotoxins produced in the gut, toxins that are ingested (exotoxins) also adversely affect the liver. The liver functions to detoxify and rid the body of toxins. When the liver is overburdened, whether from an excessive amount of toxins or from a buildup of fat and the ensuing inflammation, the function of the liver becomes compromised. Humans encounter many more environmental toxins on a daily basis than they did in the past, so the liver is working harder than ever. Lessening this toxic burden is an important step in supporting optimal liver health.

Certain medications may cause NAFLD. Some of these include:[30]

- Glucocorticoids (steroids)
- Synthetic estrogen
- Aspirin
- Amiodarone
- Tamoxifen
- Tetracycline
- Methotrexate
- Perhexiline maleate
- Antiviral agents

Family history of diabetes or NAFLD may be found in NAFLD patients. Where specific genes are concerned, certain gene polymorphisms are thought to be associated with the progression of fatty liver to NASH.[31] This is currently being studied. Environmental influences seem to play the major role in NAFLD development, however.

What Are the Signs and Symptoms?

In most people, NAFLD does not move past the fatty liver stage, which is usually not associated with any symptoms. However, some people do experience the following symptoms:

- Fatigue
- Weight loss
- Upper right abdominal pain or discomfort

How Is It Diagnosed?

Tests used to help diagnose NAFLD include:

- Blood tests – liver function tests, and to rule out viral hepatitis
- Imaging tests – ultrasound, CT scan, MRI
- Liver biopsy – tissue sample of liver

Since there are no specific tests for NAFLD, diagnosis is partially based on the exclusion of other liver diseases.[34] Liver function abnormalities, particularly increased transaminase levels, are the first sign of NAFLD, but further testing is needed to confirm NAFLD because increased transaminase levels may be found in other liver diseases, and normal transaminase levels can be found in NAFLD.[35] Ultrasound is usually the next step because it is a relatively harmless test which can show liver fat accumulation. CT scan or MRI may be preferred in some cases, however. The liver biopsy is the best test for confirming NAFLD. It can also detect the severity of the disease.[36]

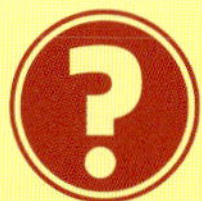

Did You Know

It is estimated that NAFLD affects 24 percent of Americans, almost five percent of children[32] and 65 percent of those over age 65.[33]

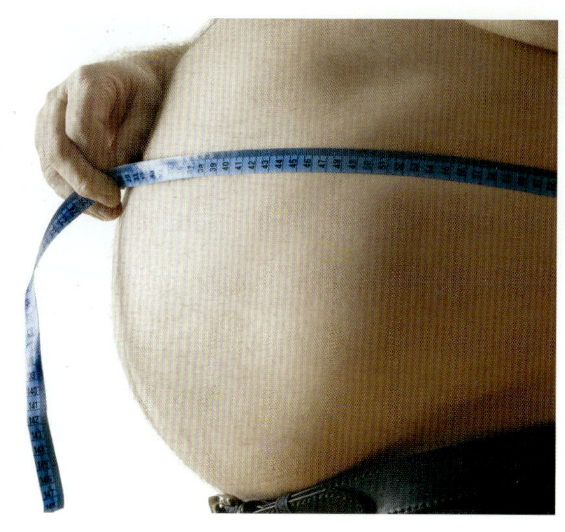

Natural health practitioners may also suggest a comprehensive stool analysis (CSA) (see the Appendix), helpful to determine underlying causes of fatty liver such as bacterial imbalance, fungal infection or yeast overgrowth.

What Is the Standard Medical Treatment?

There is really no standard treatment for NAFLD. Treatment depends on the contributing factors for the individual patient. The following recommendations are made according to the patient's history:

- Lose weight – when obesity is a factor
- Healthy diet – this is recommended for everyone
- Exercise – to encourage overall health
- Control diabetes – when diabetes is a factor
- Avoid toxins – this will help to protect the liver and is recommended for everyone

In overweight and obese people, gradual weight loss can help to reduce liver enzyme levels and insulin levels.[37] Rapid weight loss, however, can be detrimental, as it may worsen liver disease.

Drugs may be prescribed depending on what factors underlie each patient's NAFLD. Medications to treat insulin resistance may be prescribed, as well as medications for lowering triglycerides or cholesterol.

In the most severe of cases, liver transplant may be necessary, but, even in these cases, NAFLD may develop in the transplanted liver.[38]

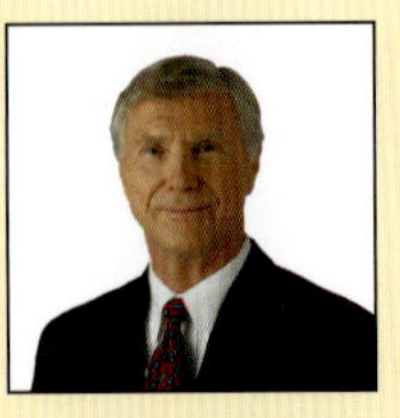

Dr. Smith's Comments

There are approximately 70 million Americans with NAFLD (non-alcoholic fatty liver disease) and about 20 percent of them have NASH (non-alcoholic steatohepatitis) which translates into about 14 million Americans who will likely end up with cirrhosis due to chronic liver inflammation leading to either liver transplant or death. These conditions are already at epidemic proportions, and will bankrupt the country and overload the operating rooms if we don't change our diet, sleep and exercise, improve elimination, and decrease stress and toxic exposures.

It is interesting that the medical profession has chosen to call fat in the liver NAFLD or NASH (NAFLD often progresses to NASH). I guess it is nice to know alcohol doesn't have anything to do with it, since that creates enough problems on its own. However, the diet that creates NAFLD/NASH can be as dangerous as too much alcohol. An acronym that would better state the truth would be BDBBTLSFLD. I know it's a little long, but it tells it like it is: Bad Diet, Bad Bacteria, Terrible Life Style, Fatty Liver Disease (Bad Diet Disease for short). Bad Diet Disease includes too much of the following: saturated and trans fats, simple carbs such as: white pasta, bread, cereal, excess sugar (it's in everything), liquid sugars in soft drinks, sugar- and fat-loaded coffee, junk snack foods, candies and desserts loaded with high fructose corn syrup. Remember that your mitochondria breathe in your oxygen to make ATP for you, which is your energy currency. If you choose to eat a diet with excess saturated fats, your mitochondria are likely to make excess hydrogen peroxide and damage themselves, thereby knocking out your own energy and your ability to function normally or to repair anything.[39]

We would be remiss in our Bad Diet list to not also include pesticides/herbicides (atrazine), plastics (bisphenol A), flavorings, food additives, and genetically modified (GM) foods. This would be the short list. To see the rest of the list, visit the middle 70 percent of the aisles of most any grocery store laden with tasty non-foods and drinks. It is usually the periphery of the store that contains real food like vegetables, sprouts, fruits, meats, seafood, eggs, dairy, seeds, nuts and whole grains. Unfortunately, unless you go to a local health food store, you could still be in danger of eating mostly GMO foods and minimal organic foods. I think we are at a time when people will choose to live near stores supplying organic foods.

The Bad Diet is one of the best ways to increase total body inflammation which, in turn, promotes fat storage. Fat produces at least 10 hormones which are released and cause more inflammation, creating a vicious cycle that promotes further fat storage. When fat storage is excessive, it may first fill the fat cells (adipocytes) under the skin in the abdominal cavity. The extra fat in the blood (in the form of free fatty acids) can then be stored in cells of the muscles, pancreas, heart, blood vessel walls, and liver. Fat in these cells may seriously disrupt normal function, which is known as lipotoxicity.
In other words, high blood levels of free fatty acids

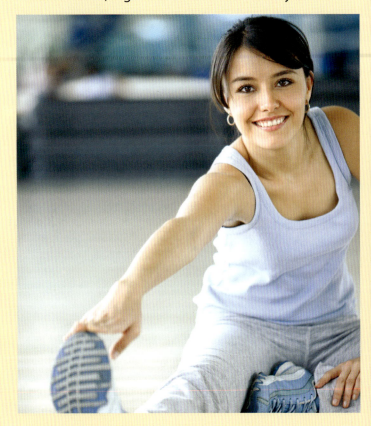

are converted into increased intracellular triglycerides that crowd the cell and create chronic cellular dysfunction and injury. This process can account for many manifestations of the metabolic syndrome,[40] which often leads to NAFLD.

Bad bacteria, or just too much bacteria, especially in the small bowel, is another major factor in increasing hepatic free radicals and inflammation leading to NAFLD/NASH. There are studies that have shown both increase in intestinal permeability and small intestinal bacterial overgrowth (SIBO) in patients with NAFLD and NASH.[41] Overgrowth of Candida and bacteria in the gut produces alcohol which is easily converted into acetaldehyde which travels from the gut to the liver through the portal vein and creates cellular changes like that seen with NAFLD.

Another bacterial connection involves eating a high-saturated-fat diet which causes the intestinal bacteria to release their cell wall lipopolysaccarides (LPS), as well as other endotoxins. Their first stop is the liver where they create inflammation, and then on to the entire circulation where they create endothelial dysfunction (blood vessel wall dysfunction, and leaking), creating the so called "leaky vessel" syndrome.

As one might expect, treating with probiotics has been shown to improve NAFLD and lower NF-kB activity (major nuclear transcription factor for inflammation) after four weeks of therapy.[42]

Early diagnosis and treating people with the correct diet and lifestyle changes is essential. In addition to being overweight with a large belly (waist/hip ratio less than 0.8 for women and 0.9 for men), an abdominal ultrasound or an MRI spectroscopy will usually make the diagnosis of fat in the liver. The blood tests include: cholesterol/HDL, triglyceride/HDL, and apo B/apo A-I ratios. These ratios give a clearer view of the overall lipid status of the patient, and serve as tools to monitor progress with diet and lifestyle changes. The lifestyle changes include exercise, stress reduction, sleep, proper elimination, appropriate supplementation with extra antioxidants, and detoxification. These will be essential if we are to reverse this epidemic.

Since some people may not be clearly overweight, and many overweight people may not have NAFLD/NASH, it is important to do the blood tests and check the blood pressure for early signs of the conditions. The pattern follows closely to that of metabolic syndrome and type 2 diabetes with: high blood pressure, abdominal obesity, high cholesterol, high triglyceride, high LDL, low HDL, lipoprotein imbalances, and elevated blood sugar and/or insulin levels.

As soon as it is apparent that the patient is headed toward metabolic syndrome or NAFLD/NASH, the diet should be changed. There is data to support the DASH diet or the Mediterranean diet, which includes: vegetables, whole fruit, whole unprocessed grains, legumes, low sodium foods, lean cuts of meat and fish, and increased omega-3 fatty acid intake and olive oil. This diet alone may reverse the problem if done early enough. The HOPE program also plays an important part here with high fiber, essential oils with the right balance of omega-6/omega-3, probiotics, and enzymes. Omega-3 and 6 fats help to remove liver fat through speeding up metabolism.

However, if the person waits too long, and has gone too far with advanced metabolic syndrome, and dangerous levels of NAFLD/NASH, pharmaceutical drugs or gastric bypass will be necessary to prevent progression to cirrhosis.

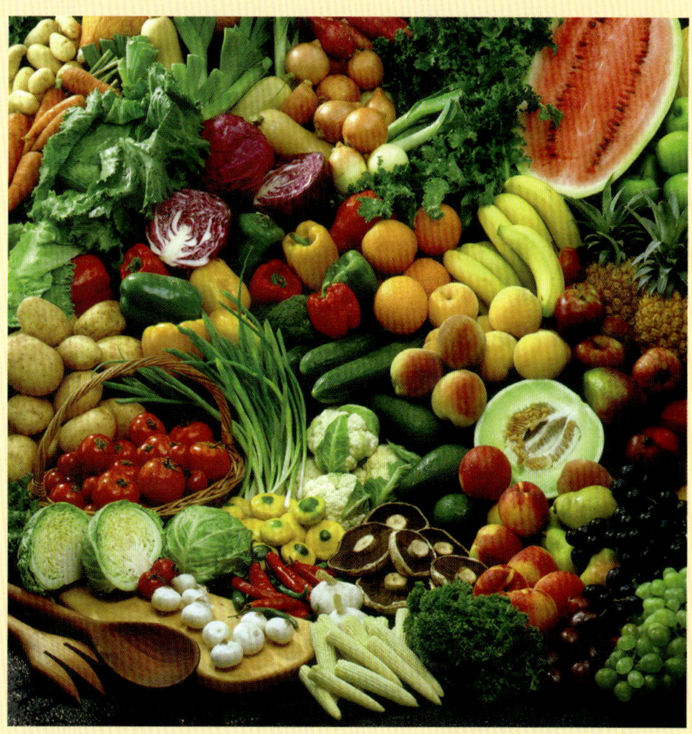

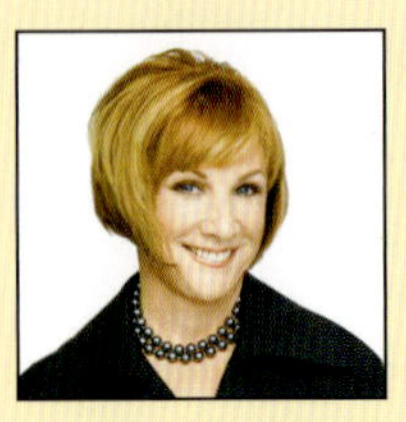

Brenda's Bottom Line

In my experience, people who have fatty liver also have a major Candida overgrowth that compromises the liver. This gut imbalance created by Candida overgrowth results in an overburdened liver because toxins from the gut are transported directly to the liver. I strongly recommend that everyone with this condition follow a complete cleansing program that includes a Candida cleanse, in addition to eating a Candida diet for three to six months. (See the Appendix for more information.)

Fatty liver is one of the gateway conditions between digestive function and other conditions like metabolic syndrome, diabetes and cardiovascular disease. The good news is that this condition can be reversed. Correcting any digestive dysfunction through diet and supplementation, and maintaining a healthy weight through exercise and lifestyle changes, can go a long way to healing fatty liver, and, thus, preventing these more serious health conditions.

Recommended Testing

- Comprehensive stool analysis (CSA) (See the Appendix.)

Diet

- Follow the Candida Diet (see the Appendix) for three to six months.
- Next, follow the Fiber 35 Eating Plan. (See the Appendix.) Include plenty of fruits and vegetables.
- Watch protein intake (especially animal sources) if ammonia levels are high. If you do eat animal protein, limit to small quantities of poultry and fish.
- Watch fats, especially fried foods, saturated and trans fats. If the liver is too damaged, it may not be able to handle fat-soluble vitamins like A, D, E and K, except in small amounts.
- Keep refined carbohydrates (sugar, white bread, white pasta, white rice, etc.) out of the diet. Carbohydrate consumption should be in the form of vegetables and whole grains.
- Do not overeat. Eat small meals more frequently.
- Do not consume alcohol (most important!).

Lifestyle

- Medications can be stressful for the liver. Take with caution.
- Do not become constipated. Use the LifeStep (see Resource Directory) for proper elimination posture.
- Do not smoke, and avoid second-hand smoke.
- Clean up your environment, as all chemicals and toxins can affect liver function.

Complementary Mind / Body Therapies

- Stress can be a major component of this disease, so find ways to reduce it with therapies such as meditation, yoga, deep breathing, massage, biofeedback, or music therapy.
- Colon hydrotherapy is beneficial to remove toxins.

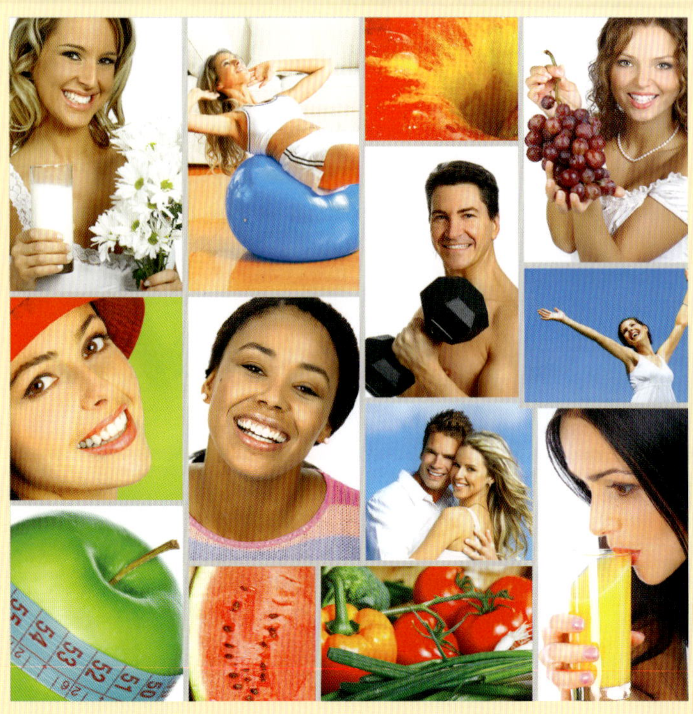

Recommended Nutraceuticals	Dosage	Benefit	Comments
Critical Phase	Daily maintenance recommendations should also be taken during this phase unless otherwise indicated.		
Total Body Cleanse	See Appendix	Encourages elimination and detoxification.	Herbal formula should support the seven channels of elimination.
Liver Detox	This should follow the Total Body Cleanse. See Appendix	Encourages detoxification involving the liver.	Should contain milk thistle seed extract containing silymarin, phosphatidylcholine, selenium and herbs.
Helpful			
SAMe	180 mg daily	Helps improve liver function.	Do not use if you have bipolar disorder or are taking antidepressants.
L-Glutamine Powder with Gamma Oryzanol	5 grams twice daily	Essential for maintaining the health and integrity of the intestinal lining.	Added gamma oryzanol may help relieve pain associated with gastrointestinal complaints.
High Potency Multi-vitamin/mineral	Follow directions on label	Provides needed nutrients that may be deficient.	Powder or liquid formulation would be helpful as it is easier assimilated and absorbed.
Antioxidant Supplement	Use as directed	Protects tissue from damage.	You can purchase a high-potency antioxidant formulation from most health food stores.
Daily Maintenance			
Critical Liver Support Formula	Use as directed	Enhances liver detoxification.	Should include milk thistle seed extract containing silymarin, N-acetyl-cysteine, alpha lipoic acid and L-glutathione.
Fiber	4-5 grams twice daily	Helps produce healthy bacteria levels and good elimination.	Use in conjunction with high fiber diet to reach 35g daily.
Digestive Enzymes	Take with meals	Helps digest and absorb nutrients from food to reduce liver stress.	If low stomach acid is found, find a formula that contains hydrochloric acid.
Omega-3 Fatty Acids	At least 2 grams daily of EPA/DHA combination	Reduces inflammation.	Look for a concentrated, enteric coated fish oil.
Probiotics	30 - 80 billion culture count twice daily	Restores bacterial balance and pH of colon and promotes regularity.	Look for high amount of bifidobacteria, the main beneficial bacteria in colon.

See further explanation of supplements in the Appendix

Pancreatitis

What Is It?

The pancreas is a large gland located behind the stomach and close to the duodenum (upper portion of the small intestine). Pancreatitis involves inflammation of this gland. When functioning properly, the pancreas secretes digestive enzymes (exocrine function) and releases the hormones glucagon and insulin, which regulate blood sugar levels (endocrine function). Pancreatitis primarily affects the exocrine pancreas, but, in severe chronic cases, the endrocrine pancreas may also be affected.

There are two types of pancreatitis: acute and chronic. The onset of symptoms is sudden in acute pancreatitis and, while the attack may be severe, or even life-threatening, recovery is usually complete without permanent damage to the pancreas. Chronic pancreatitis, on the other hand, involves continuous low-grade persistent inflammation and scarring of the gland, resulting in permanent damage and impaired pancreatic function.

The enzymes produced by the pancreas serve the purpose of breaking down food into its component parts. Lipase breaks fat down into fatty acids; amylase breaks carbohydrates down into glucose; and protease splits proteins into amino acids. These powerful digestive enzymes normally become active only within the cavity (lumen) of the bowel, where they are sealed off from the rest of the body.[1] However, in pancreatitis, a process of auto-digestion occurs as pancreatic enzymes are activated within the gland itself, and leak out into adjacent tissue causing severe tissue damage.

What Causes It?

Alcoholism, alcohol abuse, gallstones or other gallbladder diseases are the major causes of pancreatitis. Gallstones may be able to block the flow of pancreatic juice from the pancreatic duct, trapping digestive enzymes in the pancreas. The result is inflammation of the gland and leakage of enzymes. Over-consumption of alcohol can result in premature activation of pancreatic enzymes.

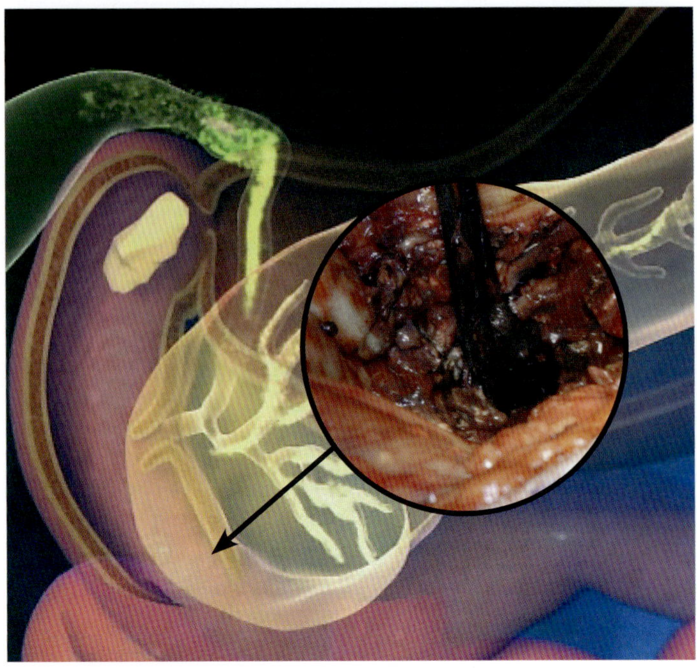

Endoscopic image of diseased pancreas

Other causes and factors contributing to pancreatitis may include:

- Viral infection (hepatitis A or D, Epstein-Barr virus, mumps, coxsackie B, mycoplasma pneumonia, Campylobacter)
- Hyperparathyroidism (metabolic disorder causing elevated levels of calcium in the blood)
- Hyperlipidemia (metabolic disorder involving high concentrations of fat circulating in the blood)
- Traumatic injury (or surgery) to the abdomen
- Excess iron in the blood
- Hypothermia (accidental exposure to low temperatures)
- Kidney transplants
- Certain medications
- Leaky gut

Among the medications linked to pancreatitis are thiazide diuretics, antibiotics (sulfonamides, salazopyrine, tetracycline), high-dose estrogens, corticosteroids, several immunosuppressive drugs, azathioprine, divalproex and the chemotherapy drug 6-MP.[2-4]

In children, pancreatitis may be associated with some of the factors listed above (mumps, abdominal trauma, viral illnesses and medications), as well as cystic fibrosis, hemolytic uremic syndrome, Kawasaki disease and Reye's syndrome.[5] In some cases of pancreatitis, the cause is unknown.

Pancreatitis is most likely to affect alcoholics, people who abuse alcohol and people with gallstones and other gallbladder problems. Those suffering from the conditions listed above or taking the drugs listed above are also at increased risk for developing the disease. Also at increased risk are women with a history of several pregnancies, and people who go on crash diets.[6]

Pancreatitis affects more men than women, presumably due to the fact that more men abuse alcohol. Onset of symptoms usually occurs between the ages of 30 and 40.[7] In some cases, the disease may be inherited.[8]

Leaky gut, or intestinal permeability, may be an underlying feature of pancreatitis. Leaky gut has been associated with an increase in bacterial toxins, organ failure and even death in people with acute pancreatitis.[9] Because leaky gut leads to an increase of toxins in the bloodstream, it is very important to heal the intestines. (See the Leaky Gut Syndrome section for more information on this condition.)

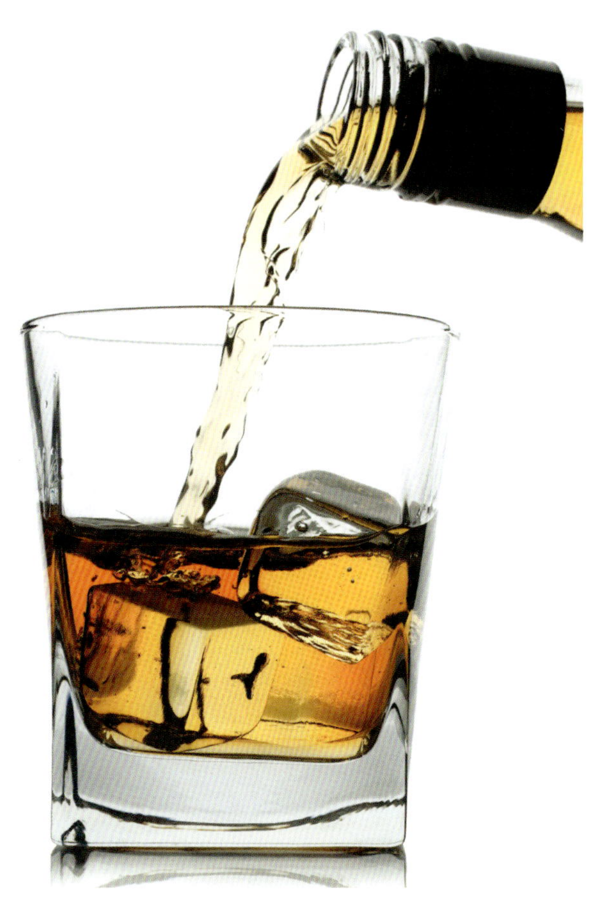

What Are the Signs and Symptoms?

The most prominent symptom of acute pancreatitis is pain above the naval that may spread across the abdomen and to the back. The pain of acute pancreatitis often comes on suddenly and intensely, but it may be mild in the beginning and gradually increase in severity. It is usually worse when lying down or moving, and tends to diminish upon sitting up and leaning forward. Other symptoms of acute pancreatitis may include:

- Nausea/vomiting
- Fever
- Mild jaundice (yellow tint to skin and whites of the eyes)
- Fatty (clay-colored) stools
- Anxiety
- Chills
- Sweating
- Weakness
- Abdominal swelling/gas
- Increased pulse rate

The symptoms of chronic pancreatitis may be similar to those of pancreatic cancer, and indeed pancreatitis can lead to pancreatic cancer.

Symptoms of chronic pancreatitis are much the same as those of the acute variety, except for the fact that some level of pain tends to linger, interspersed with episodes of acute pain. In some rare cases of chronic pancreatitis, pain may be entirely absent. It is possible that pain may disappear as the condition advances, and the pancreas loses its ability to make enzymes. Repeated episodes of gallbladder infection and gallstones are often involved in chronic pancreatitis.

Complications of acute pancreatitis may include the following:[10]

- Low blood pressure
- Heart failure
- Kidney failure
- ARDS (adult respiratory distress syndrome)
- Ascites (accumulation of fluid in the abdomen)
- Cysts or abscesses in the pancreas

Did You Know

- Pancreatitis affects approximately 50,000 to 80,000 people in the United States each year, and is a common reason for people to be admitted to the hospital.
- In about 30 percent of cases, no cause can be found.
- Approximately 10 percent of patients with alcohol-related acute pancreatitis develop chronic pancreatitis.
- Pancreatitis caused by heavy drinking is likely to recur if drinking continues.

Complications of chronic pancreatitis may include:[11]

- Obstruction of the small intestine or bile duct
- Pancreatic insufficiency, leading to diabetes (from damage to insulin-producing cells in the pancreas)
- Fat malabsorption (and accompanying weight loss)
- Ascites
- Pancreatic pseudocysts (fluid collections), which may become infected
- Blood clots in the splenic (related to the spleen) vein
- Pancreatic cancer

Severe cases of pancreatitis can involve bleeding into the pancreas (leading to shock and sometimes death), dehydration, infection, cysts, and serious tissue and organ damage as enzymes and toxins enter the bloodstream.

How Is It Diagnosed?

Blood tests may be done to identify abnormal enzyme levels. Blood levels of the carbohydrate-digesting enzyme amylase may be elevated in pancreatitis as a result of leakage of the enzyme into the blood when the gland is inflamed. Blood levels of the fat-digesting enzyme lipase may likewise be elevated, while trypsinogen levels may be low. Pancreas function tests may be ordered to confirm the diagnosis of pancreatitis. Evidence of malabsorption may be found through a test for fecal fat. Changes in blood levels of calcium, magnesium, potassium, sodium and bicarbonate are typically seen with pancreatitis, as are elevated sugar and fat levels in the blood.

Abdominal X-rays, ultrasound, or CT scan may also be performed to provide images of the upper abdomen. These tests may show inflammation and swelling, as well as reveal gallstones and obstruction of bile flow, if present. Endoscopic retrograde cholangio-pancreatography (ERCP) is a procedure done under anesthesia that uses a gastroduodenal endoscope with special dye-injecting capabilities. The endoscope is placed through the mouth, esophagus, stomach, and into the duodenum. The tip of the scope is then placed into the opening of the common bile duct and pancreas duct (just inside the ampulla of Vater) in the duodenum. Next, dye is injected into the ducts and pictures are taken to show the anatomy of the bile and pancreatic ducts and their branches. This can be very helpful in finding stones, strictures (narrowed areas), leaks and even cancer. The endoscopist can then simultaneously use the scope to remove stones, dilate strictures, and place either permanent or temporary stents in the ducts to control damaged areas that demonstrate leaks. The risks of ERCP include anesthesia, bleeding, and pancreatitis in about five percent of the cases.

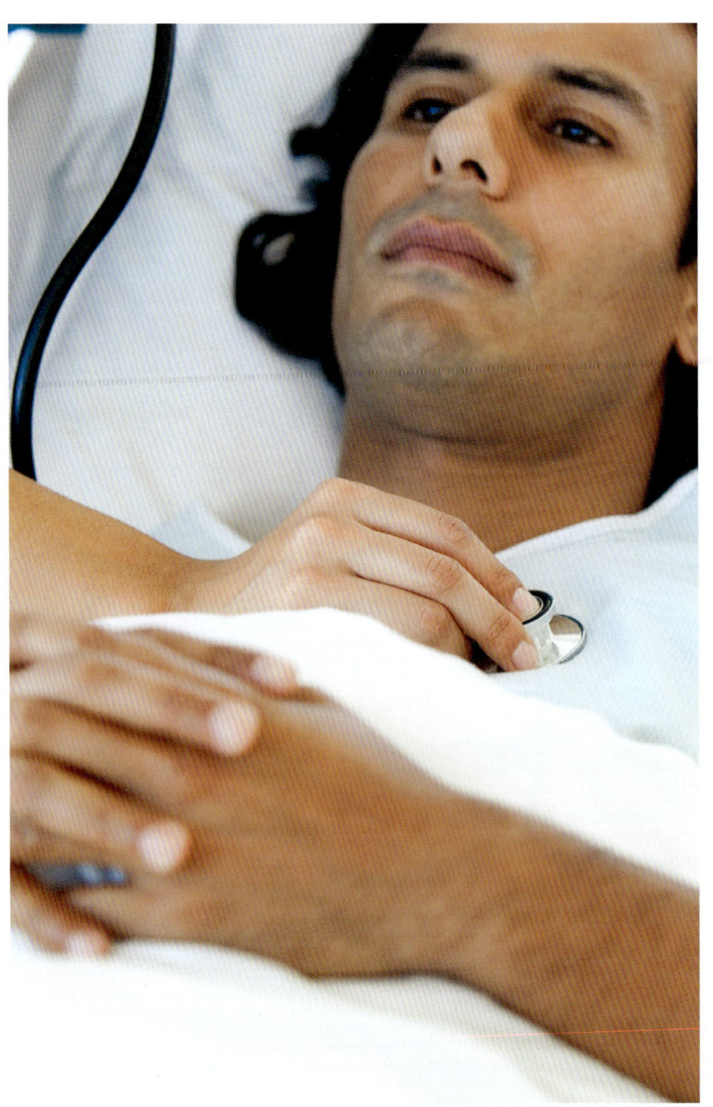

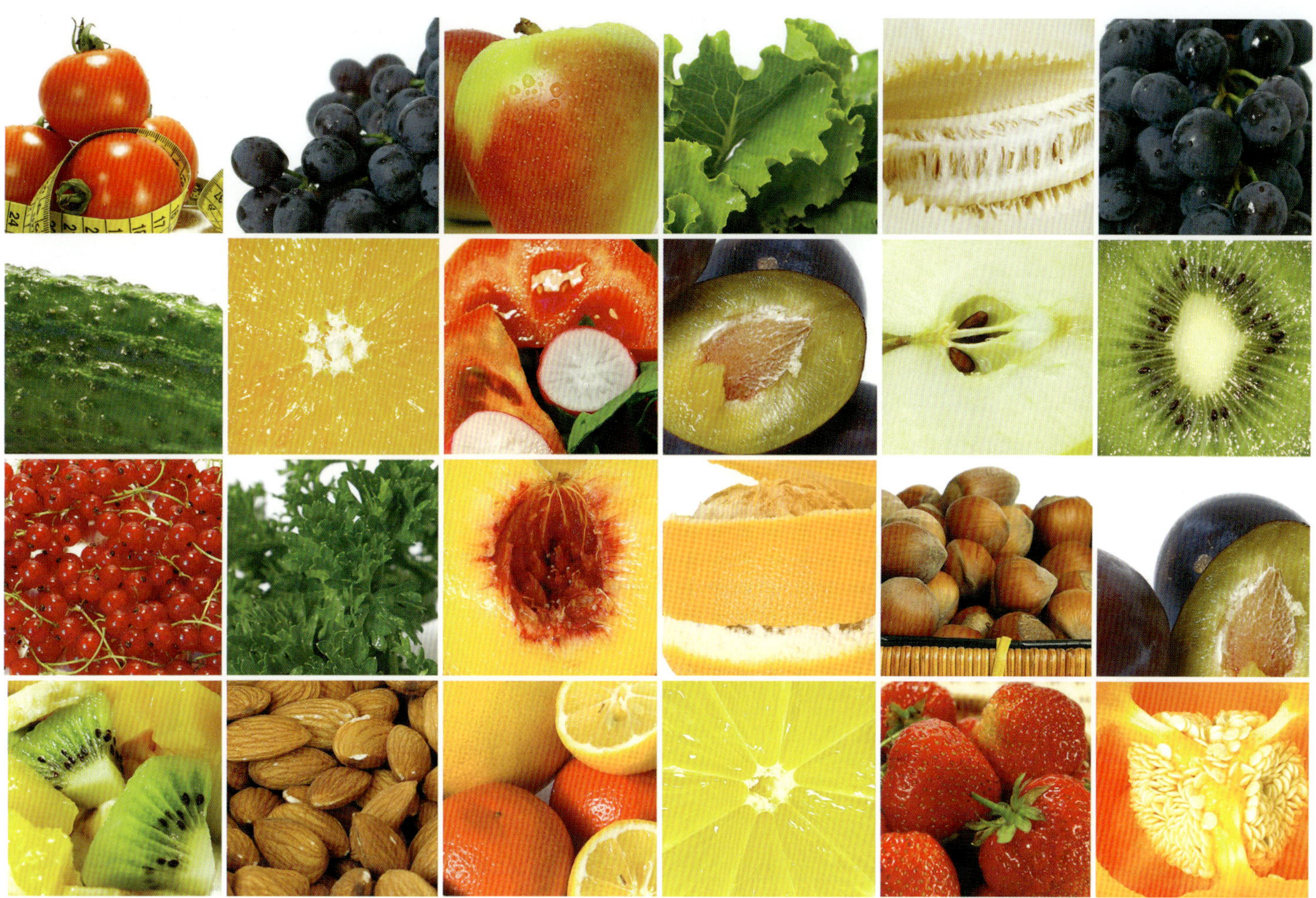

Another noninvasive option is the use of magnetic resonance cholangio-pancreatography (MRCP). With this noninvasive, awake procedure, the patient drinks contrast material, and magnetic resonance imaging (MRI) is done over the upper abdomen. The information obtained with MRCP is considered to be as accurate as ERCP, but with less danger.

In either case, when the information is obtained regarding stones, strictures, or leaks of the ducts, it is a great medical advance that these problems may now be solved endoscopically rather than with major surgery.

In fact, the whole approach to pancreatitis has been revolutionized by this approach. Today, a patient with pancreatitis will likely undergo imaging studies which may show a leak in the main pancreatic duct. If this is the case, the endoscopist could place a stent in the pancreatic duct, which could block the leak, and still allow pancreatic juice to flow into the duodenum. This procedure prevents the leaking pancreatic juice from damaging adjacent structures, and speeds healing and recovery from pancreatitis as well.

What Is the Standard Medical Treatment?

An attack of pancreatitis will typically last only a few days, though it can last much longer. The patient is typically hospitalized, and, in an effort to rest the pancreas, no food will be given by mouth for a few days in mild cases. Circulation will be supported with intravenous fluids. In severe cases, IV feeding may be necessary for three to six weeks while the pancreas heals.

For chronic pancreatitis, analgesics or nerve blocks will likely be used for pain relief rather than risk use of potentially addictive narcotics. High doses of pancreatic enzymes may also help control pain by reducing the secretion of juices from the pancreas. These exogenous enzymes will help rest the pancreas, and also correct its underproduction of enzymes assisting the body in digestion of food once a normal diet is resumed. Pancreatic extract may also be used in the long term. It can help correct greasy stools and weight loss resulting from underproduction of digestive enzymes and malabsorption of fat. If gallstones are blocking ducts, the gallbladder will likely be removed.

In severe cases, or if complications such as infection, cysts, or bleeding occur, surgical intervention may be necessary. Surgery will be necessary to drain the pancreas if it is infected or necrotic. If diabetes has developed, blood sugar levels will be controlled with insulin. Dietary and lifestyle modifications may be recommended. These typically include:

- No alcohol
- No smoking
- Reduction of fat in the diet
- Reduction of sugar in the diet
- Correction of underlying disorders (such as gallbladder disease and metabolic disorders)
- No large meals
- Use of digestive enzyme supplements

By adhering to the above recommendations, most patients with acute pancreatitis will be able to prevent it from becoming chronic. Additional measures, such as supplementation with antioxidant nutrients, may also assist toward this end.

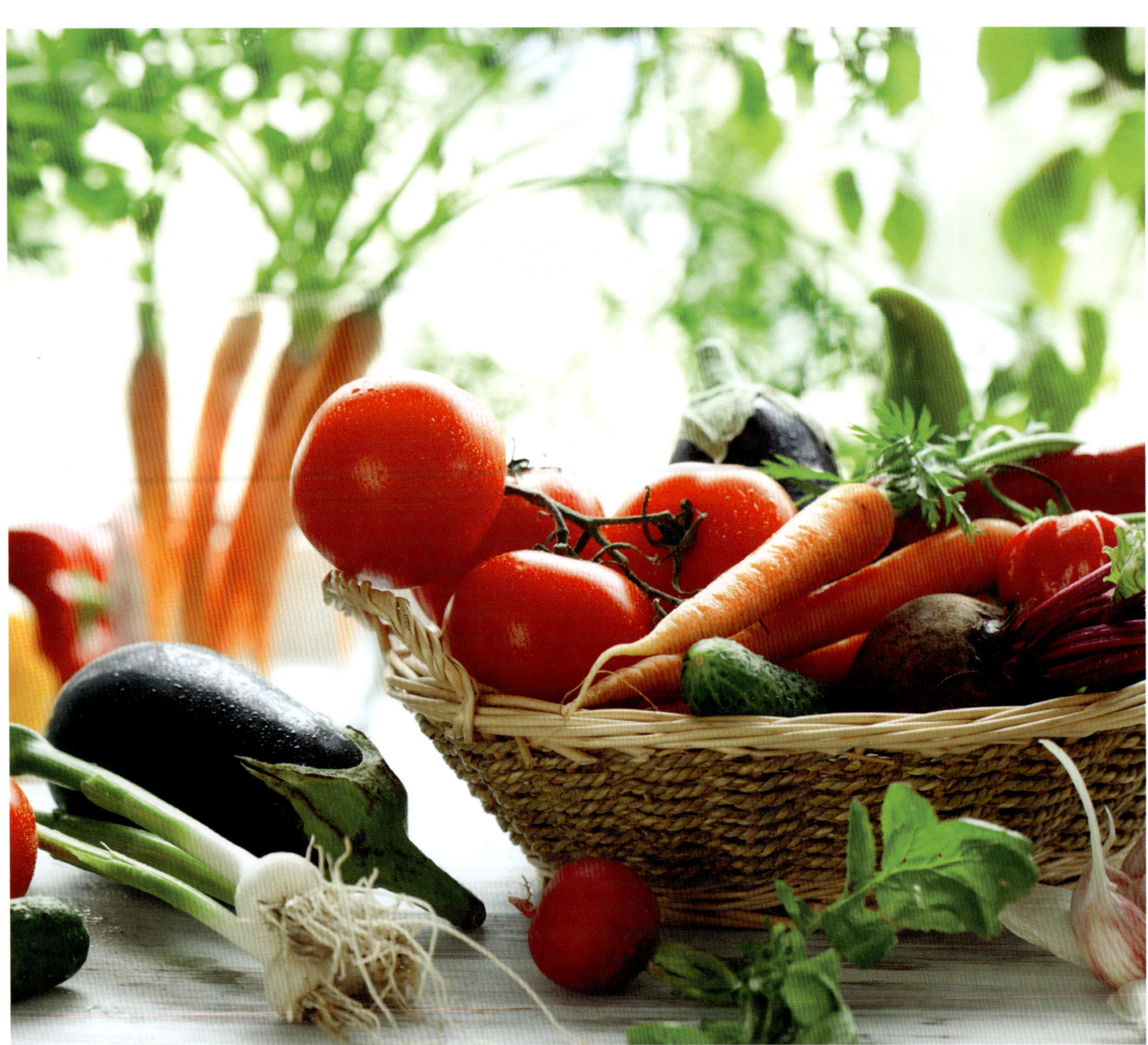

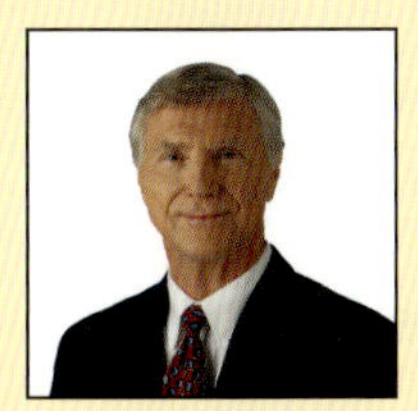

Dr. Smith's Comments

I have occasionally seen patients who had severe pancreatitis secondary to small gallstones that became lodged in the end of the common bile duct at the ampulla of Vater, which disrupts the flow of pancreatic juice, as well as bile. Usually patients recover within a few days and have the problem corrected with laporoscopic cholecystectomy. In some cases, however, the pancreatitis can be severe and even lead to death. This is one reason to consider cholecystectomy if there are multiple small stones.

Some patients are very sensitive to alcohol consumption, which is probably the major cause of pancreatitis. In some of these cases, there are genetic defects that do not allow for the production of inhibitory proteins, which keep the pancreas from prematurely releasing its enzymes. This would be like having too sensitive of a trigger on a gun. The inappropriate release of the enzymes can cause the pancreas to digest itself, ranging from a mild to fatal condition.

Autoimmune chronic pancreatitis has become an important clinical problem, and is easily confused with pancreatic cancer. This misdiagnosis can lead to removal of part or all of the pancreas instead of medical treatment with anti-inflammatory steroids.
This condition, again, can be due to auto-antibodies. Such antibodies are produced in response to unrecognized, partially digested food or microbial products from leaky gut syndrome. It is these auto-antibodies that cross react with pancreatic tissue (which they view as foreign tissue) and cause major damage to the pancreatic cells and ducts.

Finally, chronic pancreatitis can be due to toxic and/or infected bile washing into the pancreatic duct causing inflammation. It is easy to see, as mentioned before, that healing the leaky gut and liberal use of antioxidants and natural anti-inflammatories could be beneficial.

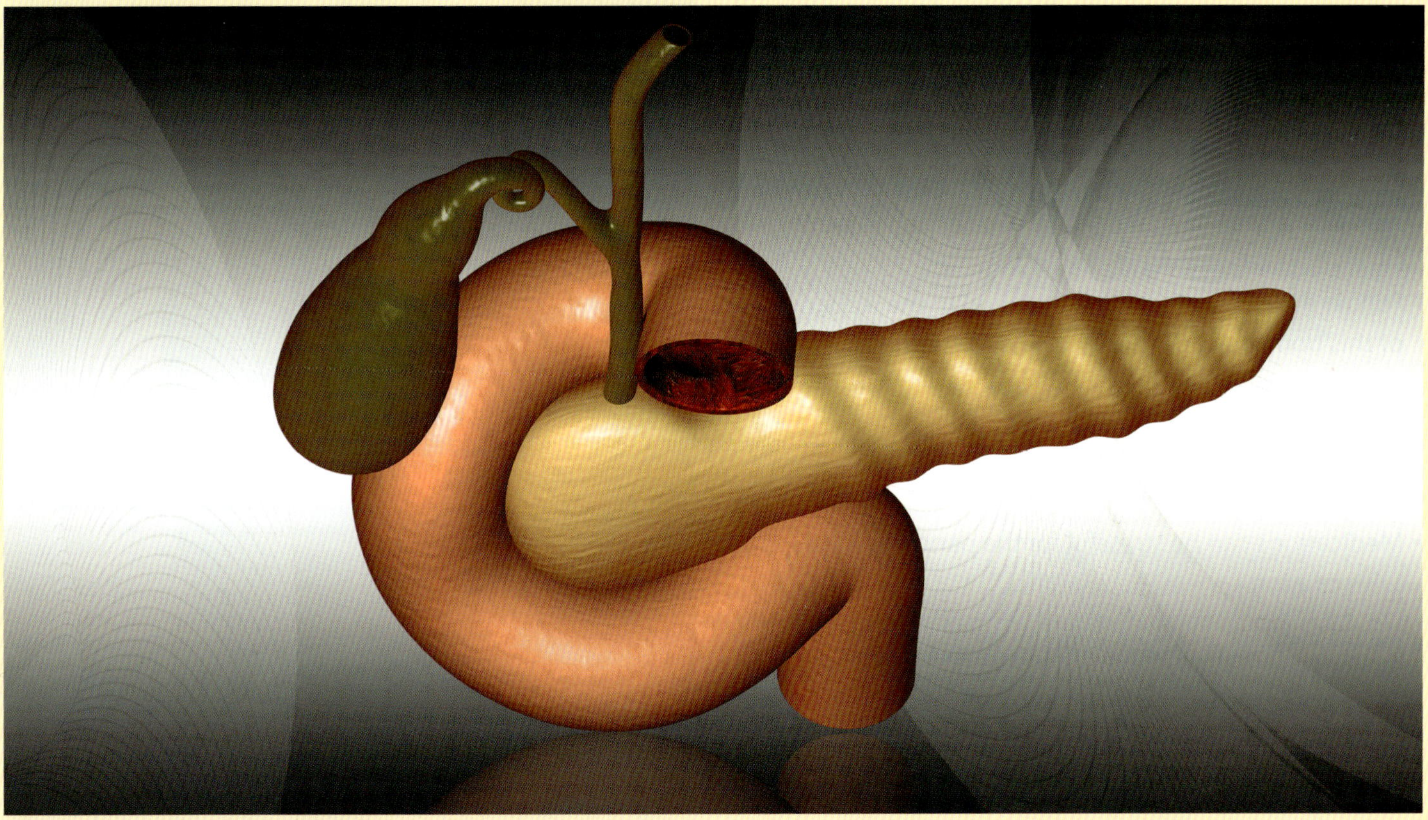

Illustration of pancreas and gallbladder

APPENDIX

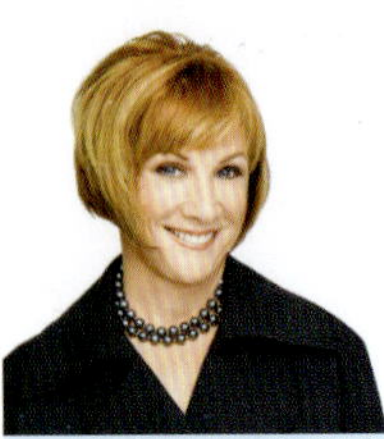

Recommended Testing

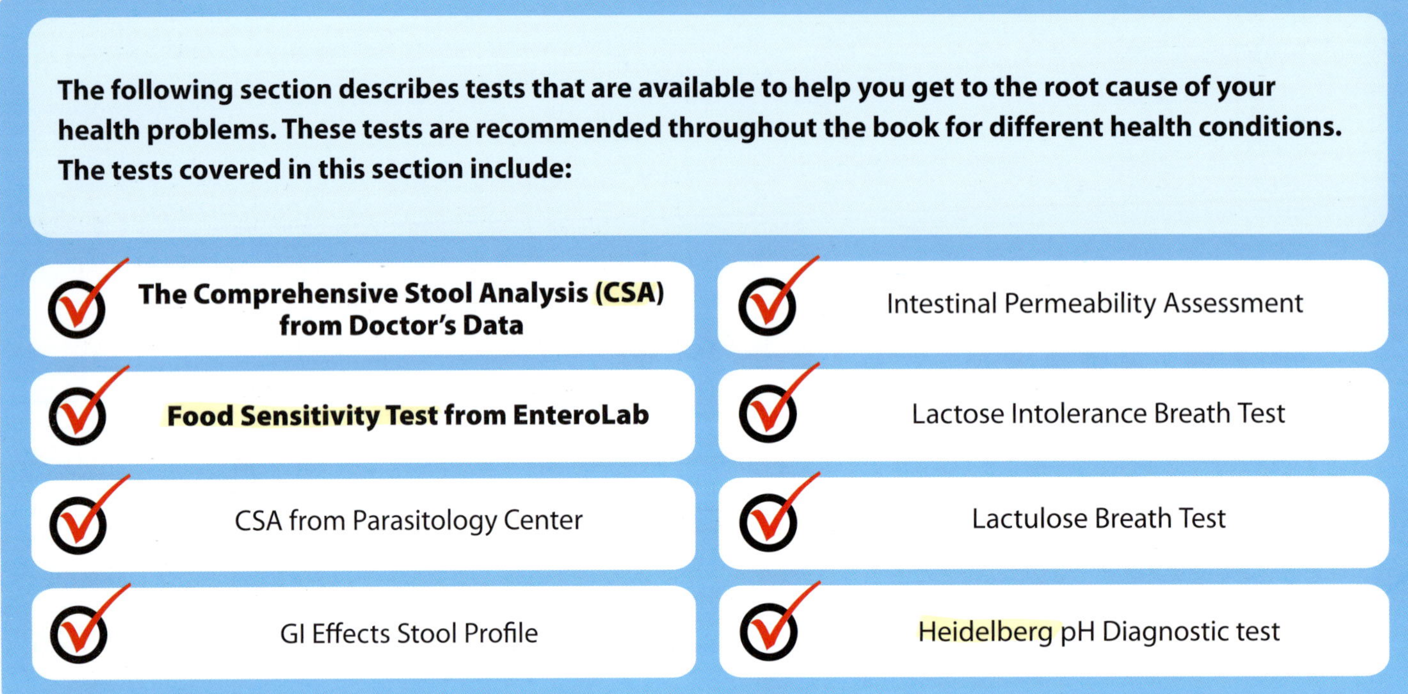

The following section describes tests that are available to help you get to the root cause of your health problems. These tests are recommended throughout the book for different health conditions. The tests covered in this section include:

- **The Comprehensive Stool Analysis (CSA) from Doctor's Data**
- **Food Sensitivity Test from EnteroLab**
- CSA from Parasitology Center
- GI Effects Stool Profile
- Intestinal Permeability Assessment
- Lactose Intolerance Breath Test
- Lactulose Breath Test
- Heidelberg pH Diagnostic test

Of these tests, I would like to highlight the first two, the Comprehensive Stool Analysis (CSA) from Doctor's Data, and the Food Sensitivity Test from EnteroLab. These two tests are critical to the reversal or management of all the conditions in this book.

The CSA is the test I use to determine what is going on in the gut. I would not hesitate to say this test would be helpful for anyone wishing to manage their health long-term, even if they have not exhibited symptoms of any kind. The CSA gives a good baseline picture of your health in a similar way as preventive blood work does. This test will show a gut imbalance even before symptoms develop. Because gut imbalance can lead to so many health conditions, correcting this imbalance is essential, even before health conditions arise. In cases where the person has already developed a health condition, this test is a must. This test will give you a picture of the health of your entire body. Each of the conditions in this book may begin with an imbalance in the gut.

It is amazing the amount of people who go to doctor after doctor with an enormous amount of testing and money spent without ever finding out what is wrong. The important part of my message, and the message in this book, is about looking to the gut first for the solution to your health problems, as well as preventively to keep yourself healthy for life.
When I consult with people who have chronic health challenges, I always request they do the CSA, as it provides a direct way for me to help them. This test takes away the guess work! When you address gut health, the pathway to healing the body just happens.

The second test I highly suggest for people struggling to find the answer to ANY health problem is the EnteroLab food sensitivity test. If there is anyone to thank for his/her work in this field, it is Dr. Fine at EnteroLab. Dr. Fine's work is saving the lives of many people, myself included. He has made it possible for people to go directly to the EnteroLab website to

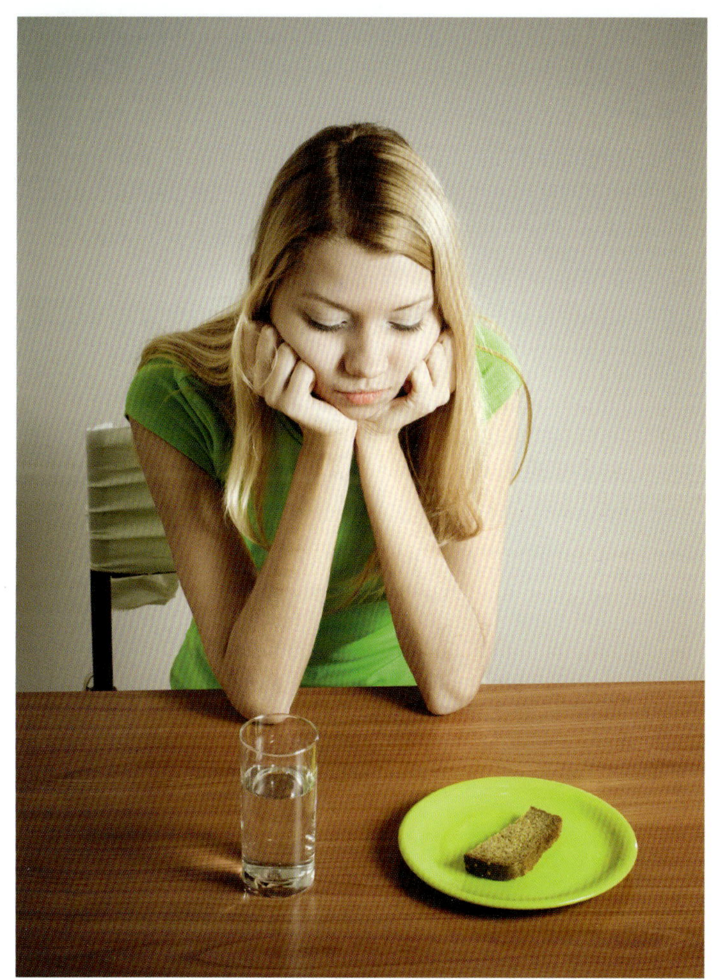

Food sensitivities are an underlying factor in many health conditions.

order the test directly. You can also have your genes tested to see if you are genetically predisposed to these food sensitivities. With many people I work with, I insist they take this test, which is critical to getting to the bottom of many disease conditions.

People often have chronic health problems due to the fact that the gut becomes out of balance. But what causes that imbalance? In many cases, food sensitivity. The most common food sensitivities are to gluten and dairy. Here is where allopathic medicine is missing the boat—a person can have an intolerance or sensitivity to gluten that has not yet progressed to celiac disease. A blood test is used to detect celiac disease, but the gluten reaction occurs in the intestine. Immune complexes will only be found in the blood after significant damage to the intestine has occured. Detecting food sensitivity before this damage occurs is key. That is why the stool sensitivity test is so important. This is a very hard concept to get across.

Many people suffer from chronic health problems due to the fact that they regularly consume foods that create an immune response in the gut that they may not feel directly, but that occurs daily. Over time this food reaction slowly creates an imbalance in the ratio of good to bad bacteria in the gut, creating inflammation and then leaky gut. The leaky gut proteins (from gluten or dairy) enter the bloodstream and circulate throughout the body, creating more inflammation and even autoimmunity.

Here is the best advice I can give anyone: Stop looking for the solutions to symptoms—look at your inner terrain. You will find the real source of health in your gut. Then you can heal from the inside out. Read on for more information about the the tests recommended throughout this book.

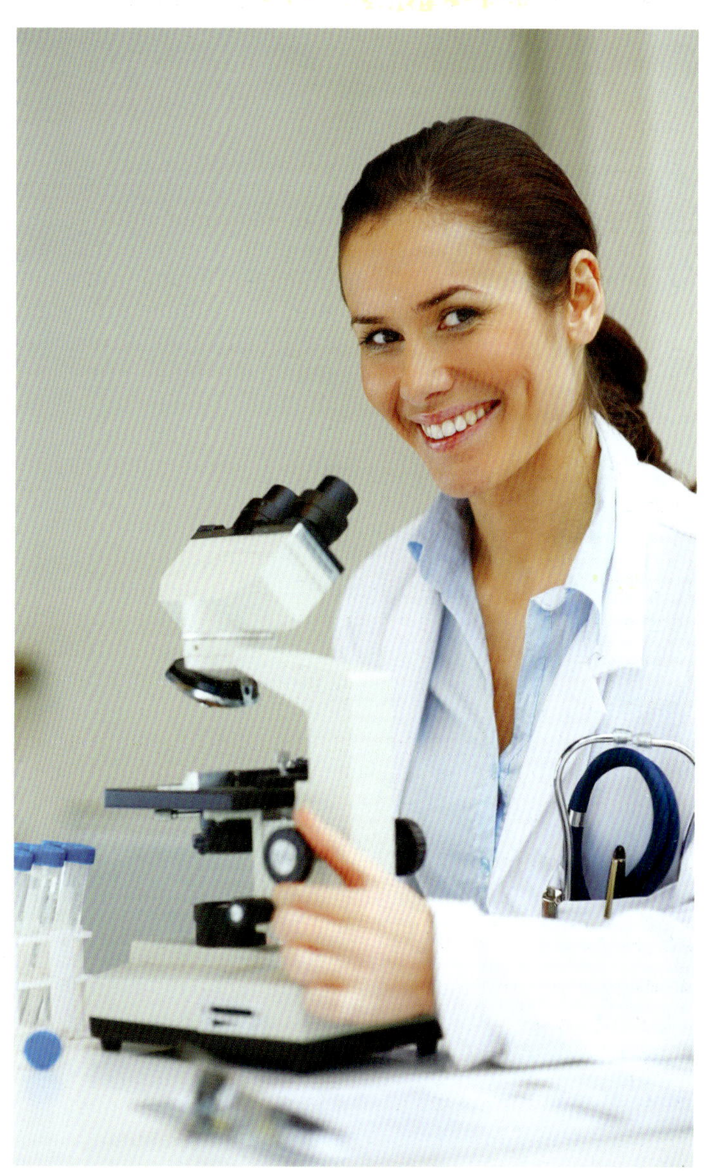

The Comprehensive Stool Analysis or CSA from Doctor's Data

(also available with Parasitology to detect parasites) The CSA is an invaluable noninvasive diagnostic assessment that permits practitioners to objectively evaluate the status of beneficial and imbalanced commensal microflora including Lactobacillus and Bifidobacterium species, Clostridium species, pathogenic bacteria, yeast/fungus and parasites.

Inflammation can significantly increase intestinal permeability and compromise assimilation of nutrients. The CSA determines the extent of inflammation, whether caused by pathogens or inflammatory bowel disease (IBD), and can be assessed and monitored by examination of the levels of biomarkers such as lysozyme, lactoferrin, white blood cells and mucus. These markers can be used to differentiate between inflammation associated with potentially life-threatening inflammatory bowel disease (IBD), which requires life-long treatment, and less severe inflammation that can be associated with the presence of invasive pathogens. Since the vast majority of secretory IgA (sIgA) is normally present in the GI tract where it prevents binding of pathogens and antigens to the mucosal membrane, it is essential to know the status of sIgA in the gut; sIgA is the only bona fide marker of humoral immune status in the GI tract.

The CSA also supplies information regarding the efficiency of digestion and absorption from the measurement of the fecal levels of elastase (pancreatic exocrine sufficiency), muscle and vegetable fibers, carbohydrates, and steatocrit (percent total fat).

The CSA is offered online at www.labtestingdirect.com The test kit is shipped directly to your home, and does not require a lab visit. A stool sample is sent to the lab, and results are mailed to your home.

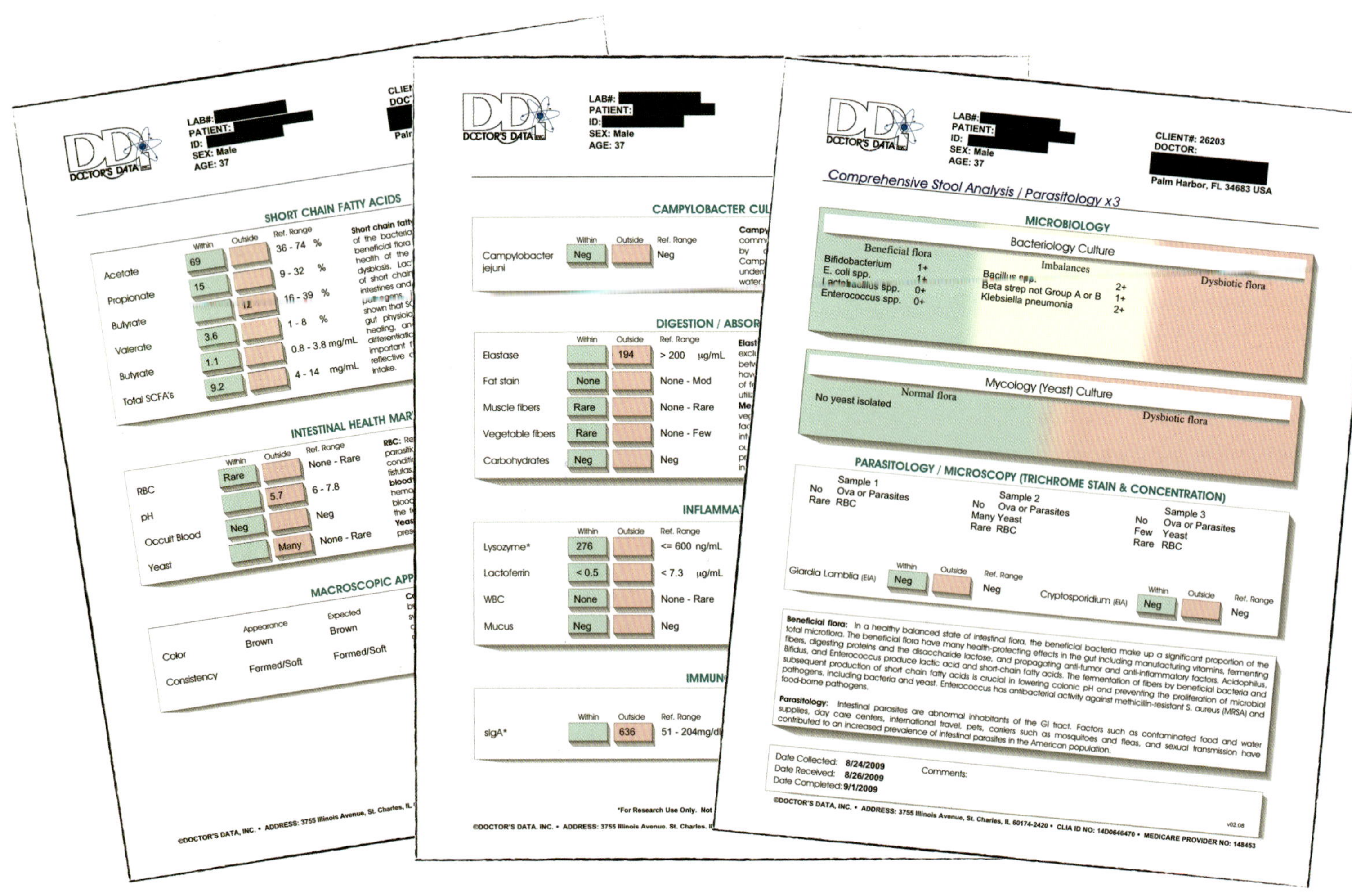

DOCTOR'S DATA
LAB#:
PATIENT:
ID:
SEX: Male
AGE: 37

SHORT CHAIN FATTY ACIDS

	Within	Outside	Ref. Range
Acetate	69		36 - 74 %
Propionate	15		9 - 32 %
Butyrate		12	16 - 39 %
Valerate	3.6		1 - 8 %
Butyrate	1.1		0.8 - 3.8 mg/mL
Total SCFA's	9.2		4 - 14 mg/mL

INTESTINAL HEALTH MAR

	Within	Outside	Ref. Range
RBC	Rare		None - Rare
pH		5.7	6 - 7.8
Occult Blood	Neg		Neg
Yeast		Many	None - Rare

MACROSCOPIC APP

	Appearance	Expected
Color	Brown	Brown
Consistency	Formed/Soft	Formed/Soft

©DOCTOR'S DATA, INC. • ADDRESS: 3755 Illinois Avenue, St. Charles, IL

DOCTOR'S DATA
LAB#:
PATIENT:
ID:
SEX: Male
AGE: 37

CAMPYLOBACTER CUL

	Within	Outside	Ref. Range
Campylobacter jejuni	Neg		Neg

DIGESTION / ABSOR

	Within	Outside	Ref. Range
Elastase		194	> 200 µg/mL
Fat stain	None		None - Mod
Muscle fibers	Rare		None - Rare
Vegetable fibers	Rare		None - Few
Carbohydrates	Neg		Neg

INFLAMMA

	Within	Outside	Ref. Range
Lysozyme*	276		<= 600 ng/mL
Lactoferrin	< 0.5		< 7.3 µg/mL
WBC	None		None - Rare
Mucus	Neg		Neg

IMMUN

	Within	Outside	Ref. Range
sIgA*		636	51 - 204mg/dl

*For Research Use Only. Not

©DOCTOR'S DATA, INC. • ADDRESS: 3755 Illinois Avenue, St. Charles, I

DOCTOR'S DATA
LAB#:
PATIENT:
ID:
SEX: Male
AGE: 37
CLIENT#: 26203
DOCTOR:
Palm Harbor, FL 34683 USA

Comprehensive Stool Analysis / Parasitology x3

MICROBIOLOGY

Bacteriology Culture

Beneficial flora
Bifidobacterium 1+
E. coli spp. 1+
Lactobacillus spp. 0+
Enterococcus spp. 0+

Imbalances
Bacillus spp. 2+
Beta strep not Group A or B 1+
Klebsiella pneumonia 2+

Dysbiotic flora

Mycology (Yeast) Culture

Normal flora
No yeast isolated

Dysbiotic flora

PARASITOLOGY / MICROSCOPY (TRICHROME STAIN & CONCENTRATION)

Sample 1: No Ova or Parasites, Rare RBC
Sample 2: No Ova or Parasites, Many Yeast, Rare RBC
Sample 3: No Ova or Parasites, Few Yeast, Rare RBC

	Within	Outside	Ref. Range
Giardia Lamblia (EIA)	Neg		Neg
Cryptosporidium (EIA)	Neg		Neg

Beneficial flora: In a healthy balanced state of intestinal flora, the beneficial bacteria make up a significant proportion of the total microflora. The beneficial flora have many health-protecting effects in the gut including manufacturing vitamins, fermenting fibers, digesting proteins and the disaccharide lactose, and propagating anti-tumor and anti-inflammatory factors. Acidophilus, Bifidus, and Enterococcus produce lactic acid and short-chain fatty acids. The fermentation of fibers by beneficial bacteria and subsequent production of short chain fatty acids is crucial in lowering colonic pH and preventing the proliferation of microbial pathogens, including bacteria and yeast. Enterococcus has antibacterial activity against methicillin-resistant S. aureus (MRSA) and food-borne pathogens.

Parasitology: Intestinal parasites are abnormal inhabitants of the GI tract. Factors such as contaminated food and water supplies, day care centers, international travel, pets, carriers such as mosquitoes and fleas, and sexual transmission have contributed to an increased prevalence of intestinal parasites in the American population.

Date Collected: 8/24/2009
Date Received: 8/26/2009
Date Completed: 9/1/2009
Comments:

©DOCTOR'S DATA, INC. • ADDRESS: 3755 Illinois Avenue, St. Charles, IL 60174-2420 • CLIA ID NO: 14D0646470 • MEDICARE PROVIDER NO: 148453

Gluten Sensivity Stool and/or Gene Panel from EnteroLab

EnteroLab has developed a unique screening test for gluten sensitivity, and dietary yeast, cow's milk, and chicken egg sensitivity. The test is more sensitive and specific than tests in current use (U.S. patent issued; International patents pending). Their method utilizes stool rather than blood as the testing substrate. The rationale of using stool rather than blood for testing food sensitivity is that immunologic reactions to proteins in the diet that cause these reactions are centered within the intestinal tract and not in the blood. These tests allow a person to find food sensitivities before intestinal damage becomes severe.

Tests are offered online at www.enterolab.com The test kit is shipped directly to your home, and does not require a lab visit. A stool sample is sent to the lab, and the results are mailed to your home.

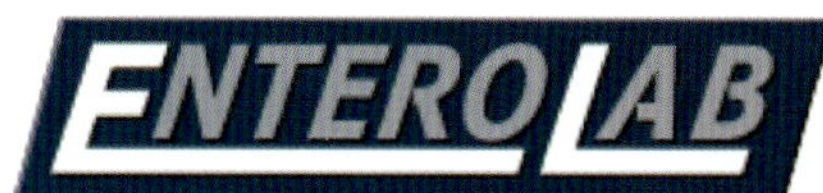

Final Laboratory Report

Date: 11/18/2009

Name: Sample Report

A) Gluten Sensitivity Stool and Gene Panel Complete *Best test/best value
Fecal Anti-gliadin IgA: 33 Units

Fecal Anti-tissue Transglutaminase IgA: 60 Units

Quantitative Microscopic Fecal Fat Score: Less than 300 Units

Fecal Anti-casein (cow's milk) IgA: 9 Units

HLA-DQB1 Molecular analysis, Allele 1: 0202

HLA-DQB1 Molecular analysis, Allele 2: 0301

Serologic equivalent: HLA-DQ 2,3 (Subtype 2,7)

Interpretation of Fecal Anti-gliadin IgA (Normal Range is less than 10 Units): Intestinal antigliadin IgA antibody was elevated, indicating that you have active dietary gluten sensitivity. For optimal health, resolution of symptoms (if you have them), and prevention of small intestinal damage and malnutrition, osteoporosis, and damage to other tissues (like nerves, brain, joints, muscles, thyroid, pancreas, other glands, skin, liver, spleen, among others), it is recommended that you follow a strict and permanent gluten free diet. As gluten sensitivity is a genetic syndrome, you may want to have your relatives screened as well.

Interpretation of Fecal Anti-tissue Transglutaminase IgA (Normal Range is less than 10 Units): You have an autoimmune reaction to the human enzyme tissue transglutaminase, secondary to dietary gluten sensitivity.

Interpretation of Quantitative Microscopic Fecal Fat Score (Normal Range is less than 300 Units): Provided that dietary fat is being ingested, a fecal fat score less than 300 indicates there is no malabsorbed dietary fat in stool indicating that digestion and absorption of nutrients is currently normal.

Interpretation of Fecal Anti-casein (cow's milk) IgA (Normal Range is less than 10 Units): Levels of fecal IgA antibody to a food antigen greater than or equal to 10 are indicative of an immune reaction, and hence immunologic "sensitivity" to that food. For any elevated fecal antibody level, it is recommended to remove that food from your diet. Values less than 10 indicate there currently is minimal or no reaction to that food and hence, no direct evidence of food sensitivity to that specific food. However, because 1 in 500 people cannot make IgA at all, and rarely, some people can still have clinically significant reactions to a food antigen despite the lack of a significant antibody reaction (because the reactions primarily involve T cells), if you have an immune syndrome or symptoms associated with food sensitivity, it is recommended that you try a strict removal of suspect foods from your diet for up to 12 months despite a negative test.

Interpretation Of HLA-DQ Testing: Although you do not possess the main HLA-DQB1 genes predisposing to celiac sprue (HLA-DQB1*0201 or HLA-DQB1*0302), HLA gene analysis reveals that you have two copies of a gene that predisposes to gluten sensitivity (any DQ1, DQ2 other than by HLA-DQB1*0201, or DQ3 other than by HLA-DQB1*0302). Furthermore, HLA-DQ2 genes other than by HLA-DQB1*0201 can be associated with celiac sprue in rare cases. Having two copies of a gluten sensitive gene means that each of your parents and all of your children (if you have them) will possess at least one copy of the gene. Two copies also means there is an even stronger predisposition to gluten sensitivity than having one gene and the resultant immunologic gluten sensitivity may be more severe.

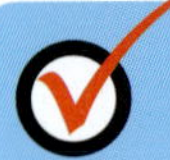

Comprehensive Stool Analysis from Parasitology Center

For cases in which parasites are specifically suspected, the best stool analysis comes from Dr. Amin at the Parasitology Center. The analysis tests fecal, blood, tissues and skin specimens to diagnose and taxonomically identify human and animal-borne parasitic organisms and agents of medical and public health importance. These include over 40 species of protozoan (single-celled organisms), cysts and trophozoites, eggs and other stages of metazoans (multiple-celled parasites like roundworms, tapeworms, flukes, and other parasitic organisms) that may be found in biological specimens, e.g., fecal, blood, tissues, and skin.

This test is offered online at www.parasitetesting.com The test kit is shipped directly to your home, and does not require a lab visit. A stool sample is sent to the lab, and the results are mailed to your home.

GI Effects Complete Stool Profile from Metametrix

The GI Effects Profile uses DNA analysis to identify microbiota including anaerobes in the stool, a previously immeasurable area of the gut environment. DNA assessment is specific and accurate, avoids the pitfalls of sample transport, reports results as specific numbers, and is more sensitive than classic laboratory methods. In addition to much more comprehensive bacteriology, mycology, and parasitology assessments, GI Effects Profiles report drug resistance genes, antibiotic and botanical sensitivities, gliadin-specific sIgA, Elastase1, plus other inflammation, digestion, and absorption markers. The test does not measure live microorganisms, however, which is one major difference between this stool test and the Comprehensive Stool Analysis.

This test is offered online at www.labtestingdirect.com The test kit is shipped directly to your home, and does not require a lab visit. A stool sample is sent to the lab, and the results are mailed to your home.

Intestinal Permeability Assessment from Genova Diagnostics

The Intestinal Permeability Assessment is a noninvasive assessment of small intestinal absorption and barrier function in the bowel. The small intestine uniquely functions as a digestive/absorptive organ for nutrients as well as a powerful immune and mechanical barrier against excessive absorption of bacteria, food antigens, and other macromolecules. Both malabsorption and increased intestinal permeability (leaky gut) are associated with chronic gastrointestinal imbalances as well as many systemic disorders.

Increased permeability of the small intestine can:

- Increase the number of foreign compounds entering the bloodstream.
- Allow bacterial antigens capable of cross-reacting with host tissue to enter the bloodstream, leading to auto-immune processes.

Healing HOPE Testimonial

"Years ago my mom and I came to the conclusion that we were both having symptoms of a parasite problem. I felt toxic and looked it. I was always constipated with a bloated lower tummy, bad acne problems, mucus in my stool and an occasional itchy rectum. I was always anxious or fatigued and was dealing with major bruxism.

So the two of us got together and did some research on all the books we could find for natural herbal parasitic combinations or single herbs used for the expelling of parasites. We crossed referenced our lists and made one list, then drove to a few natural health food stores. The only product we found to best match our list was your Parasite Cleanse. So we purchased it. The results were wonderful.

Since then I tell all my friends and family about it. I currently work in a natural health food store and to anyone coming to me looking to do a cleanse or who suspects they are dealing with parasites, I explain to them why I feel this is a excellent product to contribute to their cleansing process."
– Tilla

- Enhance the uptake of toxic compounds that can overwhelm the hepatic detoxification system and lead to an overly sensitized immune system.

The Intestinal Permeability Assessment directly measures the ability of two non-metabolized sugar molecules to permeate the intestinal mucosa. The patient drinks a premeasured amount of lactulose and mannitol. The degree of intestinal permeability or malabsorption is reflected in the levels of the two sugars recovered in a urine sample collected over the next six hours.

This test is offered online at www.labtestingdirect.comThe test kit is shipped directly to your home, and does not require a lab visit. A stool sample is sent to the lab, and the results are mailed to your home.

Lactose Intolerance Breath Test from Genova Diagnostics

This simple, noninvasive test detects lactose intolerance, a condition affecting more than 50 million Americans. Proper detection enables effective treatment of lactose maldigestion and malabsorption, to help alleviate chronic symptoms of bloating, gas, diarrhea and abdominal pain. This test measures the levels of methane and hydrogen in the breath, which can determine how well lactose is digested. The test demonstrates increases in hydrogen and methane

arising from bacterial fermentation of undigested lactose, which show up in the breath within one to two hours after exposure.

This test is offered online at www.labtestingdirect.com The test kit is shipped directly to your home, and does not require a lab visit. A stool sample is sent to the lab, and the results are mailed to your home.

Lactulose Breath Test (Bacterial Overgrowth of the Small Intestine) from Genova Diagsnostics

This test measures levels of hydrogen and methane in the breath for a period of three hours after ingesting lactulose. This simple, noninvasive test detects bacterial overgrowth in the small intestine, a common condition that often underlies chronic symptoms of maldigestion and malabsorption, including bloating, gas, diarrhea, irregularity, and abdominal pain.

Normally, far fewer bacteria inhabit the small intestine than the ample growth found in the colon. Gastric acid secretion and intestinal motility keep the small intestine relatively free of bacteria. A wide range of abnormalities and malfunctions, however, can encourage bacteria to multiply in the small intestine. The most common causes relate to a decrease in the production of hydrochloric acid or pancreatic enzymes, thereby creating a unsterile environment for the small intestine.

This test is offered online at www.labtestingdirect.com The test kit is shipped directly to your home, and does not require a lab visit. A stool sample is sent to the lab, and the results are mailed to your home.

Heidelberg pH Diagnostic Test

The Heidelberg pH Diagnostic System is a state-of-the-art diagnostic tool for measuring the pH levels in the digestive tract. The Heidelberg pH capsule is a technically advanced micro-electronic diagnostic tool that can accurately diagnose a patient who may have hypochlorhydria, hyperchlorhydria, achlorhydria, pyloric insufficiency and heavy mucus. When the Heidelberg pH capsule is activated and administered to the patient, the pH capsule will measure, and transmit the pH Levels and the re-acidification time of the stomach's parietal cells.

Unlike other pH tests, which require the use of an invasive nasal-gastric tube, or a standard endoscopic procedure, which in many cases may traumatize the patient, the Heidelberg pH Diagnostic test is accurate and noninvasive, and very user- and patient-friendly. The pH capsule is similar to the size of a vitamin capsule.

To find a doctor who can perform this test, visit www.phcapsule.com

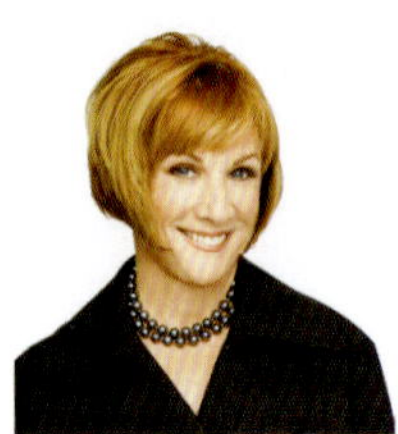

Fiber 35 Eating Plan

There was a time when we all naturally ate a high-fiber diet. We ate fresh foods from the farm, either our own or one nearby. But in the early 1900s, the processing and packaging of food became an enormous growth industry. Almost overnight, we went from eating fresh foods to eating processed foods. Just as quickly, our rates of obesity and chronic diseases—like heart disease, diabetes and cancer—skyrocketed. Today, the processed food industry is the largest industry in the world. Unfortunately, most of the fiber and other crucial nutrients are processed out of our diet.

Busy with my own life, I too fell prey to the ease and availability of processed food, which lead to weight gain, fatigue, impaired digestion and more. But as I learned about the incredible benefits of fiber, I added more into my own diet and not only saw my health improve, but I also lost 15 pounds. This inspired me to create the Fiber35 Diet and write the *Fiber35 Diet* book, a New York Times best-seller.

The reason Fiber 35 is not just a weight loss plan, but a healthy eating plan for life, is the ever-declining digestive health of the aging population. For example, over 50 percent of people will develop diverticulosis as they age, usually a result of lack of dietary fiber. Diverticulosis involves the pocketing of the colon, placing the person at risk for diverticulitis, as well as cancer. I have noticed over the years that people do not have a clue about how much fiber they eat. As I lecture around the country people tell me about digestive conditions they think have developed suddenly. Most of these conditions take years to develop, however. Years of lack of fiber creates an out-of-balance digestive tract, both structurally—as with diverticulosis and hemorrhoids—and functionally—as with bacterial imbalance. Soluble dietary fiber is fermented in the gut, leading to increases in the friendly gut bacteria. It acts like your internal fertilizer.

Healing HOPE *Testimonial*

"I want to thank you for saving my life. I have been on the Fiber 35 Diet for 5 months. I weighed 250 pounds and now I'm 185 pounds. I have lost 65 pounds from the diet and I can't stop now. I have been on a lot of diets and they never worked like this one. I have not been happy when I was fat but now I'm happier than ever. Thank you again."

– Lisa

People have two misconceptions about fiber. The first is the false belief that if a person has a bowel movement every day, then they have enough fiber in their diet. Wrong. **The amount of a bowel movement is just as important as frequency.** Think about how long your colon is—about 5 feet. One-third of that is the length of the descending colon (about a foot and a half) and that is the total amount of bowel elimination you should have everyday. This may occur all in one bowel movement, or split between two to three. The second thing people are confused about is what 35 grams of fiber looks like in a daily diet. Most people think if they eat a salad everyday they're getting enough fiber. Guess again! The average salad (unless you add in extra ingredients like beans) is about 4 grams of fiber. I know that I, myself, have to eat a fiber bar with 10 grams of fiber to reach my 35 grams daily. It can be difficult to get enough fiber from only the diet, even when you're trying.

Not only have thousands of people lost weight on this easy program, they have healed their bodies with a diet of fresh, wholesome, high-fiber foods. Fiber 35 is much more than a weight loss plan, it's a lifetime eating system that will help you have more energy, better digestion and nutrient absorption, and keep you and your family free from chronic diseases that plague our society.

Fiber 35 Optimum Eating Plan

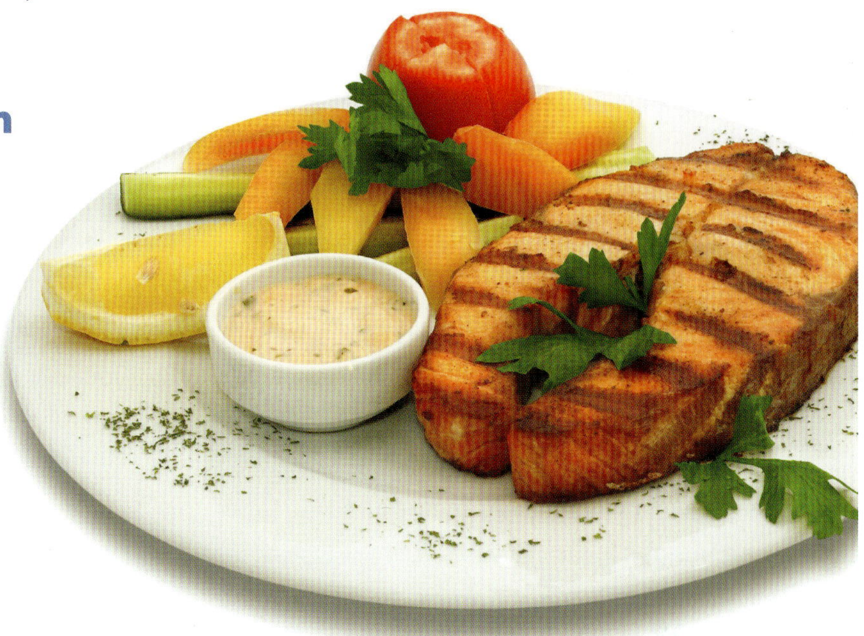

1. Lean Protein
2. Fats
   - healthy oils
   - nuts and seeds
   - dairy (moderate consumption)
3. Carbohydrates/at least 35 grams of fiber per day for life
   - fruits
   - vegetables
   - legumes/beans
   - grains
   - fiber supplements

When you follow the above Optimum Nutrition Food Choices, your daily diet will consist of approximately:

- **25% Protein.** Two or three servings (3-4 ounces per serving) of poultry, fish, and red meat (use sparingly).
- **25% Fat.** Two to three servings of seeds and/or nuts, totaling 1 ounce daily, healthy oils (1-3 tablespoons daily); ¼ avocado; lean proteins.
- **50% Complex Carbohydrates.** Six to eight servings of fruits, vegetables, legumes; two or three servings of whole grains (1/2 cup = one serving).

The 4 Ways Fiber Helps You Lose Weight

While a daily dose of fiber provides myriad health benefits, it is also an indispensable calorie-free weight loss tool. When incorporated into your diet, fiber can help you lose weight in four important ways:

- **Fiber will help curb your appetite.** Controlling your appetite is the key to weight loss. Fiber stimulates cholecystokinin (CCK), a hormone that sends a message to your brain that you are full. Fiber promotes and prolongs the elevation of CCK in the blood, which makes you feel full for longer periods of time.
- **Fiber will actually eliminate calories from the food you eat.** Research shows that people who consume a high-fiber diet tend to excrete more calories in their stool. This ***Fiber Flush Effect*** occurs because fiber helps to block the absorption of calories consumed and lead those calories out of the body. One recent study actually found that for every gram of fiber we eat, we eliminate 7 calories. That means that if you eat at least 35 grams of fiber each day over a period of one month, you'll eliminate 7,595 calories (7 x 35 = 245 calories x 31 days = 7,595 calories).
- **Fiber foods are low energy-density foods.** Because high-fiber foods typically have a very low energy density (the number of calories in a particular volume of food), eating them allows you to eat a larger volume of food without consuming as many calories.
- **Fiber slows down the rate at which your body converts carbohydrates into sugar.** High-fiber foods help normalize blood glucose levels by slowing down the time it takes food to leave the stomach and delaying the absorption of glucose (blood sugar) from a meal.

The Fiber 35 Eating Plan – Calories and Fiber

In addition to following a healthy diet and exercising regularly, clinical research has proven that reducing the amount of calories you consume every day is the key to losing weight. The good news is that it has never been easier! While eating fewer calories every day may seem challenging at first, the Fiber 35 Eating Plan provides a nutritious and satisfying plan designed to support you every step of the way.

With the Fiber 35 Eating Plan, eating fewer calories no longer means going hungry or eating foods that don't satisfy your hunger. In fact, it will be just the opposite—you'll be eating five to six times daily, enjoying wholesome meals and snacks that include plenty of fruits, vegetables, whole grains, nuts and legumes. Within weeks, eating the right foods for your body will have become second nature, and you will be on your way to achieving healthy weight management for life.

As part of the Fiber 35 Plan program, you will make a note of everything you eat and drink each day. This will help you keep track of how many calories and grams of fiber you consume. For example, most women should eat between 1,500 and 2,000 calories per day, as this is how much fuel the body needs (on average) to maintain a healthy metabolic rate.

Considering that a pound of fat equals 3,500 calories, you must eat 3,500 fewer calories than your body needs over a given period of time if you want to lose one pound. That means that if every day you ate one less calorie than your body required, it would take 3,500 days (or 9.58 years) to lose one pound. The good news is that with the Fiber 35 Diet you can lose weight much faster than that!

Just How Many Calories Do You Need?

When we discuss how many calories we need per day, we are actually talking about how many calories our cells need to function optimally. Although caloric needs differ from one person to another, food manufacturers base the nutritional information on their labels on a 2,000 calorie diet. This represents the caloric intake of the average person. To achieve success with the Fiber 35 Eating Plan, it is important to determine how many calories you need each day to maintain your weight, and there are several things that may influence that number:

- *Weight*
- *Gender*
- *Activity Level*

The mathematical formula created to help you determine your personal daily caloric needs takes into account the variables listed above and is calculated using two other variables: your metabolic rate (MR), and the amount of energy expended during physical activity.

To get an idea of your daily caloric needs, it helps to complete the calculations on the following page.

By using a simple formula based on how many pounds you want to lose, you will be able to calculate your **Reduced Calories Goal (RCG).** Once you have calculated your RCG, you will then determine your daily caloric needs using a simple formula based on your **Resting Metabolic Rate (RMR)** and the amount of energy you expend during physical activity.

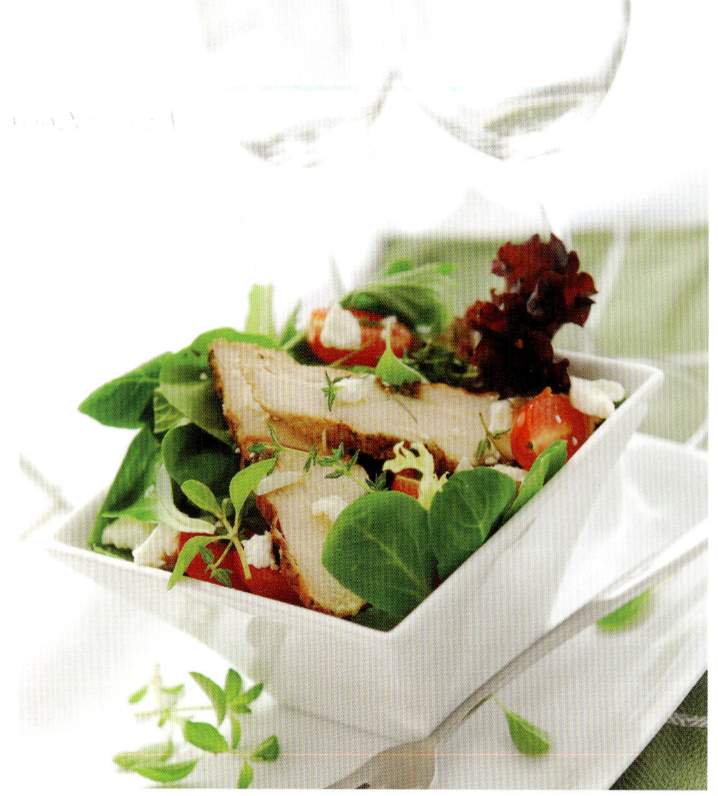

Calculating Your Caloric Requirements

Step One:

To establish how many pounds you want to lose, multiply that number by 3,500 (every pound of fat equals 3,500 calories). This will determine the number of calories you will need to restrict over a given period of time to lose your desired amount of weight. To calculate your personal formula, use the space below. If you want to use this eating plan **to maintain your current weight, begin with Step Two.**

1. Enter your weight loss goal in pounds: [ ]
2. Multiply your weight loss goal in pounds by 3,500: [ ]

This is called your **Reduced Calories Goal**, or RCG.

Step Two:

The next step is to simply calculate your **daily personal caloric needs,** which takes into account two variables: your **Resting Metabolic Rate,** or RMR, and the amount of energy expended during physical activity.

1. Calculating your RMR:

- For Women: Current weight in pounds x 10 = RMR [ ]
- For Men: Current weight in pounds x 11 = RMR [ ]

2. Calculating your energy expenditure:

- RMR number x 0.2 = Activity Calories (sedentary lifestyle)* = [ ]
- RMR number x 0.3 = Activity Calories (moderately active)* = [ ]
- RMR number x 0.4 = Activity Calories (very active)* = [ ]

Add the results of 1 and 2 above to determine the total number of calories you potentially burn in a day to maintain your current weight:

[ ] + [ ] = [ ] **EMR (Estimated Metabolic Rate)**

(RMR) **(Activity calories)**

Once you have calculated your **Reduced Calories Goal** and your **Estimated Metabolic Rate**, all that is left is to set your Daily Calorie Goal for each phase of the Fiber 35 eating plan. To do so, follow the instructions provided in the next section.

The 3 Phases of the Fiber 35 Eating Plan

The Fiber 35 Diet offers a personalized solution tailored to your specific weight loss goal. A gradual three-phase approach takes the stress out of dieting and lets you progress at your own pace from a period of accelerated weight loss to a lifetime of healthy weight maintenance. In each phase, it is essential to consume at least 35 grams of fiber every day.

Phase 1: Accelerated Weight Loss. During this phase, you will reduce the amount of calories you consume by up to 1,000 calories per day, but you should not consume fewer than 1,200 calories each day. In Phase 1 you will eat 5 to 6 times daily to maintain a healthy metabolism (the rate at which your body naturally burns calories). Although Phase 1 is the most restrictive phase of the diet, don't give up hope—it is during this phase that you will lose the most weight! Phase 1 can last from 2 to 4 weeks, depending on your personal weight loss goal.

Here is how to set your Daily Calorie Goal goal for Phase 1. This calculation provides the number of calories you can eat per day. For example, if your EMR was 2,500 calories per day, you would subtract 1,000 from that number, making your Phase 1 Daily Calorie Goal 1,500.

Insert your EMR here	-1,000 =	Phase 1 Daily Calorie Goal
Do not consume fewer than 1,200 calories a day.		

Phase 2: Moderate Weight Loss. During this phase, you will reduce the amount of calories you eat by up to 500 calories while continuing to eat 5 to 6 times daily. As in Phase 1, do not consume fewer than 1,200 calories each day. Phase 2 has no definite end point, and you may stay in this phase for as long as necessary to reach your desired weight.

Insert your EMR here	-500 =	Phase 1 Daily Calorie Goal
Do not consume fewer than 1,200 calories a day.		

Phase 3: Lifetime Weight Maintenance. Once you have reached Phase 3, you will have attained your weight loss goal. Congratulations—the Fiber 35 Eating Plan is now a way of life! At this point, you will continue to eat 5 to 6 times daily and incorporate at least 35 grams of fiber into your daily diet. You will also need to recalculate your EMR based on your new weight and set your Daily Calorie Goal for this phase. In Phase 3, you will begin to gradually increase your caloric intake and add more full meals into your diet.

Helpful tips for each phase:

- Exercise regularly (3 times per week for 30 minutes)
- Keep a journal of everything you eat and drink to help you record calorie and fiber intake
- Do not consume fewer than 1,200 calories each day
- Consume at least 35 grams of fiber every day
- Do not eat after 7:30pm
- Eat 5 to 6 times per day
- Drink plenty of water

Fiber 35 Recipes: A Typical Diet

Breakfast Recipe

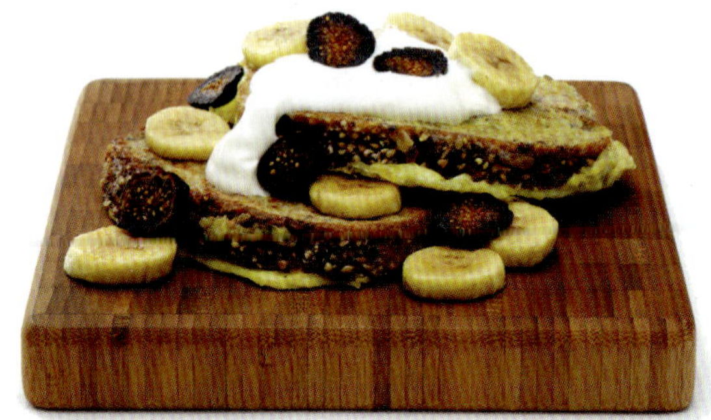

Multigrain French Toast with Yogurt and Bananas
serves two (6g fiber/serving)

1 whole egg and 1 egg white, lightly beaten
¼ teaspoon real vanilla
Pinch of salt
Pump spray olive oil
4 slices of nutty organic whole grain bread
½ cup banana, sliced
2 medium figs, sliced
6 ounces of plain yogurt

Combine eggs, vanilla, and salt in a bowl large enough to lay 1 piece of bread in it flat.
Preheat a skillet to medium and spray with oil.

Set 2 pieces of bread in your egg mixture, coating both pieces well on all sides.
Hold the bread in the egg mixture to soak up roughly half of the egg.
Place the bread into the heated skillet and cook until slightly golden brown on both sides. Repeat for the remaining 2 pieces of bread.
Plate the French toast then top with a big spoonful of yogurt, banana and fig slices.

Note: Whole grain breads vary in nutritional content. Make sure to use whole grain bread, not just a multigrain.

Nutrition Facts: Serving size, 2 slices—calories 295, fiber 6 g, protein 14 g, fat 7 g, saturated fat 3 g, carbohydrate 47 g, cholesterol 104 g, sodium 400 mg, sugars 22 g.

Snack Recipe

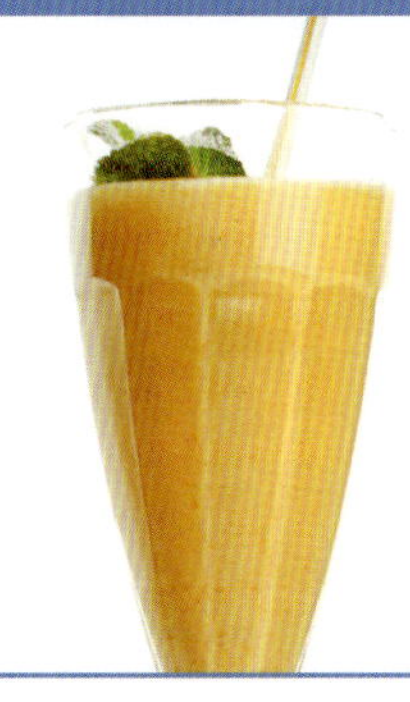

Orange Pineapple Crave
serves one (10g fiber/serving)

Fiber 35 vanilla shake mix
½ cup frozen pineapple chunks
4 ounces orange juice
4 ounces almond milk

Usinging an electric blender on medium setting, blend all ingredients together and serve in tall glass.

Nutrition Facts: One serving—calories 280, fiber 10 g, protein 20 g.

Lunch Recipe

Seafood, Spinach, and Orange Salad
serves four (6g fiber/serving)

12 cups baby spinach leaves, stems removed, loosely packed
3 navel oranges, halved
1 large red or yellow bell pepper
12 ounces cooked shrimp or fresh lump crabmeat
8 very thin slices of red onion
1 cup freshly squeezed orange juice
Juice of 1 lime
¼ teaspoon turmeric
1 teaspoon marjoram
1 ½ tablespoons olive oil
Freshly ground black pepper
1 lime cut into quarters (optional)

Divide the spinach among four dinner plates. On top of the spinach, arrange the oranges and bell pepper. On top of that arrange the shrimp or crab. Separate onions into rings and arrange over shrimp or crab.

In small bowl, swish together orange juice, lime juice, turmeric, marjoram, and olive oil; season to taste with fresh pepper. Spoon the dressing over each salad. Salads can be garnished with fresh lime quarters.

Note: Whole grain breads vary in nutritional content. Make sure to use whole grain bread, not just a multigrain.

Nutrition Facts: Serving size, ¼ recipe—calories 245, fiber 6 g, protein 20 g, fat 7 g, saturated fat 1 g, carbohydrate 29 g, cholesterol 67 mg, sodium 327 mg, sugars 18 g.

Snack Recipe

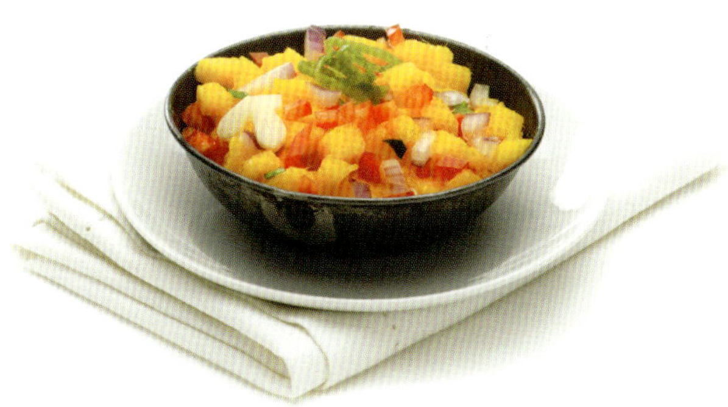

Tortilla Chips and Salsa

1 ounce blue corn tortilla chips (15 chips) and
2 ounces (4 tablespoons) homemade salsa

Homemade Salsa (1g fiber/serving)

2 large tomatoes, seeded and chopped
1 serrano or jalepeño pepper, chopped
⅓ cup chopped green onion
2 tablespoons chopped fresh cilantro
2 tablespoons fresh lime juice
¼ teaspoon salt

Mix all ingredients well and chill.

Chips Nutrition Facts: Calories 150, fiber 3 g, protein 3 g. Salsa Nutrition Facts: Serving size, 2 ounces—calories 13, fiber 1 g, protein 1 g, fat 0 g, saturated fat 0 g, carbohydrate 4 g, cholesterol 0 mg, sodium 100 mg, sugars 2 g.

Dinner Recipe

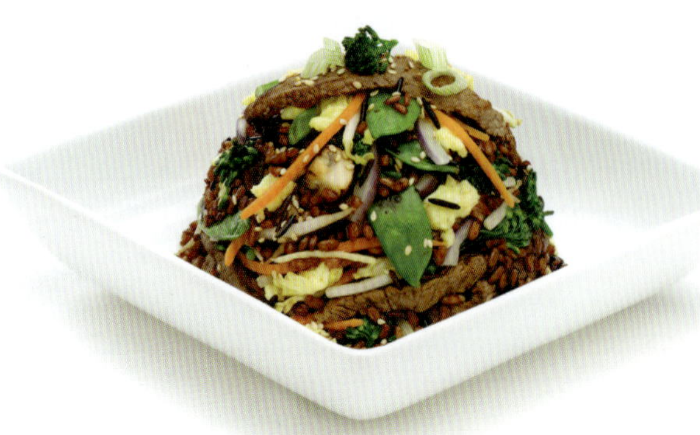

Beef and Vegetable Fried Rice
serves two (4g fiber/serving)

2 tablespoons peanut oil
¼ pound beef, any cut, sliced into thin strips
1 rib celery, cut lengthwise
¼ cup bean sprouts
12 snow peas
¼ cup cremini* mushrooms
5 broccoli florets
¼ cup carrots, julienned
1 radish, sliced
1 teaspoon ginger, grated
2 cloves garlic, chopped
1 cup brown rice, cooked
2 teaspoons low-sodium soy sauce
½ teaspoon sesame seed oil
1 egg, beaten
1 teaspoon sesame seeds

Put into a large skillet or wok, at high heat, 1 tablespoon peanut oil and the beef. Sauté beef until done. Set beef aside. Add remaining peanut oil and all vegetables, ginger, and garlic and stir frequently for about 3–4 minutes or until vegetables are tender-crisp. Add rice, soy sauce, and sesame oil and stir frequently to keep rice from sticking. Remove from heat and add cooked beef. Place in serving bowl or plate. Return pan to medium heat and cook egg quickly, whisking with fork. Add cooked egg to beef mixture. Garnish with sesame seeds.

Note: * A dark brown mushroom with a round cap

Nutrition Facts: Serving size, 1/2 recipe—calories 437, fiber 4 g, protein 20 g, fat 26 g, saturated fat 6 g, carbohydrate 32 g, cholesterol 120 g, sodium 275 mg, sugars 3 g.

Dessert Recipe

Carrot Spice Snack Cake
serves twelve (2g fiber/serving)

½ cup liquid honey
3 tablespoons cooking oil
2 eggs
1 cup spelt flour
½ teaspoon sea salt
¾ teaspoon baking soda
1 teaspoon baking powder
1 teaspoon cinnamon
1 teaspoon fresh grated nutmeg
2 cups grated carrots
¼ cup applesauce (unsweetened)
¼ cup chopped walnuts
7 ounces unsweetened
crushed pineapple
Cooking spray

Using a mixer, beat honey, cooking oil, and eggs together until well blended. Add flour, salt, baking soda, baking powder, cinnamon, and nutmeg; mix well. Fold in carrots, applesauce, nuts, and pineapple. Spray an 8- by 8-inch ungreased pan with cooking spray. Add cake mixture to pan. Bake in preheated oven for 50–60 minutes.

Nutrition Facts: One serving (¼ cake)—calories 124, fiber 2g, protein 3g.

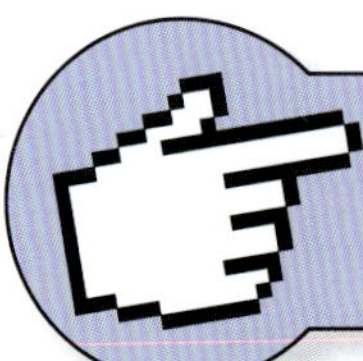

Get started online. It's FREE! Visit www.Fiber35Diet.com to sign up today and enjoy exclusive member benefits.

The Fiber35 Diet

Nature's Weight Loss Secret

The revolutionary way to
lose weight,
improve health,
prevent disease,
have more energy
and stay slim!

Brenda Watson, C.N.C.
with Leonard Smith, M.D.

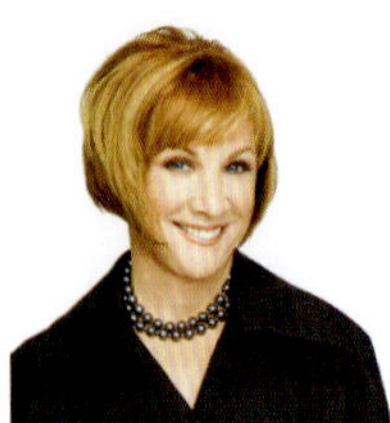

CANDIDA DIET

I learned about Candida overgrowth from Dr. William Crook in the early 90s. I worked with a medical doctor who treated patients who were very ill, and often, financially spent. We used Dr. Crook's Candida Questionnaire (found on the following pages) for people who could not afford stool analysis.

Today, the prevalence of Candida overgrowth is even more severe than it was just two decades ago. The widespread presence of antibiotics in our food and water, and prescribed by doctors, is out of hand. In addition, the overuse of proton pump inhibitors (PPIs) for acid reflux is similarly out of control. These drugs are creating a Candida epidemic that Dr. Crook called a "silent epidemic" back in the 90s.

Today, conventional medicine still does not recognize Candida overgrowth as a valid health condition unless it presents as oral thrush. Thanks to the more progressive natural health practitioners and holistically minded doctors, the comprehensive stool analysis (CSA) is a great baseline test that shows you what is going on "on the inside." (See the Recommended Testing section.)

Some people choose to take prescription antifungals for Candida overgrowth, which may be necessary in severe cases. One mistake these people often make, however, is falling back into their old diet and lifestyle habits. Unless you heal your leaky gut so that your friendly bacteria can adhere to the intestinal lining and re-establish, the Candida overgrowth will recur.

I recommend a natural antifungal Candida Cleanse be taken for a minimum of three months (even for people who are also taking a prescription antifungal). In addition, rebuilding the leaky gut with nutrients for the intestinal lining, re-establishing the beneficial gut bacteria with probiotics, and replacing nutrients by providing the body with digestive enzymes are all a part of maintaining a healthy gut to avoid recurrence of Candida overgrowth. If followed correctly, this program of Candida elimination takes about a year. After the program, it is still necessary to watch your sugar intake.

Candida – the Unfriendly Yeast

Candida organisms are commensal (neutral) yeasts when present in small amounts in the digestive tract. When these potentially pathogenic yeasts begin to proliferate, creating an imbalance in the ratio of good to bad microflora (a condition known as dysbiosis), it can lead to a host of other health problems. (See the Candidiasis section.) When the gut flora is in balance, the beneficial microflora greatly outnumber the potentially pathogenic microflora, essentially keeping them in check.

Candida overgrowth in the gut releases toxins, increases inflammation and perforates the lining of the intestine, all of which lead to the development of leaky gut. Leaky gut, intestinal inflammation and dysbiosis all contribute to the development of each of the health conditions described in this book by allowing toxins and bacteria to enter into the bloodstream, creating systemic inflammation that spreads throughout the body. Bringing the gut back into balance is essential for maintaining optimal health. Eliminating Candida overgrowth is an important step in this process.

To determine whether Candida overgrowth is present, there are two options. The first option involves testing for gut imbalances, including Candida overgrowth, with a CSA. If it is not possible to do a CSA, the second option is to fill out the Candida questionnaire on the following pages to determine if you might have Candida overgrowth. This questionnaire is very effective at identifying people with Candida overgrowth. The first questionnaire is for adults, the second is for children.

Yeast Questionnaire – ADULT

Section A – History

Circle the number next to the questions to which you answer "yes," then add all the circled numbers, and write the total in the box at the bottom.

Have you taken tetracycline or other antibiotics for acne for 1 month or more? 50

Have you, at any time in your life, taken other "broad spectrum" antibiotics for respiratory, urinary or other infections for 2 months or more, or for shorter periods, 4 or more times in a 1-year span? 50

Have you taken a broad spectrum antibiotic drug —even a single dose? 6

Have you at any time in your life, been bothered by persistent prostatitis, vaginitis, or other problems affecting your reproductive organs? 25

Have you been pregnant...
- 2 or more times? 5
- 1 time? 3

Have you taken birth control pills for...
- more than 2 years? 15
- 6 months to 2 years? 8

Have you taken prednisone, or other cortisone-type drugs by mouth or inhalation
- for more than 2 weeks? 15
- for 2 weeks or less? 6

Does exposure to perfumes, insecticides, fabric shop odors, or other chemicals provoke...
- moderate to severe symptoms? 20
- mild symptoms? 5

Are your symptoms worse on damp, muggy days or in moldy places? 20

If you have ever had athlete's foot, ringworm, jock itch or other chronic fungus infections of the skin or nails, have such infections been...
- severe or persistent? 20
- mild or moderate? 10

Do you crave sugar? 10

Do you crave breads? 10

Do you crave alcoholic beverages? 10

Does tobacco smoke really bother you? 10

Total Score for Section A:

Section B – Major Symptoms

For each symptom that is present, enter the appropriate number on the adjacent line:

If a symptom is occasional or mild, score 3 points
If a symptom is frequent or moderately severe, score 6 points
If a symptom is severe and/or disabling, score 9 points

Total the scores for this section, and record them in the box at the bottom of this section.

Fatigue or lethargy .... _____
Feeling of being "drained" .... _____
Poor memory .... _____
Feeling "spacey" or "unreal" .... _____
Inability to make decisions .... _____
Numbness, burning or tingling .... _____
Insomnia .... _____
Muscle aches .... _____
Muscle weakness or paralysis .... _____
Pain and/or swelling in joints .... _____
Abdominal pain .... _____
Constipation .... _____
Diarrhea .... _____
Bloating, belching or intestinal gas .... _____
Troublesome vaginal burning, itching or discharge .... _____
Prostatitis .... _____
Impotence .... _____
Loss of sexual desire or feeling .... _____
Endometriosis or infertility .... _____
Cramps and/or other menstrual irregularities _____
Premenstrual tension .... _____
Attacks of anxiety or crying .... _____
Cold hands or feet and/or chilliness .... _____
Shaking or irritability when hungry .... _____

Total Score for Section B:

Section C – Minor Symptoms

For each symptom that is present, enter the appropriate number on the adjacent line:

If a symptom is occasional or mild, score 3 points
If a symptom is frequent or moderately severe, score 6 points
If a symptom is severe and/or disabling, score 9 points
Total the scores for this section, and record them in the box at the bottom of this section.

Drowsy .... _____
Irritable or jittery .... _____
Lack of coordination .... _____
Inability to concentrate .... _____
Frequent mood swings .... _____
Headaches .... _____
Dizzy/loss of balance .... _____
Pressure above ears...feeling of head swelling .... _____
Tendency to bruise easily .... _____
Chronic rashes or itching .... _____
Psoriasis or recurrent hives .... _____
Indigestion or heartburn .... _____
Food sensitivity or intolerance .... _____
Mucus in stools .... _____
Rectal itching .... _____
Dry mouth or throat .... _____
Rash or blisters in mouth .... _____
Bad breath .... _____
Foot, hair or body odor not relieved by washing .... _____
Nasal congestion or post-nasal drip .... _____
Nasal itching .... _____
Sore throat .... _____
Laryngitis, loss of voice .... _____
Cough or recurrent bronchitis .... _____
Pain or tightness in chest .... _____
Wheezing or shortness of breath .... _____
Urinary frequency, urgency or incontinence .... _____

Total Score for Section C:

Grand Total:

The total score will help you and your physician decide if your health problems are yeast-connected. A comprehensive history and physical examination are also important. In addition, laboratory studies, X-rays, and other types of tests may also be appropriate.

Scores for women will be higher, as seven items in this questionnaire apply exclusively to women, while only two apply exclusively to men.

If your total score for all three sections above was less than 60 for a woman or less than 40 for a man, then you are less likely to have a problem with candida. However, if you scored higher than this, then you may wish to consider lifestyle and dietary changes, as well as a detoxification and cleansing program, all of which may help you feel healthy and more energetic.

IF YOUR SCORE IS	YOUR SYMPTOMS ARE
180 (women) 140 (men)	Almost certainly yeast connected
120 (women) 90 (men)	Probably yeast connected
60 (women) 40 (men)	Possibly yeast connected
below 60 (women) below 40 (men)	Probably no yeast connected

Yeast Questionnaire – CHILD

Circle appropriate point score for questions you answer "yes."
Total your score and record it at the end of the questionnaire.

1. During the two years before your child was born, were you bothered by recurrent vaginitis, menstrual irregularities, premenstrual tension, fatigue, headache, depression, digestive disorders of "feeling bad all over?" 30
2. Was your child bothered by thrush? (Score 10 if mild, score 20 if severe or persistent) 10/20
3. Was your child bothered by frequent diaper rashes in infancy? (Score 10 if mild, 20 if severe or persistent) 10/20
4. During infancy, was your child bothered by colic and irritability lasting over 3 months? (Score 10 if mild, 20 if moderate or severe) 10/20
5. Are his/her symptoms worse on damp days or in damp or moldy places? 20
6. Has your child been bothered by recurrent or persistent "athlete's foot" or chronic fungus infections of his skin or nails? 30
7. Has your child been bothered by recurrent hives, eczema or other skin problems? 10
8. Has your child received:
   (a) 4 or more courses of antibiotic drugs during the past year? Or has he received continuous "prophylactic" courses of antibiotic drugs? 80
   (b) 8 or more courses of "broad-spectrum" antibiotics during the past 3 years? 50
9. Has your child experienced recurrent ear problems? 10
10. Has your child had tubes inserted in his ears? 10
11. Has your child been labeled "hyperactive?" (Score 10 if mild, 20 if moderate or severe) 10/20
12. Is your child bothered by learning problems (even though his early developmental history was normal)? 10
13. Does your child have a short attention span? 10
14. Is your child persistently irritable, unhappy and hard to please? 10
15. Has your child been bothered by persistent or recurrent digestive problems, including constipation, diarrhea, bloating or excessive gas? (Score 10 if mild, 20 if moderate, 30 if severe) 10/20/30
16. Has he/she been bothered by persistent nasal congestion, cough and/or wheezing? 10
17. Is your child unusually tired or unhappy or depressed? (Score 10 if mild, 20 if servere) 10/20
18. Has your child been bothered by recurrent headaches, abdominal pain or muscle aches? (Score 10 if mild, 20 if severe) 10/20
19. Does your child crave sweets? 10
20. Does exposure to perfume, insecticides, gas or other chemicals provoke moderate to severe symptoms? 30
21. Does tobacco smoke really bother him? 20
22. Do you feel that your child isn't well, yet diagnostic tests and studies haven't revealed the cause? 10

TOTAL SCORE:

Yeasts possibly play a role in causing health problems in children with **scores of 60 or more.**
Yeasts probably play a role in causing health problems in children with **scores of 100 or more.**
Yeasts almost certainly play a role in causing health problems in children with **scores of 140 or more.**

CANDIDA DIET

Candida need sugar to survive, obtaining it from the simple carbohydrates and sugars present in food that passes through the digestive tract. In order to eliminate Candida, these foods must be avoided for a period of at least three months. In addition, if any food allergies or sensitivities are present, those foods should also be avoided.

The Candida Diet features an abundance of fresh organic vegetables, whole grains, and lean organic easy-to-digest fish and poultry. Among the vegetables, the diet emphasizes those low in starch (primarily leafy greens), though the starchy vegetables (lima beans, peas, potatoes, etc.) may be eaten in small amounts.

There is no set rule about duration of this diet, though it should be followed for at least three months. The severity of the Candida overgrowth and how much "cheating" is done will also dictate how long an individual stays on the diet. Generally speaking, when symptoms have subsided, foods may be slowly added back, starting with fruits, then grains, and finally, dairy products if desired. Add foods back one at a time. If old symptoms return, or gas and bloating occur with a reintroduced food, it may be necessary to eliminate that food indefinitely, for this is a sign that the body has a sensitivity to it, or that the yeast has been reactivated. Use of a food diary is helpful for this stage.

Once the Candida Diet has been established, you may want to do an anti-Candida cleanse that includes antifungal herbal formulas. See the Candida Cleanse for more information. To support the gut during this process, it is important to replace the beneficial bacteria with probiotics.

The following recommendations outline which foods can be eaten and which foods should be avoided. Finally, recipes for a sample day on the Candida Diet are included.

FOODS TO ENJOY

Breakfast foods:

Yeast-free, gluten-free breads made from brown rice flour, buckwheat flour, millet flour, potato starch, etc.

Fruit choices – granny smith apples, grapefruit, berries (strawberries, blueberries, blackberries)

Butter (preferably organic), ghee (clarified butter)

Eggs (organic are best)

Whole-cooked gluten-free grains as cereal (millet, buckwheat, kamut, etc.)

Turkey bacon or turkey sausage

Snacks:

If dairy tolerant, plain, organic yogurt, unsweetened kefir (contains very little milk sugar, usually safe)

Pumpkin or sunflower seeds

Nut butters, like almond butter (raw, should be refrigerated)

Celery sticks, broccoli, zucchini, yellow squash, any green vegetables

Brown rice cakes

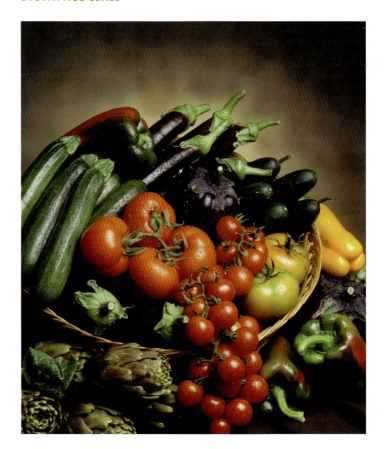

Vegetables:

Non-starchy vegetables, raw or steamed – EAT PLENTY!

Shiitake mushrooms

Vegetables juices (only green juices with lemon or granny smith apples to taste)

Red skinned potatoes (not brown) in moderation

Whole grains:

Gluten-free grains – millet, quinoa, wild rice, brown rice, amaranth, buckwheat, arrowroot, sorghum, teff, flax, nut flours (corn and soy if not sensitive)

Yeast-free grain cereals that are unsweetened

Quinoa or rice pasta

Dairy substitutions:

Rice milk, almond milk, hemp milk

Rice, almond cheeses

If dairy tolerant, goat milk, goat cheeses, goat kefir

Proteins:

Lean meats – beef, chicken, turkey, buffalo, lamb (organic is best, grass fed when available)

All fish – deep sea white fish, salmon and sardines are particularly beneficial

Beans – sprout your beans before cooking them

Nuts – avoid peanuts and pistachios, soak nuts in water

Condiments:

Liquid amino acids in place of soy sauce

Cold-pressed olive oil, flax oils, coconut oil

Raw apple cider vinegar

All spices (as tolerated) – garlic, tumeric, ginger, sea salt, etc.

Beverages:

Drink at least ½ your weight in ounces of water daily, lemon or lime may be added

Herbal teas (chamomile, peppermint, pau d'arco, etc)

Green tea is a great coffee substitute

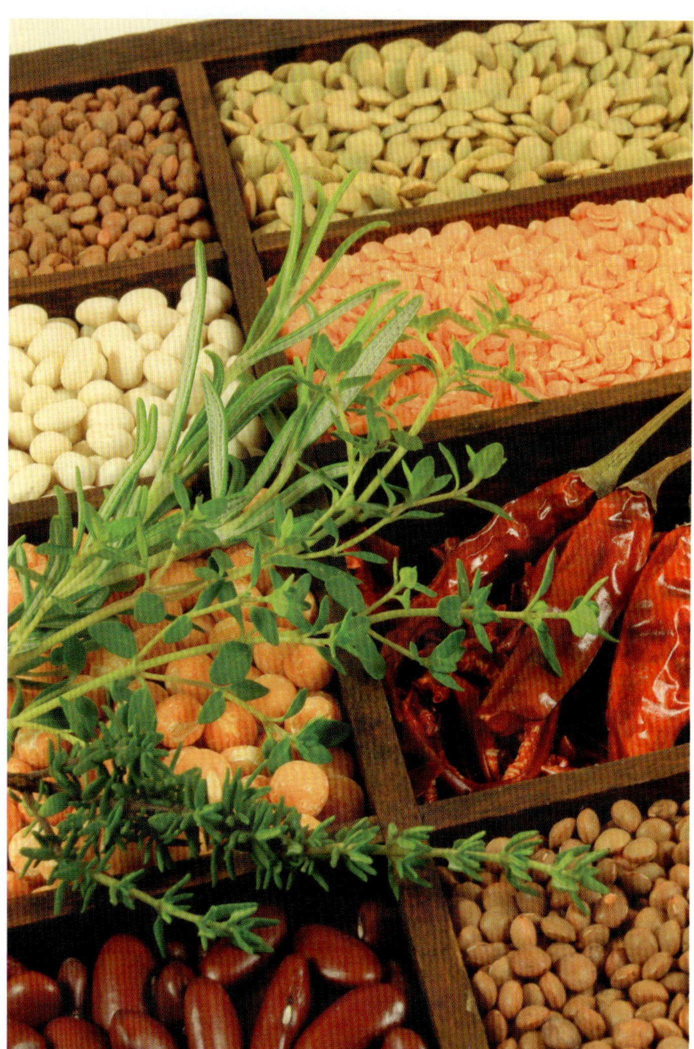

Sparkling or soda water

Vegetable juices (see vegetables above)

Sweeteners:

Lo han and stevia are extraordinarily sweet natural sugar substitutes

FOODS TO AVOID

Sugars and artificial sweeteners:

Table sugar, honey, fructose, molasses, maple syrup, corn syrup, etc., and any foods containing these

Limit grains:

During the first week or two, all grains should be eliminated.

Gluten-free grains many be added after that

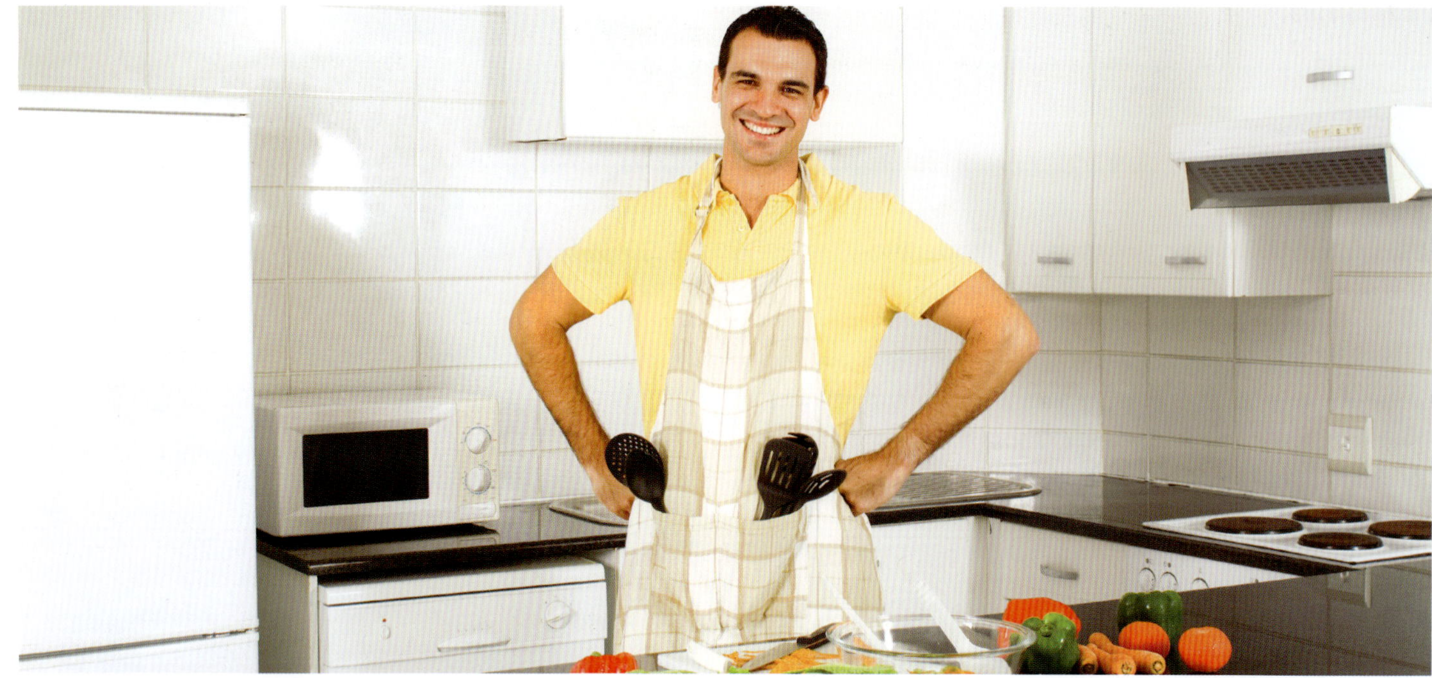

Preparing your own meals will help ensure that you're eating the right foods.

Fruits and fruit juices:

Most fruits and fruit juices have a high sugar content

Yeast-containing foods:

Most breads, rolls and crackers

Beer and wine

Sauerkraut, vinegars (found in many foods – check the label), soy sauce, Worcestershire sauce, horseradish, pickles, relish, green olives, dry roasted nuts

Mushrooms and cheese:

Contain mold or yeast

Peanuts and peanut-containing products:

Have high aflatoxin content, a carcinogenic mold

Most dairy products:

See exceptions under "Foods to Enjoy"

Pickled, smoked or dried meat, fish, poultry

If extremely sensitive, avoid or limit coffee, tea, pepper, many spices, tobacco, which tend to acquire mold or yeast in drying process.

YEAST-FREE AND/OR GLUTEN-FREE BRANDS

Food for Life
Glutino
Bob's Red Mill
Breads from Anna
Chebe bread
Ener-G
Pacific Bakery
Kinnikinnick Foods
Smart Snacks
Arrowhead Mills
Kinnikinnick
Pamela's Products
Mary's Gone Crackers
Quinoa Corp
Ian's
Udi's

These brands and more can be found online or at your local health food store. Store clerks can also help you find yeast- free foods.

Breakfast Recipe

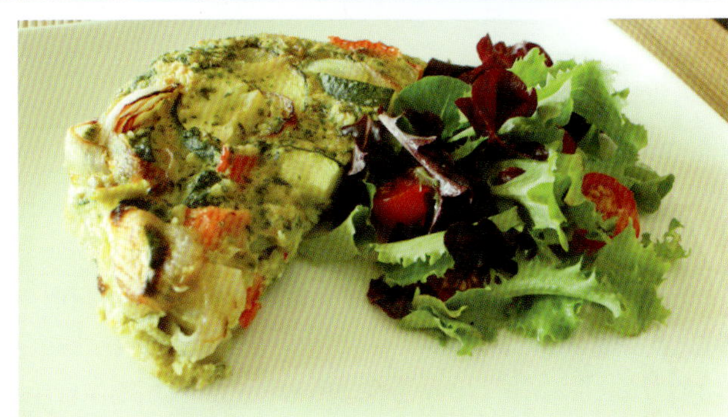

thecandidadiet.com

Vegetable Quiche

serves two

1 bell pepper
2 red onions
½ zucchini
3 eggs
1 clove garlic
Pine nuts (a handful)
Fresh basil leaves (a handful)
3 Tbsp olive oil
Green salad leaves
Preheat oven to 180C.

Chop vegetables and panfry with 1 ½ tbsp olive oil on medium heat for 3-4 minutes, then add to a well oiled ovenproof dish.

Add basil, garlic, pine nuts and eggs to the food processor. Now pour over the vegetables and bake for 25 minutes or until firm in the centre. Serve with green salad.

Lunch Recipe

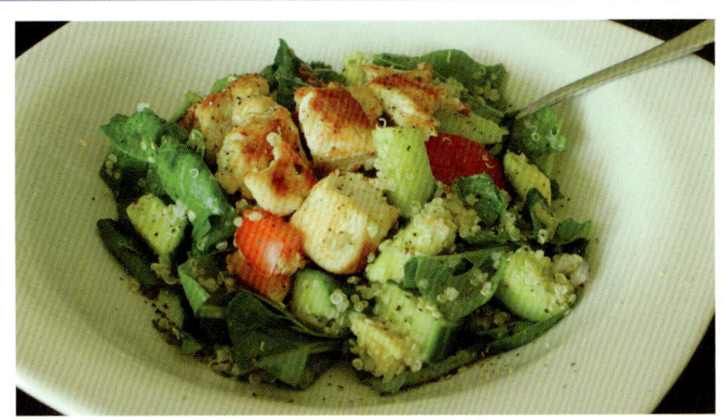

thecandidadiet.com

Chicken Quinoa Salad

serves four

1 chicken breast
⅔ cup of cooked quinoa
2 cups of spinach
2 medium tomatoes
½ a cucumber
1 avocado
2 shallots
1 garlic clove
Juice of ½ lemon
2 tablespoons olive oil
Salt and pepper to taste

Cook the quinoa as directed. Chop up chicken, pan-fry until cooked, about 5 minutes. Now chop up the veggies, toss everything in a bowl and serve.

Snack Recipe

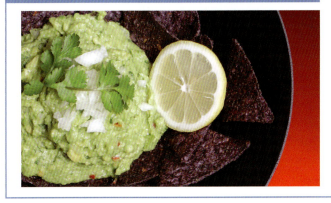

Delicious Guacamole

serves four

2 avocados
1 tomato
½ onion
1 clove garlic, grated
Lemon/lime juice, fresh

This is a quick and easy 10-minute recipe that will impress houseguests and is all-natural and healthy for your skin. Just chop and mash up all the ingredients in a bowl, then throw a couple of sprigs of cilantro on top for presentation.

Dinner Recipe

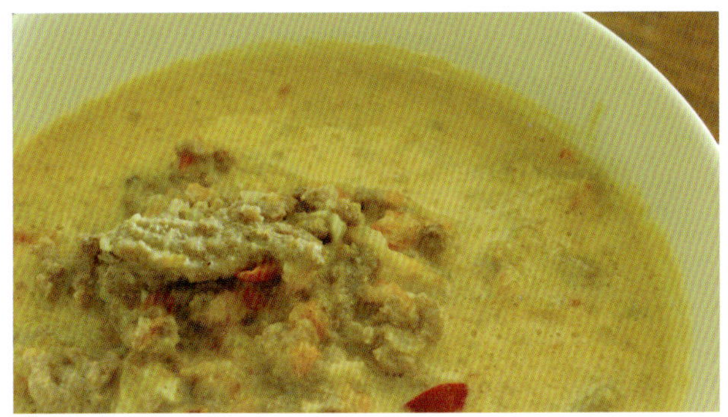

thecandidadiet.com

Lamb Coconut Curry

serves two

500 mg minced lamb
4 medium tomatoes, chopped
1 medium onion
1 can coconut milk
2 cloves garlic
1 tablespoon coconut oil
1 chili pepper (seeds removed)
½ teaspoon cayenne pepper
½ teaspoon turmeric powder
½ teaspoon curry powder
Salt to taste

Chop up the onions, garlic and chili pepper - you can use your food processor to save time. Add them to a frying pan with the lamb and a tablespoon of coconut oil for 5 minutes. Then add all the other ingredients, and simply leave it to simmer for 30 minutes on a low heat.Serve with wild or brown rice (optional).

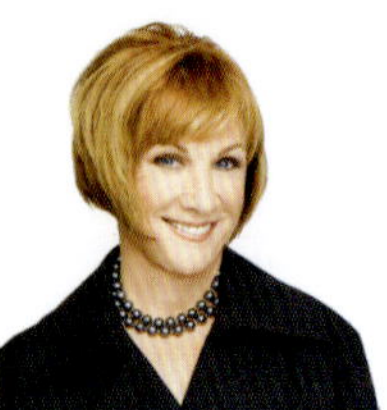

Steps of Cleansing

When I began cleansing for my own health in the late 80s, it was a labor-intensive, time-consuming process of fasting and juicing that involved a lot of down-time. Later when I began to educate the public about cleansing I realized that most people were not willing or able to do such an intensive program.

The only cleansing products available on the market were colon cleanses made from psyllium fiber. I don't recommend this fiber, however, because it can be irritating for people with a sensitive colon. Cleansing was changing at this time because people were not able to spend so much time and effort on the process. Products were developed that took a total-body approach, supporting all the organs of elimination, not just the colon.

I began to educate the public on this new approach to cleansing over a period of about two to three years. One thing I noticed was that people were still confused about cleansing programs. It was then that I realized the program needed to be organized into steps.

Let me explain a little more about how I developed the Steps of Cleansing. When I developed the first program on internal cleansing, it was focused on parasite elimination. The product had been heavily researched, as I had used the formula for years in my digestive care clinics before entering the natural products industry for the health food store market. Once the product was on the market, some consumers called who had reactions like headache, or flu-like symptoms.

In my digestive care clinics, anyone taking this kind of formula would have also done colon hydrotherapy before or during the cleanse. Now, people were purchasing the product from a health food store without having cleansed before. I soon realized what was happening. People who had not first addressed cleansing of the seven channels of elimination experienced these cleansing reactions because of what is known as "die off." Die off occurs when harmful organisms die in the intestines and give off toxins. This is also known as a Herxheimer reaction. I responded by formulating a Total Body Cleanse program and always suggest people take it before any type of microbial cleansing, whether for parasites or Candida. This is very important in the process of healing.

As I continued to lecture and consult, and as the science around cleansing developed, I formulated more targeted cleansing programs for the liver and kidneys, as well as specific heavy metal detoxing programs. I put these all programs into a step-by-step process so they could be utilized over a time period to make the program easier for people to follow, as well as thorough enough to prepare the body for deeper cleansing. Please remember that it takes time for the body heal from the inside out.

My hope, for you, is that the Steps of Cleansing program is a transformative program for your health. It needs to be incorporated into a full program of healthy eating, exercise and plenty of water intake. I suggest a Total Body Cleanse program for 30 days. From there, the Steps of Cleansing can be tailored to your health condition. My programs are not about quick results, but more about the long-term benefit of good health.

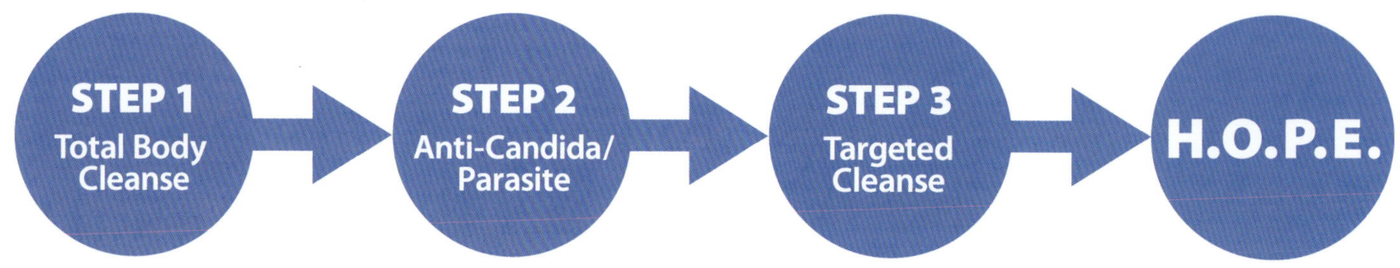

The Process of Detoxification & Elimination

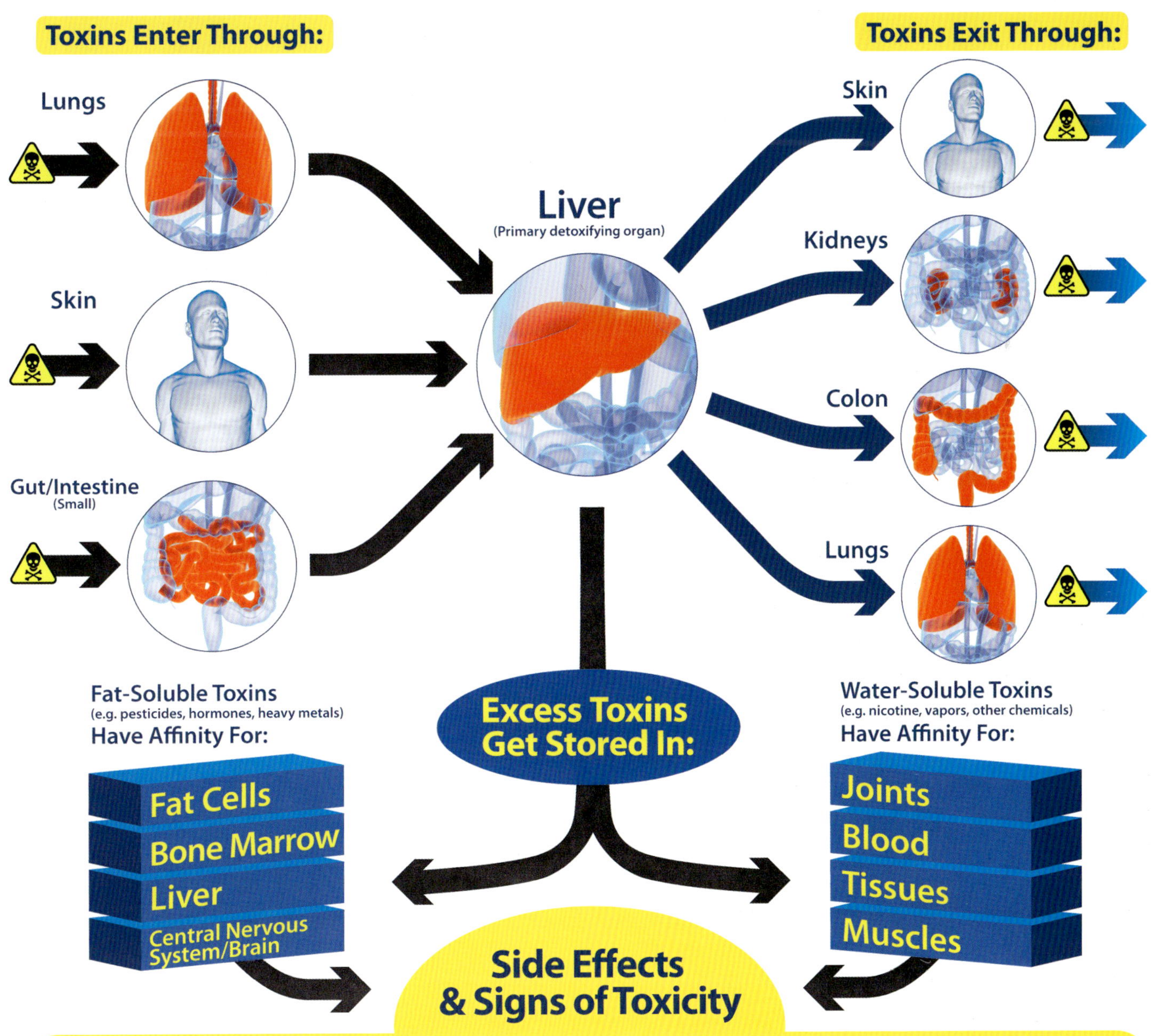

Side Effects & Signs of Toxicity

acne/skin rashes • allergies • arthritis/joint pain • autoimmune disorders • cardiovascular disease chronic fatigue • constipation • diabetes • diarrhea • fibromyalgia • headaches hormone imbalance • inflammatory disorders • IBS • neurologic disorders • obesity/overwieght

STEPS OF CLEANSING

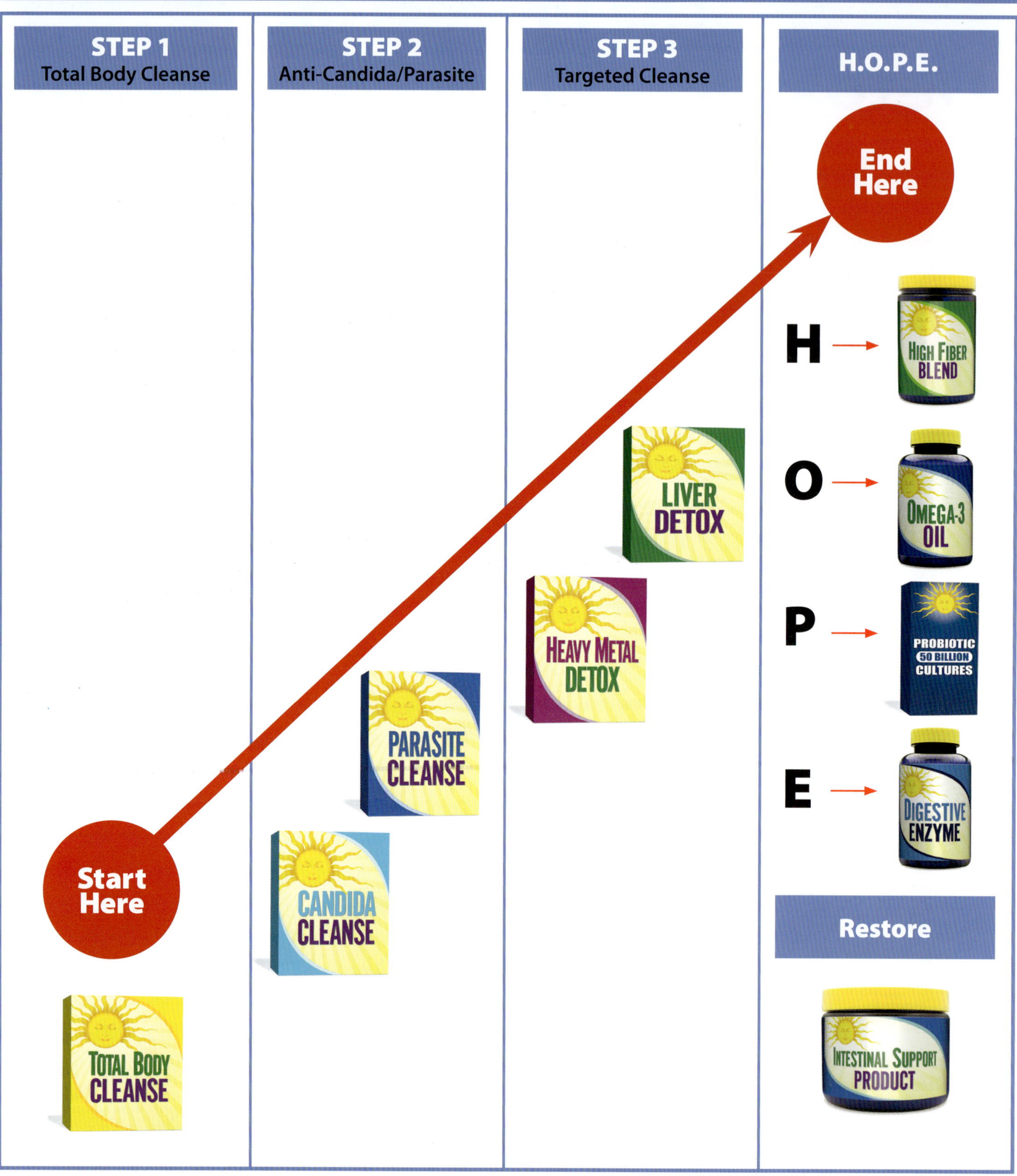

For optimal results: Maintenance products: H.O.P.E. **H**igh fiber, **O**il, **P**robiotics and **E**nzymes should be used for each cleanse.

Step One: **Total Body Cleanse**

Supports all seven channels of elimination for a comprehensive initial cleanse: Liver, lungs, skin, kidneys, blood, lymphatic system and colon.

Step Two: **Elimination of Microorganisms with Candida Cleanse or Parasite Cleanse**

Supports the elimination of parasites and other intestinal microbes, as well as yeast overgrowth (Candida).

Step Three: **Targeted Cleanse with Liver Detox, Kidney Detox or Heavy Metal Detox**

Specifically supports detoxification of the liver and kidneys and elimination of heavy metals in the body.

Step One: Total Body Cleansing

Since most of us in today's world lead busy, stressful lives, it is of utmost importance to keep the cleansing program as simple as possible. There are two areas to address when beginning a total body cleanse: The first focuses on the cleansing of the colon, while the second targets the remaining channels of elimination—liver, blood, lymph, skin, kidneys and lungs—supporting them with herbs and nutraceutricals. This is total body detoxification. When the liver is overburdened with toxins, the load is passed on through blood and lymph circulation to other organs of elimination: colon, kidneys, lungs and skin. It is therefore wise to begin a general cleanse that is designed to support all of these organs simultaneously, with special emphasis on the liver and colon. General cleanse kits are easy to use and are available in a variety of programs—first-time cleanses, 30-day cleanses, rapid cleanses and even liquid cleanses. Such kits should include herbs that provide support for all organs and systems of elimination. Included in an effective herbal cleansing formula would be ingredients such as:

Milk thistle – stimulates bile secretion, acts as an antioxidant, and strengthens the cells of the liver to protect them.
Dandelion – stimulates bile and acts as a gentle laxative.
Beet – helps reduce damaging fats in the liver.
Artichoke leaf – stimulates secretion of bile and protects cells of the liver.
Mullein, an expectorant – helps expel mucus from the lungs.
Burdock – helps purge toxins that cause skin conditions.
Corn silk – a diuretic to flush the kidneys.
Red clover – a blood purifier and expectorant.
Larch gum – a blood purifier and expectorant.

Among other colon cleansing herbs, a total body cleanse formula should contain cape aloe, rhubarb, burdock or triphala to stimulate intestinal peristalsis, and magnesium hydroxide to regulate water in the bowel. **It is very important that the colon functions properly or it will not be capable of eliminating toxins from the liver.** These toxins will then recirculate, creating more of a problem. Colon-cleansing formulas like this should be taken in the evening before bed. Kits containing these herbs that address both colon and total-body cleansing make your cleanse very easy to perform.

Fiber is also important in a cleansing program. Cleansing stimulates the liver to release toxins into the bile, which is then secreted back into the digestive tract (via the gallbladder). It is necessary to ingest extra fiber for these toxins to be absorbed and removed through bowel elimination. One of the best fiber supplements is flax, as it is about 50 percent soluble and 50 percent insoluble fiber. Soluble fiber absorbs the toxins, and insoluble fiber sweeps the colon. Flax is also available in organic (pesticide-free) form, which is a plus. Unless severe constipation is an issue, never do a cleansing program without adding fiber for support to pick up and eliminate the toxins. If constipation is an issue, fiber can be added after bowel elimination is regulated.

Step Two: Elimination of Microorganisms

For many people, an underlying cause of their health problems is a dysbiotic (imbalanced) microflora in the digestive tract caused by an overgrowth of either Candida or parasites. For these people, a Candida or Parasite Cleanse should be undertaken to help eliminate these harmful microorganisms and rebalance the digestive tract.

Candida Cleanse

This would be a formula that helps the body to eliminate Candida overgrowth. It should be a two-part formula that includes a capsule formula along with a liquid herbal tincture. The product should combine a broad spectrum of natural anti-fungals, including:

Uva ursi

Calcium undecylenate

Neem leaf

Olive leaf

Berberine sulphate

Oregano leaf

Oregano grape root

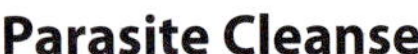

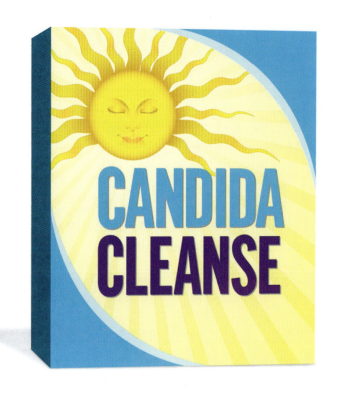

Parasite Cleanse

This formula will help support the body's elimination of parasitic overgrowth. Look for a two-part formula that includes a capsule formula along with a liquid herbal tincture. The product should combine natural antimicrobial herbs including:

Wormwood

Garlic

Cloves

Undecylenic acid

Grapefruit seed extract

Pumpkin seed

Pippali

Quassia

Rosmary and thyme

In more severe cases, these programs may be repeated up to three times consecutively. The Candida Diet should be followed during these programs to maximize the benefits of the program.

Other supplements that should be taken during these cleansing programs include:

A parasite or Candida-specific enzyme formula that targets the degradation of these harmful microorganisms.The enzymes are taken on an empty stomach so that they reach the intestines.

Probiotics to replenish the friendly bacteria that have been out of balance. This is a very important part of the protocol for establishing and maintaining intestinal balance. The probiotic should be taken at least two hours apart from the anti-parasite or anti-Candida supplements.

Fiber supplement, to support bowel regularity and to help absorb any microbial toxins that are produced during the "die-off" of parasites and yeast. Look for a fiber that contains flax seed, oat bran and acacia fiber for a good mix of soluble and insoluble fibers.

Omega oils to lubricate the intestines and provide anti-inflammatory support. Purified fish oil, or a mix of omega oils (with omega-3, 5, 6, 7, 9) is best. Look for an omega oil that contains the enzyme lipase for better absorption.

If the anti-parasitic program or anti-Candida program does not seem to be working, antibiotics may be needed.

Step Three: Targeted Cleansing

Liver Detox

Liver detox formulas are designed to support liver detoxification mechanisms, while reducing the amount of detoxification stress. Due to the thousands of chemicals people encounter each day, this cleanse is recommended for everyone. A complete liver detox program would support phase I and phase II detoxification pathways of the liver, which are overworked when liver toxicity is present. This support is best achieved with antioxidants and herbs.

The two-part liver detox program should be followed for 30 days. Part I would include a combination of the following antioxidants and herbs:

NAC (N-aceytl-cysteine)

Alpha lipoic acid

Selenium

Vitamin C and E

Taurine and methionine (amino acids)

Phosphatidylcholine choline

Milk thistle, dandelion, green tea and tumeric

This antioxidant liver formula (Part I) should be accompanied by an evening formula (Part II) that includes herbs to increase bile flow. Ayurvedic medicine (from India) uses some wonderful herbs that have been quite successful in liver detoxification. They include:

Belleric myrobalan fruit (Terminalia bellerica)

Boerhavia diffusa root and herb

Eclipta alba root and herb

Tinospora conrdifolia stem

Andrographis paniculata leaf

Picrohiza kurroa root

This combination of antioxidants and herbs (Parts I and II) creates a total liver detox formula, which can be followed continuously while adhering to dietary guidelines. A good flax-fiber supplement added to this program will help absorb the toxins that are being eliminated from the liver. An important function of a Liver Detox is to stimulate bile flow, which can become stagnant over time, increasing in toxicity. Increasing bile flow helps to move toxins out of the body that are carried in bile.

Heavy Metal Detox

A heavy metal detox formula specifically supports the body's elimination of heavy metals through natural chelation and support of detoxification. The formula should be a 30-day program that includes a two-part formula. The Morning Support Formula should contain vitamins and minerals that are used to support overall body health and detoxification functions. It should include ingredients like:

Vitamin C

B vitamins

Minerals

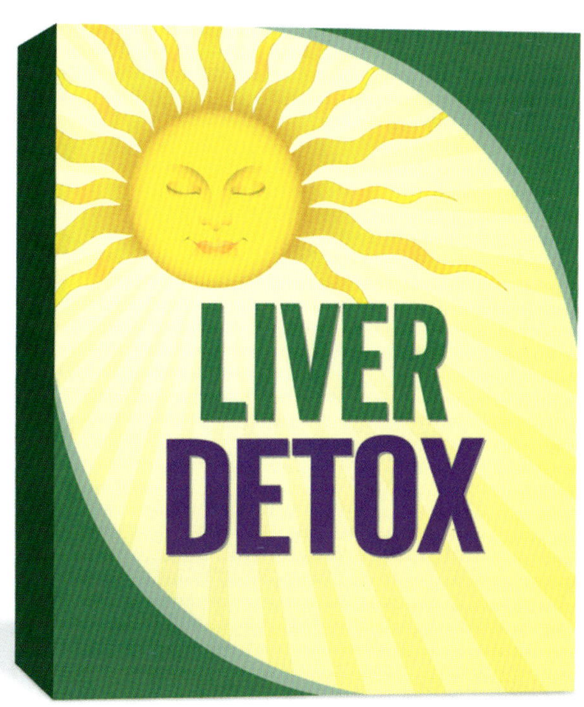

The evening formula should contain natural herbs and amino acids that have traditionally been used to support organ cleansing and natural chelation. These ingredients include:

Chlorella

Cilantro leaf

Spirulina

N-acetyl-cysteine (NAC)

Alpha-lipoic acid (ALA)

After completing these detox programs, many people feel rejuvenated and have noticeably more energy. Those who are in good health need this type of detox to stay on that path. Those with chronic health problems (especially those with liver damage), need this type of detox as part of their recovery process. The programs may be repeated for optimal results.

Total Kidney Detox

Every day, the kidneys filter several quarts of fluid from the bloodstream, allowing metabolic waste (urea) to leave the body in urine. The kidneys also adjust the body's balance of calcium, potassium, and phosphate. The bladder is a storage organ for urine that will drain through the urinary tract. The healthy urinary tract is sterile, that is, free of bacteria. When bacteria from the digestive system grow in the urinary tract, irritation to the urinary tract and bladder can occur.

A Kidney Detox formula should be a two-part blend of herbs and potassium that helps cleanse the kidneys, bladder and urinary tract. The herbs found in Part I should include:

Cranberry extract

Parsley

Dandelion

Horsetail

Stinging nettle extract

Part II should contain alkalizing compounds traditionally used to help soothe the kidneys, bladder and urinary tract, including:

Potassium

Uva ursi extract

Arbutin

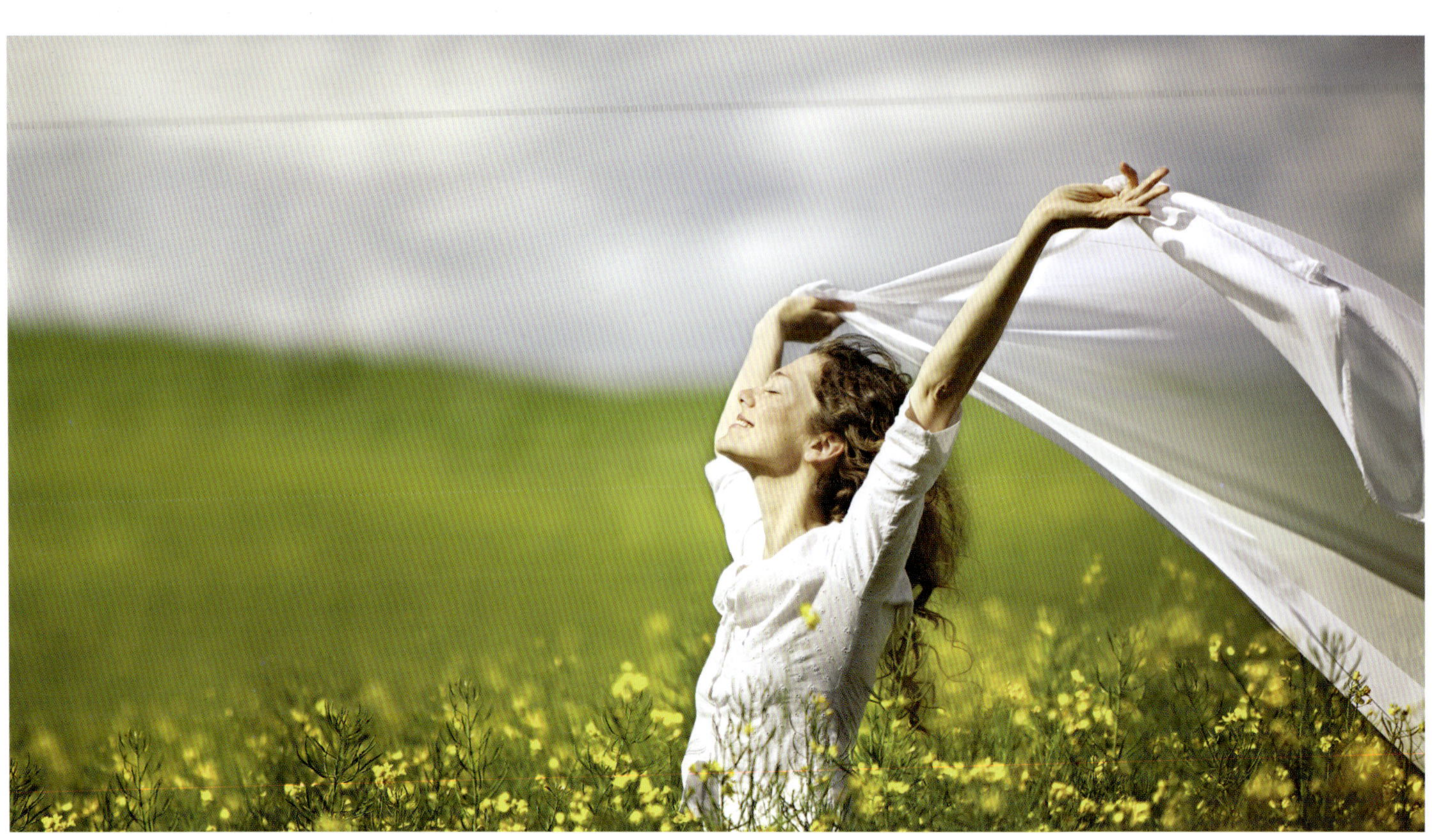

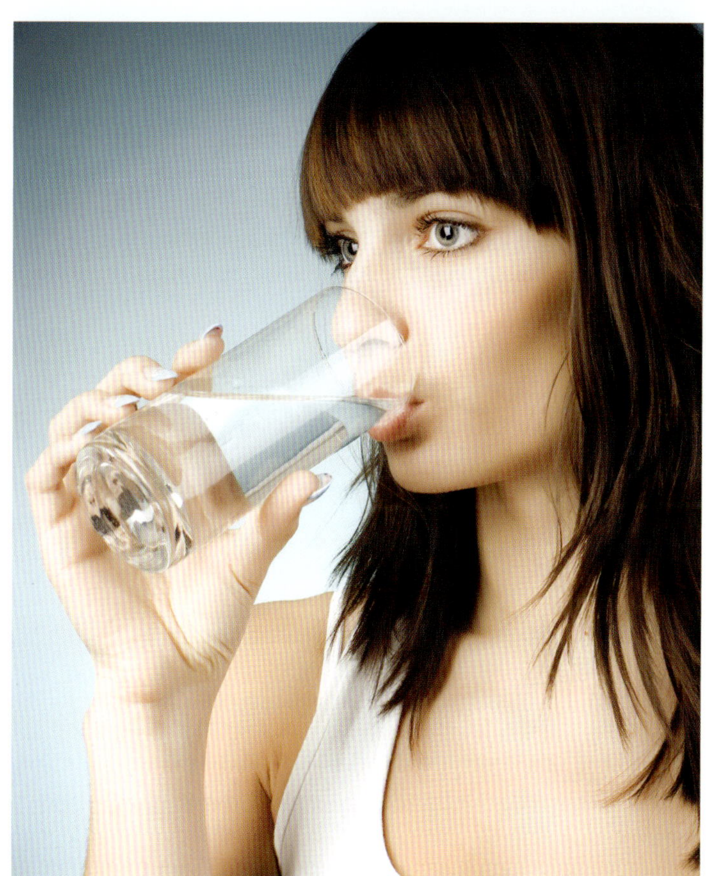

Drink plenty of water while cleansing.

Cleansing Reaction – Why do I Feel Worse?!

While the net result of a cleanse will be elimination of toxins from the body, improved health and more energy, it is quite common to feel worse before feeling better. As herbal cleansing formulas kill disease-causing microorganisms, such as Candida and parasites, toxins are released into the system. If they are released faster than the body can eliminate them, symptoms such as fever, fatigue, diarrhea, cramps, headache, increased thirst, loss of appetite, flu-like conditions, skin eruptions or irritations may be experienced. These symptoms are due to a "die-off" reaction known as the Herxheimer Reaction. It is sometimes difficult to distinguish between such a reaction and an actual illness. A natural health care practitioner can be of assistance in this regard.

Generally speaking, the Herxeimer reaction is shortlived (a day or two, but usually no longer than a week). Symptoms may range from mild to severe, depending upon the rate of cleansing. The following steps will help to avoid, reduce or eliminate a severe healing crisis.

Start at very low doses of your herbal cleansing formula—half the recommended dose (or less, if necessary), and then gradually increase to the recommended level during a 30-day period.

If liver support herbs are not present in your cleansing formula or you have a history of liver problems, support the liver with an appropriate herbal formula.

Initiate the necessary dietary modification two weeks before starting the herbal cleanse.

Get colon hydrotherapy sessions.

Increase your water intake.

Always take a fiber supplement.

A formula containing activated charcoal, bentonite clay and glucomannan will help to absorb toxins released by dying pathogens, and eliminate them with bowel movements.

A cleansing reaction, while uncomfortable to experience, is actually a sign of healing in progress. So, if the symptoms are mild and tolerable, there is no need to adjust the dosage of your herbal cleansing product. Try to resist the temptation to suppress symptoms with drugs; it will only increase the body's toxic load and halt the cleansing process.

When you start a detox or cleansing program, especially as a first-time cleanser, it is important to keep it simple. A realistic commitment is required to stay excited about creating long-term optimal health. Some detox options may not be available to you, or you may not be able to fit them into your schedule. The whole body herbal cleansing program is not a one-time affair. It is best incorporated into a prevention program at least twice a year. It is the first step toward complete detoxification. For people who have many health problems, it may be necessary to seek the services of a natural health care practitioner or physician who can design a custom program. Regardless of whether you choose this option or elect to use a pre-formulated cleanse, this is your first step in the detoxification process, the cornerstone of good health. Whichever option is chosen, clean the digestive system and support the organs of elimination before moving on to more advanced cleanses, like those that address Candida, parasites, heavy metals or liver detoxification.

A Sample Day of Total-Body Cleanse and Detox Schedule

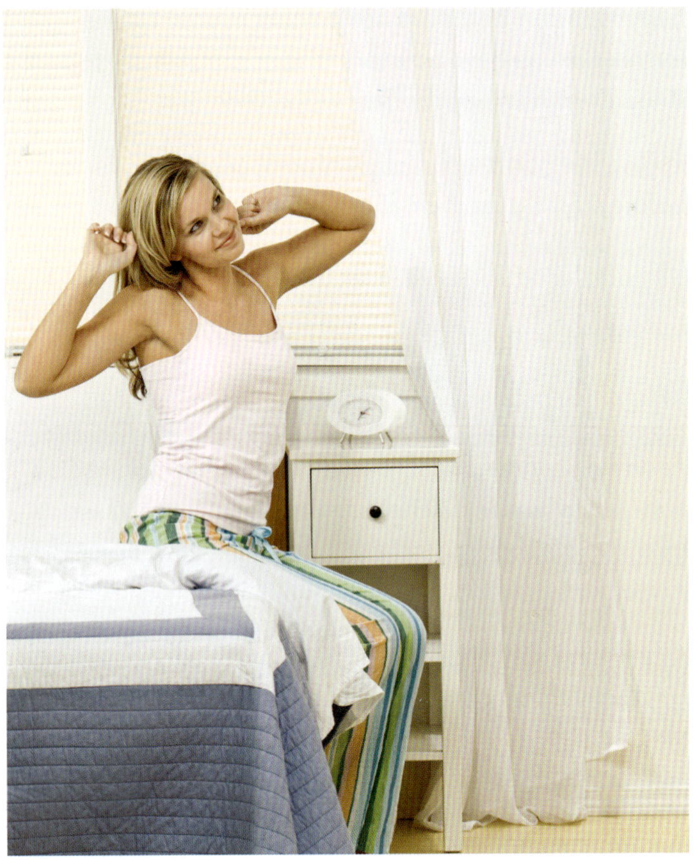

6:00 a.m. Wake up. Drink glass of room-temperature or warm fresh-squeezed lemon water. Take one dose of probiotic supplement.

6:30 a.m. 10 to 20 minutes of exercise—rebounding, bands, yoga, or cardio. Drink a glass of water during or after exercise.

7:00 a.m. Take morning dose of total-body cleanse or herbal detox product with glass of water. Dry skin brush whole body before showering.

7:30 a.m. Have a good breakfast. Choose from breakfast choices in Fiber 35 Eating Plan or Candida Diet (See the Appendix). Take enzymes and oils with the meal.

10:30 a.m. Have a fiber drink or bar. Choose from fiber choices in Fiber 35 Eating Plan.

11:00 a.m. Have one ounce liquid greens supplement with eight ounces of water, glass of fresh vegetable juice, or cup of broth.

12:30 p.m. Have lunch. Choose from lunch recipes in Fiber 35 Eating Plan or Candida Diet. Take enzymes with meal.

2:00 p.m. Have a fiber drink or bar. Choose from fiber choices in Fiber 35 Eating Plan.

3:00 p.m. Have one ounce liquid greens supplement with eight ounces of water, glass of fresh vegetable juice, or cup of broth.

5:00 p.m. Optional short exercise session (5 to 10 minutes).

6:00 p.m. Have dinner. Choose from dinner recipes in Fiber 35 Eating Plan or Candida Diet. Take enzymes and oils with meal.

7:00 p.m. Optional walk for 15 or 20 minutes.

8:00 p.m. Sauna or soak. Relax and meditate.

9:00 p.m. Take evening dose of total-body cleanse or herbal detox product and fiber supplement before bed with glass of water.

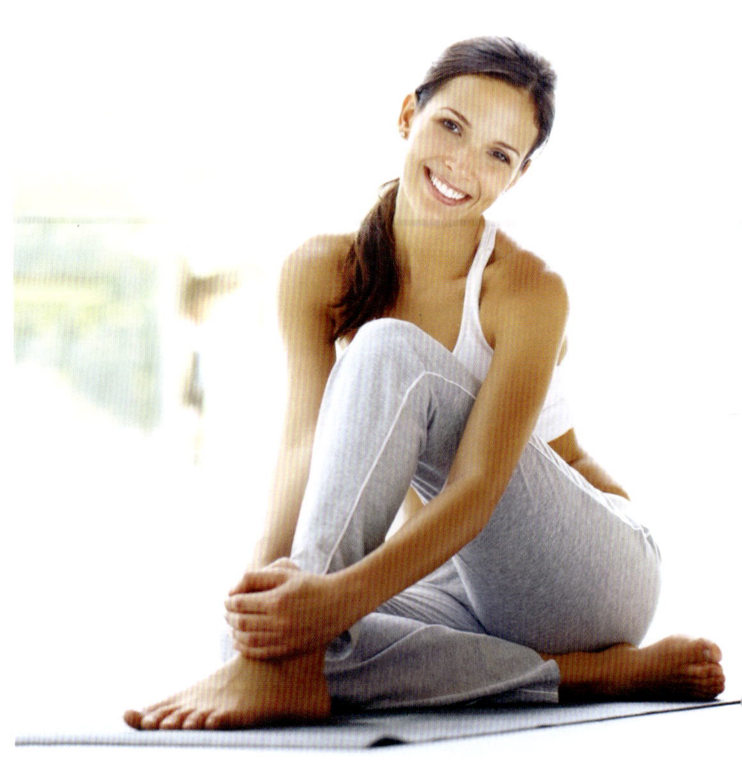

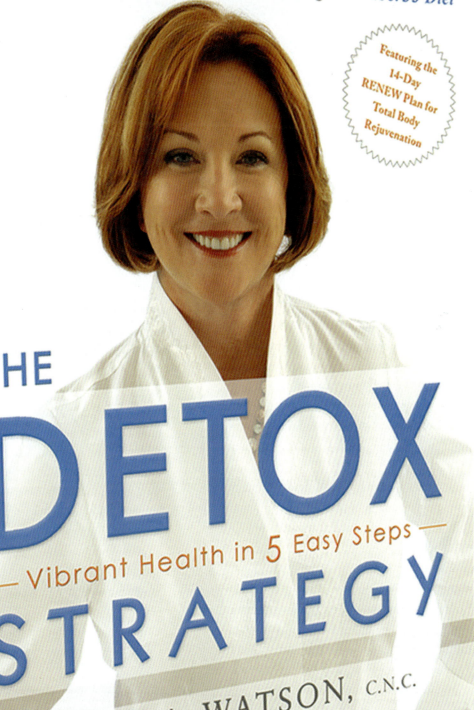

Author of The New York Times bestselling The Fiber35 Diet
Featuring the 14-Day RENEW Plan for Total Body Rejuvenation
THE DETOX
— Vibrant Health in 5 Easy Steps —
STRATEGY
BRENDA WATSON, C.N.C.
WITH LEONARD SMITH, M.D

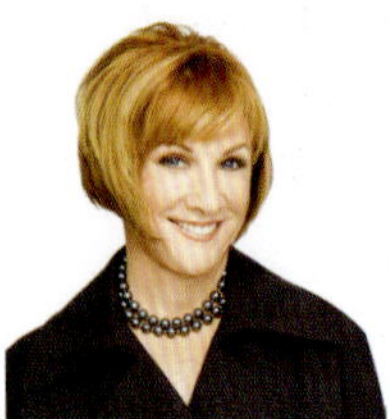

Colon Hydrotherapy

On the topic of colon hydrotherapy I would like to add my personal experience. As is common in my life, when I am ready the lesson appears. And so it was with colonics. Years ago, after I began to heal my body with diet and supplementation, I learned about colonics. Since I had many digestive problems, I thought I would give it a try. As it turned out, my health really began to turn around as I reset my digestive system with this beneficial therapy, along with herbal cleansing protocols.

As a result of this healing, I entered the field of colon hydrotherapy. I was able to work with hundreds of people over the years in a very busy alternative health clinic. I was fortunate enough to work with not only health care practitioners, but with holistic-minded MDs, which strengthened even more my belief in holistic medicine. I witnessed amazing health changes occurring to people who used natural methods of healing, and I was also humbled by the devastating effects that chronic disease and cancer can have on the body. Colonics can be a profound therapy for people.

In the state of Florida, where I live, colon hydrotherapy has been a licensed therapy since 1952. When performed by a licensed colon hydrotherapist, colonics are a safe and effective therapy. I have personally seen so many people benefit from this little-known therapy.

I never thought I would see the day when traditional gastroenterologists (GI doctors) would embrace colon hydrotherapy. But the time has finally come. One of the first digestive care clinics that I founded began receiving patients from a local GI doctor for pre-colonoscopy treatment. The positive feedback from his patients, as well as the beneficial results that he saw in their digestive tracts, are now being seen by other GI doctors as colon hydrotherapy use by mainstream medicine is increasing as an alternative to the toxic and uncomfortable pre-colonoscopy treatment.

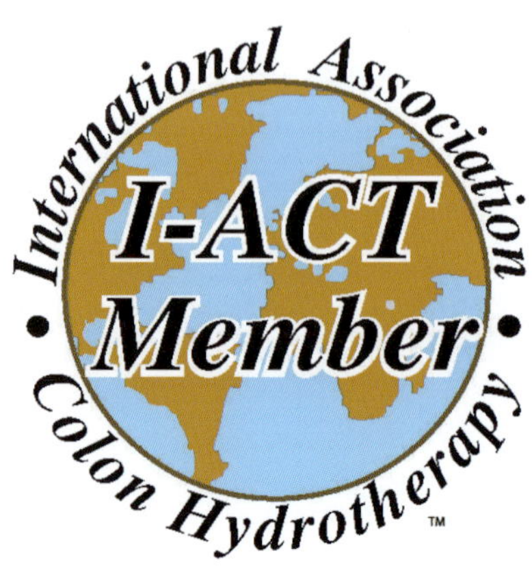

As with any treatment, whether mainstream or alternative, you must do your homework before approaching any therapy. The following information about colon hydrotherapy can help you decide whether it may be right for you. You will also learn how to find a certified colon hydrotherapist with the right equipment. Colon hydrotherapy could very well be something that helps you on the road to perfect health.

Colon hydrotherapy (also known as a colonic) is basically an extended and more complete form of enema. Both the enema and the colonic involve the infusion of water into the colon through the anal opening. However, the enema is a one-time infusion of water into the rectum. The patient takes in as much as a quart of water, holds it for a time, and then releases it directly into the toilet. In contrast, colonic treatments (now known as colon hydrotherapy sessions) involve repeated infusions of filtered, warm water into all segments of the colon by a certified colon therapist. During the course of a treatment, the patient lies comfortably on his or her back.

Colon hydrotherapists are trained to use massage techniques to help relax abdominal muscles and ensure that all areas of the colon are adequately irrigated. While the colon is filled and emptied a few times during one 45-minute session, there is no need for the client to leave the table to expel the water. The passage of the water in and out of the colon is controlled by the therapist who operates the colonic apparatus while the client lies still on the table. As the water leaves the body, it passes through a clear viewing tube, allowing both client and therapist to see what is being eliminated from the colon. In addition to fecal matter, gas bubbles, mucus and parasites are often seen.

There is no odor or health risk involved in the colonic procedure when performed properly by a trained, certified colon therapist. Therapeutic benefits of colon hydrotherapy include improved tone of colonic muscles, reduced stagnation of intestinal contents, reduced toxic waste absorption and the thorough cleansing and balancing of the colon.

Your colon can hold a great deal of waste material. That which is not eliminated promptly putrefies, adding to the toxic load of your body. Many people with "potbellies" may actually have several pounds of old, hardened fecal matter lodged within their colons. While colon hydrotherapy is not actually a weight loss procedure, it does often result in significant weight loss due to its ability to efficiently reduce the toxic burden of the large intestine. Furthermore, several ailments have been associated with colon toxicity. People with conditions in this book may benefit from colon hydrotherapy.

Colon hydrotherapy has helped many people overcome constipation. Unlike chemical laxatives, it does not encourage dependency, but rather helps to tone the bowel, gently prompting it to resume normal functioning. Your cleansing, as well as overall health, will be aided significantly by the addition of colon hydrotherapy sessions. Such therapy stimulates the liver, your body's major organ of detoxification, helping it to eliminate toxins.

Colon hydrotherapy also benefits your body's lymphatic system, for when the intestinal walls are impacted, the lymphatic system retains and continuously re-circulates cellular waste. Your lymphatic system becomes stagnant when the normally clear lymph fluid becomes thick with cellular debris, toxins, microorganisms and dietary fats. Thickened, stagnant lymph contributes to fatigue, malaise (vague feeling of illness) and weight gain, especially around the abdomen, hips and buttocks. Look for a colon hydrotherapist certified by the International Association for Colon Hydrotherapy (I-ACT). These therapists use FDA-registered equipment, disposable rectal nozzles (called speculums) and filtered water. I-ACT is the worldwide certifying body for colon hydrotherapists. The organization works in conjunction with local municipalities to regulate colon hydrotherapy by establishing standards and guidelines.

If you are able to add one or more colon hydrotherapy sessions to your cleansing regime, it can greatly facilitate your progress, and help to prevent or alleviate the symptoms associated with cleansing reactions (and with colon toxicity). Your colon therapist, following your initial session, can give guidelines about suggested frequency and duration of treatment. If colon hydrotherapy is not an option for you, enemas may be used instead. Though not as thorough as colonics, they do facilitate colon cleansing.

You can enhance your colon cleansing efforts if you stimulate the natural squatting position when you sit on the toilet to have a bowel movement. This can be done easily by elevating your feel while seated on a commode, resting them on a special platform called a LifeStep™. (See the Resource Directory.)

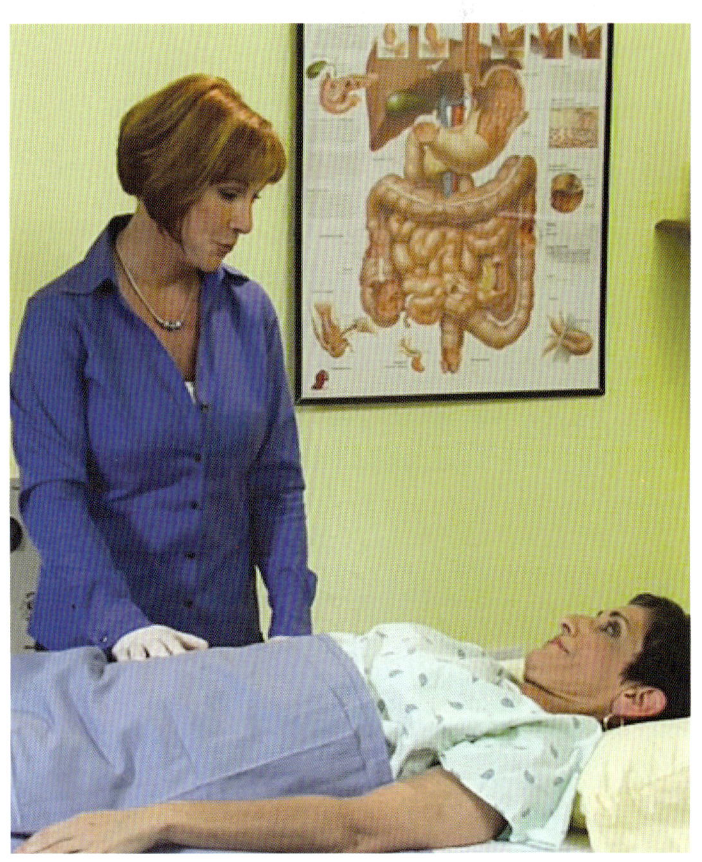

SUPPLEMENTS

The following is a description of certain supplements recommended in the book.
These products can be found in health food stores and in most places where dietary supplements are sold.

HOPE Formula

Basically, I coined the term "HOPE" from a very specific formula that I recommend to be taken daily. The HOPE Formula was designed to replace some of what the Standard American Diet (SAD) and modern living take away. I recommend the HOPE Formula be taken by everyone on a daily basis, being as important as a daily multi-vitamin/mineral. The HOPE Formula consists of:

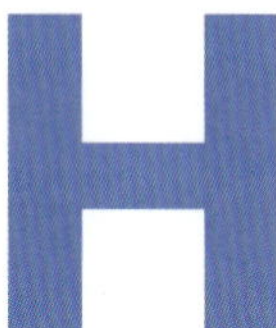

High Fiber: Dietary fiber adds bulk to the diet, which helps to strengthen and tone the colon muscles. Fiber also helps absorb and eliminate cholesterol, toxins and excess calories from the digestive tract.

Goal: At least 35 grams daily

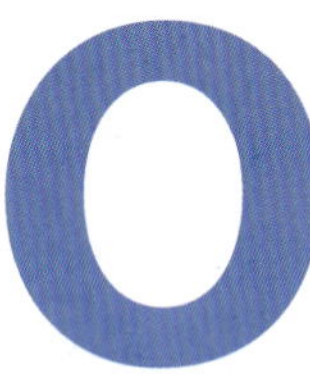

Omega Oils: Natural omega oils provide the necessary lubrication for smooth and gentle bowel elimination. The healthy oils also help nourish cells in the intestinal tract and throughout the body, relieving inflammation.

Goal: At least 3 grams daily

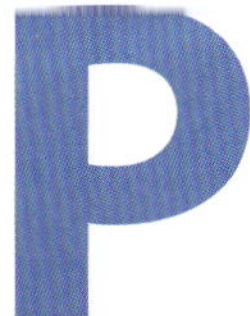

Probiotics: Beneficial probiotics promote healthy digestive and immune function by crowding out harmful bacteria in the digestive tract and promoting the growth of healthy flora. Probiotics also produce antibacterial compounds and stimulate the immune system.

Goal: 50 billion CFU (colony forming units, or culture count) daily

---

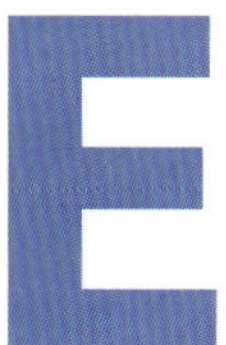

Enzymes: Digestive enzymes help break down a variety of foods such as carbohydrates, proteins, fats, sugars and dairy. They also enhance nutrient absorption from food.

Goal: Take with every meal

The following section will cover each of the four HOPE ingredients. You will learn what the ingredient is and how it contributes to good health, as well as what to look for in products containing these ingredients.

High Fiber

What is Fiber?

It used to be that fiber was thought of as one thing—roughage. But fiber actually comes in two forms. Think of fiber as one of those two-sided sponges. Soluble fiber is like the yellow part of the sponge, soaking up unwanted toxins and waste as it moves through the digestive tract. Insoluble fiber is like the green part of the sponge, helping to "scrub" the colon free of debris by removing toxins from the intestinal wall. Soluble fiber dissolves in water and leaves the stomach slowly. Insoluble fiber does not dissolve in water and travels through the intestines in much the same form as it was consumed. The natural ratio of a healthy diet is 65 to 75 percent insoluble fiber to 25 to 35 percent soluble fiber. All plant-based foods have both types of fiber.

By definition, dietary fiber includes the parts of plant foods that your body is unable to break down and absorb. This means that unlike other dietary components such as proteins, fats and carbohydrates that are ingested and absorbed, fiber passes through the body virtually intact. Fiber works to absorb and eliminate toxins and waste (including bad cholesterol) from the body, which prevents them from being reabsorbed back into the bloodstream.

The best way to receive your fiber is through a diet rich in fruits, vegetables, whole grains, legumes and other fiber-rich plant foods. Ideally, adults should consume at least 35 grams of fiber every day, but because many Americans consume less than half of that, a beneficial fiber supplement may be a convenient and easy way to provide the added fiber necessary to promote optimum health.

What to Look For in a Fiber Supplement

- Made with natural and organically grown ingredients
- Made with lignin-rich flax fiber, soluble acacia fiber or natural chia seed
- Psyllium-free to prevent cramping, gas or bloating
- Non-constipating

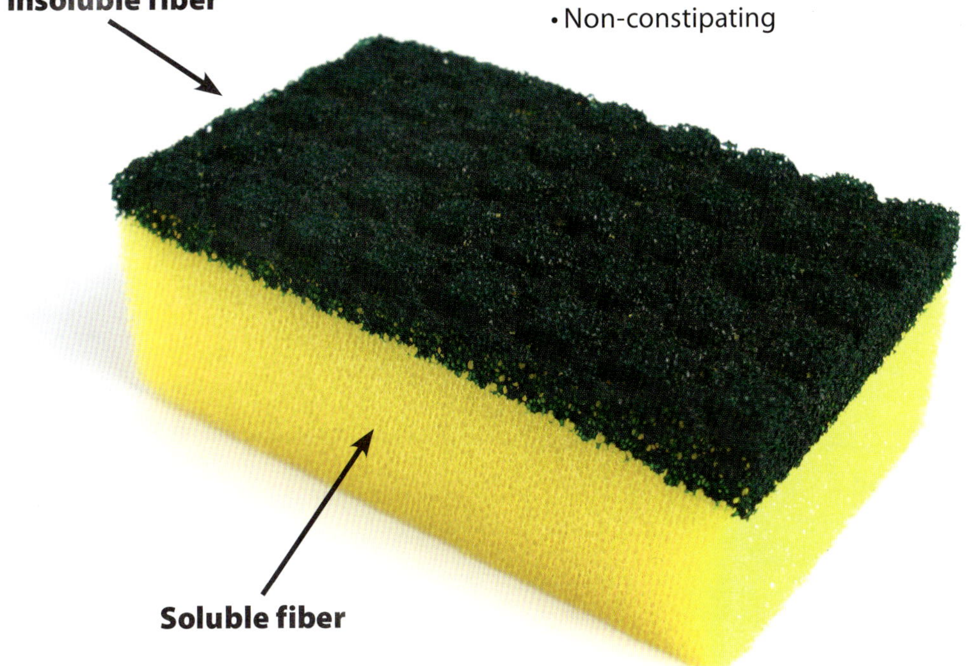

Omega Oils

What are Omega Oils?

Both omega-3 and omega-6 oils (fatty acids) are considered essential fatty acids (EFAs). Omega oils are important to your health because they cannot be produced by the body and must be obtained from the diet. Most Americans consume too many omega-6 fats and not enough omega-3 fats. What's more, it's important to consume the right omega-6 fats, which include those found in borage oil, evening primrose and black currant seed oil, all of which contain gamma linolenic acid (GLA), a "good fat" that has been shown to help reduce inflammation, like the omega-3s.

The consequences of an omega-3/omega-6 imbalance may include dry skin, brittle hair and nails, a weakened immune system, poor cognitive function, poor vision and systemic inflammation. Increasing your intake of omega-3-rich fats from fish, flaxseed oil, walnuts and some dark-green, leafy vegetables may help maintain a healthier omega 3/6 balance.

Though not considered essential, omega-5, omega-7 and omega-9 oils are also important. These omega oils are found in fish oil, as well as from pomegranate oil (omega-5), sea buckthorne oil (omega-7) and olive oil (omega-9).

There are three main types of omega-3 oils: ALA (alpha-linolenic acids) DHA and EPA:

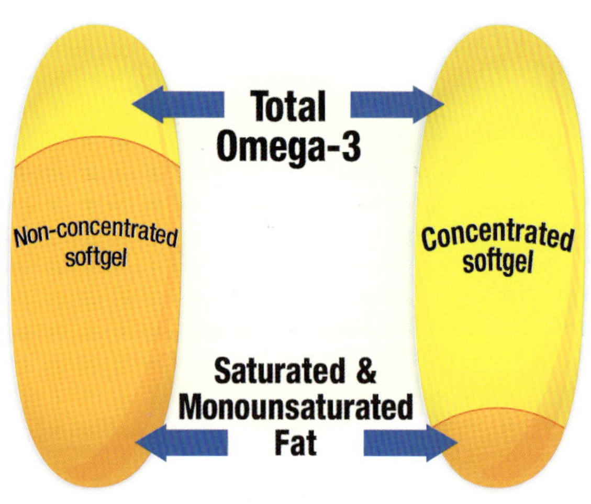

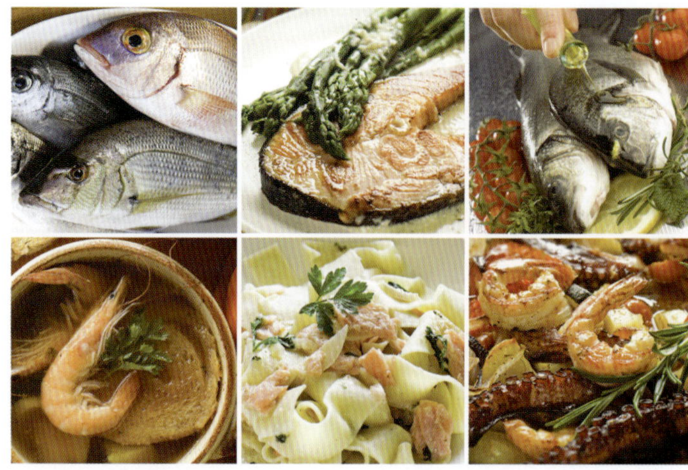

Because of the mercury content of fish, getting your omega-3's from a purified supplement is recommended.

ALA: the main omega-3 found in flaxseed, walnuts and chia seed. ALA breaks down in the body and can be converted into the next two omega-3s, EPA and DHA, but only about one to four percent of ALA is actually converted into EPA or DHA.

EPA and DHA: These two omega-3s are found almost exclusively in fish oil. They make up about 30 percent of un-concentrated fish oil. Some fish oil is purified and concentrated to maximize the amounts of these two important omega-3s. EPA and DHA are the omega-3s in fish oil that have been most studied for health benefits.

What to Look For in an Omega Oil Supplement

Potency

Most people do not realize how many softgels are needed to obtain the recommended 1 to 2 grams (1,000 to 2,000 mg) of omega-3s (EPA and DHA) daily.

To the left is an illustration of two fish oil softgels.

- The one on the left is un-concentrated, which means that it only contains one-third omega-3s. The rest of the oil in the softgel is saturated fat and other fatty acids.
- The one on the right is a concentrated fish oil, which contains a much higher percentage of omega-3 oils. Taking concentrated omega-3 fish oil will require fewer softgels to get the recommended amounts of healthy omega-3s.

Un-concentrated Fish Oil

Supplement Facts

Serving Size: **2 Soft Gels**

Amount per Serving		%DV**
Omega-3s	**Weight**	**Volume %**
EPA (Eicosapentaenoic Acid)	330 mg	18%
DHA (Docosahexaenoic Acid)	220 mg	12%
Other Omega-3s	140 mg	8%
Total Omega-3s	690 mg	38%
Oleic-Acid (Omega-9)	116 mg	6%

** Percent Daily Values (DV) are based on a 2,000 calorie diet for 1 Fish Gel.
*** Daily Value not established

Concentrated Fish Oil

Supplement Facts

Serving Size: 1 Fish Gel — Servings per Container: 60

	Amount per Fish Gel	Amount per 2 Fish Gels	%DV**
Total Omega 3•6•7•9•11	**1,100 mg†**	**2,200 mg†**	
Omega-3	880 mg	1,760 mg	***
EPA (Eicosapentaenoic Acid)	490 mg	980 mg	***
DHA (Docosahexaenoic Acid)	244 mg	488 mg	***
Omega-6	66 mg	132 mg	***
Omega-7	1 mg	2 mg	***
Omega-9	114 mg	228 mg	***
Omega-11	38 mg	76 mg	***
Lipase (activity 50 FIP)	5 mg	10 mg	***

** Percent Daily Values (DV) are based on a 2,000 calorie diet for 1 Fish Gel.
*** Daily Value not established
† The beneficial Omegas in fish oils, other than EPA & DHA, are naturally occurring and may vary seasonally by up to 10%.

Above are two Supplement Facts Panels from fish oil products. The one on the left is an un-concentrated fish oil. At first glance, reading the panel leads you to believe that you would get 690 mg of omega-3s. But notice the serving size – 2 softgels! **You would have to take double the dosage of an un-concentrated fish oil (on the left) and you would still obtain less beneficial omega-3s than one dose of a concentrated fish oil (on the right)!**

Purity and Quality

Consuming enough omega-3s from the diet by eating fish is possible, but because of the high amount of toxins like mercury, PCBs and dioxins found in fish, it is best to obtain the majority of omega-3 fats from a purified fish oil supplement that has International Fish Oil Standard (IFOS) certification. Look for the IFOS logo to be sure that you are getting a pure fish oil.

Enteric Coated, Dark Colored Fish Gelatin Softgels

Look for an enteric coated fish oil to ensure maximum absorption and minimum fishy repeat (belching). Dark colored softgels made of fish gelatin (not bovine, or pork gelatin) are the highest quality softgels. Because light can induce oxidation of the omega-3 oils, a dark softgel is recommended.

Recap: What to look for in an Omega oil Supplement

- At least 800 mg total omega-3 per ONE soft gel and a minimum of 1000 mg total omegas.
- Enteric coated softgel
- Fish gelatin, dark-colored softgel
- International purity standard (look for the IFOS logo)

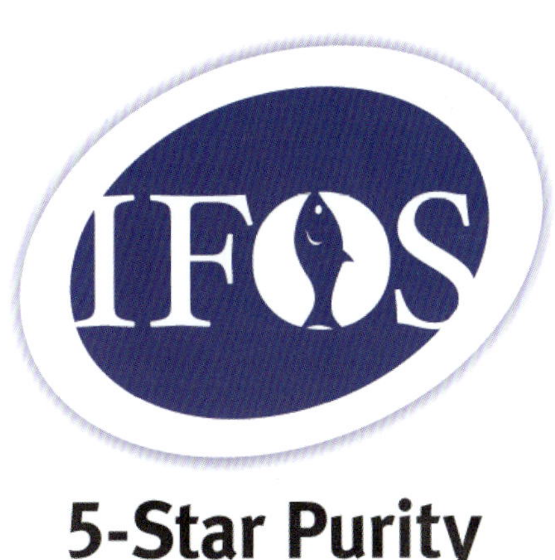

5-Star Purity Rating

Probiotics

What are Probiotics?

There are literally trillions of microorganisms in the human digestive tract. Some are beneficial, some are harmful, and some are neutral. Probiotics are the good type of bacteria that help crowd out the harmful bacteria in order to keep you healthy. This is important because more than 70 percent of your immune defense is found in your digestive tract. Probiotic literally means "for life," an appropriate name for the friendly bacteria that normally inhabit a healthy digestive tract.

Ideally, the good/neutral bacteria should greatly outnumber the harmful bacteria in your gut. However, everyday factors such as diet, stress, travel, exposure to illness and even the use of certain medications can diminish the number of healthy bacteria in the digestive tract and upset an otherwise balanced intestinal environment. This allows unhealthy microbes to flourish and may lead to intestinal issues such as inflammation, leaky gut, diarrhea and constipation, as well as a decline in healthy immune function. Taking a daily probiotic supplement can help replenish good bacteria and restore a healthy bacterial balance.

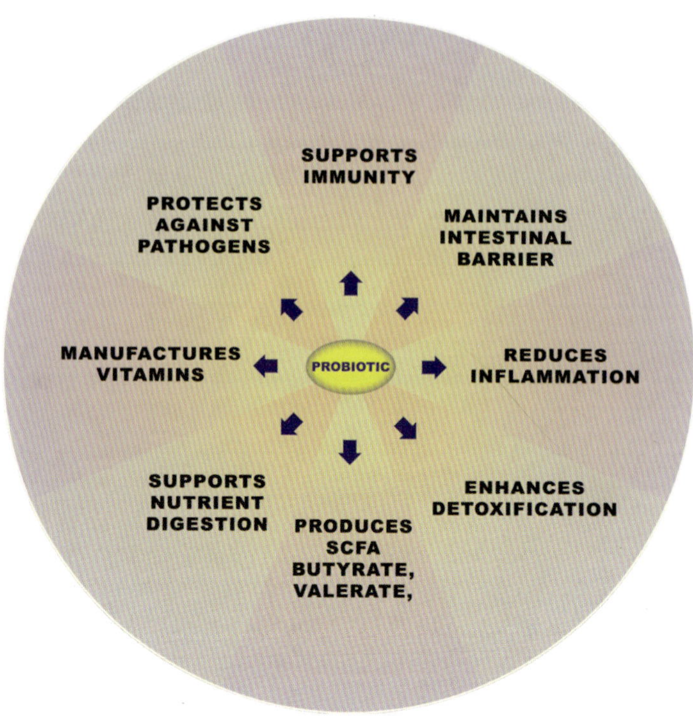

Supplement Facts

Serving Size: 1 Capsule   Servings per Container: 30

	Amount per Serving	%DV**
Ultimate Flora Critical Care Blend	470 mg	
Bifidobacterium lactis	25 billion	***
Lactobacillus acidophilus	15 billion	***
Bifidobacterium breve	2.5 billion	***
Bifidobacterium longum	2.5 billion	***
Lactobacillus casei	1.25 billion	***
Lactobacillus plantarum	1 billion	***
Lactobacillus paracasei	1 billion	***
Lactobacillus salivarius	1 billion	***
Lactobacillus rhamnosus	500 million	***
Lactobacillus bulgaricus	250 million	***
FOS (fructooligosaccharide)		***
Total Probiotic Cultures	**50 billion†**	

** Percent Daily Values (DV) are based on a 2,000 calorie diet.
*** Daily Value not established

Probiotics make up the "Gut Protection System," or GPS.

The Gut Protection System works in three ways:

- Crowds out the harmful bacteria in the gut
- Creates compounds that help to inhibit the harmful bacteria
- Communicates directly with the immune system that resides in the gut

What to Look For in a Probiotic Supplement

- High culture count (30 to 200 billion CFU per capsule)
- Multiple strains (at least 10 different strains of Lactobacillus and Bifidobacteria – the L's and the B's)
- Delayed-release delivery (effective delivery system that protects against stomach acid)
- Guaranteed potency at time of expiration, not manufacture.

Enzymes

What are Enzymes?

Enzymes play an essential role in every function in the human body, including eating, digestion and nutrient absorption, seeing, hearing, breathing, kidney and liver function, healthy elimination and more. In the digestive system, enzymes help break down foods by breaking apart the bonds that hold nutrients together. As a result, the body is able to use those nutrients for energy.

Although enzymes are typically present in raw, whole foods to assist with digestion, the majority of people do not obtain enough enzymes through diet alone. Today's diet of cooked and heavily processed foods depletes the natural enzymes from food and leads to poor digestion, as the body may not be able to completely break down foods and obtain their valuable nutrients.

Several locations in the digestive system secrete enzymes: the mouth, stomach, pancreas and cells of the small intestine. Proteins, fats and carbohydrates are the most basic foods that the body breaks down and absorbs, and the enzymes protease, lipase and amylase, respectively, are made by the body for this purpose. A healthy diet, exercise and proper detoxification will help promote healthy enzyme production in the body.

Additionally, there are several enzymes that the human body lacks, such as cellulase (the enzyme that breaks down cellulose), and phytase, the enzyme that breaks down the phytates and phytic acid we consume in our diet. Because of this deficiency, many people have difficulty breaking down certain foods such as starchy beans, legumes and nuts. Without the essential enzymes needed for proper digestion, the body may not completely break down those foods to absorb their nutrients. As a result, undigested food in the digestive tract can ferment, causing gas, bloating and other digestive difficulties.

What to Look For in a Digestive Enzyme Supplement

- High potency plant-based enzyme formula
- At least 1000,000 H.U.T. units of protease per serving
- Varied enzyme blend for full-spectrum digestion
- If you suspect you have low stomach acid, look for a formula that contains HCl

HCl self-test:

A quick test for stomach acid level involves taking a digestive enzyme with HCl at the beginning of a meal. If a burning sensation is not felt, stomach acid levels are too low. The next day, take two of the HCl enzymes at the beginning of a meal, increasing by one capsule each day until the burning sensation is felt. Once it is determined the amount of capsules it takes to induce stomach burning, the correct dosage per meal would be one less capsule. If further testing is desired, the Heidelberg pH test can be done. (See the Recommended Testing section in this Appendix.)

High-potency Digestive Enzyme

Supplement Facts

Serving Size: 1 Capsule

	Amount per Serving	%DV**
Plant-based Enzyme Blend	470 mg	
Protein Digestive Complex with *SmartZYME*		
Protease Blend	100,000 HUT	***
Papain	50,000 PU	***
Fat Digestive Complex with *SmartZYME*		
Lipase Blend	3,750 FIP = 18,750 LU	***
Carbohydrate, Fiber and Sugars Digestive Complex with *SmartZYME*		
Amylase Blend	25,000 DU	***
Cellulase Blend	3,000 CU	***
Lactase	1,200 ALU	***
Invertase	250 SU = 80 INVU	***
Glucoamylase	50 AG	***
Alpha Galactosidase	500 GAL	***
Beta Glucanase	25 BGU	***
Xylanase	550 XU	***
Hemicellulase	30 HCU	***
Pectinase w/Phytase	45 ADJU	***
Phytase	5 U	***

** Percent Daily Values (DV) are based on a 2,000 calorie diet.
*** Daily Value not established

Digestive Enzyme with HCl

Supplement Facts

Serving Size: 2 Capsules

	Amount per Serving	%DV**
Betaine HCl	440 mg	***
	423 mg	
Proprietary Digestive Blend		
Digestive Enzyme	*Activity*	
Protease *SmartZYME*	50,000 HUT	***
Amylase *SmartZYME*	10,000 DU	***
Lipase *SmartZYME*	1,000 FIP	***
Cellulase *SmartZYME*	1,000 CU	***
Proprietary Soothing Blend		
Gentian root		***
Ginger extract (4:1) root		***
Meadowsweet extract (4:1) herb		***
Peppermint leaf		***

** Percent Daily Values (DV) are based on a 2,000 calorie diet. *** Daily Value not established

Advanced Immunity Formula: Saccharomyces boulardi (S. boulardii) is a beneficial yeast that has been shown to help correct overgrowth of Candida and the diarrhea associated with overuse of antibiotics. Antibiotics do not destroy this helpful yeast, so it is particularly beneficial when taken with antibiotics. One virulent form of antibiotic-associated diarrhea (AAD) comes from Clostridium diffcile (C. diff) bacteria. S. boulardii is effective against this type of diarrhea, especially in the more difficult recurrent cases. When paired with EpiCor, a yeast fermentate ingredient, a powerful dual-action immune defense is created for seasonal immune support.

Supplement Facts

Serving Size: 2 Capsules — Servings per Container: 15

	Amount per Serving	%DV**
Advanced Immunity Blend	1,350 mg	
Saccharomyces boulardii (10 billion)†		***
Saccharomyces cerevisiae fermentate (EpiCor®)		***
Larch arabinogalactan (ResistAid™)		***

Antioxidants: Antioxidants protect cells against free radicals by neutralizing them. Free radicals are produced when food is broken down, and when certain toxins are encountered. Free radicals are molecules that are missing an electron in their outer shell, so they will grab an electron from the closest source damaging cells in the process. Antioxidants carry an extra electron that they easily donate to free radicals preventing the damage to surrounding tissues. It is important to understand that all free radical activity is not bad; it is necessary for many chemical reactions to occur and for the immune system to fight infections. Many of the immune cells produce and release free radical molecules to kill pathogenic organisms. The problem exists when there is an excess of free radicals, which come from stress, the environment, diet or from an overactive immune system. Free radical excess burdens the body with cellular dysfunction and inflammation, which can lead to a multitude of symptoms ranging from fatigue, low energy, poor digestive and mental function, generalized aches and pains to heart attacks and cancer.

Antioxidants come in many different forms, ranging from vitamins, minerals and enzymes to food.

Vitamins: vitamin C, vitamin E, vitamin A and the various carotenoids: beta carotene, alpha carotene, zeaxanthin, cryptoxanthin and lutein

Minerals: Zinc and selenium are critically important in hundreds of enzyme reactions; some of these enzymes are directly related to antioxidant production, while other enzymes, by not working correctly, allow for increased free radical activity, thereby indirectly affecting antioxidant status.

Enzymes: Glutathione reductase, superoxide dismutase and catalase are well known enzymes with antioxidant effects in the body.

Miscellaneous antioxidants include: alpha lipoic acid (very potent and a recharger of the many other antioxidants), glutathione, and amino acids N-acetyl cysteine, glycine and glutamin. (These three combine to make glutathione.) Glutathione binds heavy metals like mercury and thereby slows down oxidative stress (free radical activity).

Herbs: Pycnogenol (pine bark extract), OPCs (grape seed extract) and milk thistle extract (silymarin) help enhance liver function.

Foods: Blueberry, raspberry, cranberry, bilberry, strawberry and blackberry are just a few of the deep-colored foods that are high in antioxidants as measured by the ORAC (oxidation-reduction antioxidant capacity). At the other end of the food spectrum, there is rice bran soluble fraction containing at least 70 different measurable antioxidants.

Gas Relieving Enzyme: Plant-based enzyme formula helps break down gas-forming foods such as beans, vegetables, whole grains and pasta, which can be difficult for some people to digest. It should contain amylase, alpha galactosidase, cellulase, phytase, lipase, protease and invertase in addition to the soothing herb fennel.

Supplement Facts		
Serving Size: 2 Capsules	Servings per Container: 30	
	Amount per Serving	%DV**
Proprietary GAS STOP Blend	680 mg	
Fennel seed		***
Digestive Enzyme	*Activity*	
Amylase *SmartZYME*	20,000 DU	***
Alpha Galactosidase	1,000 GAL	***
Cellulase *SmartZYME*	3,000 CU	***
Phytase	40 FTU	***
Lipase *SmartZYME*	200 FIP	***
Protease *SmartZYME*	10,000 HUT	***
Invertase	160 INVU	***

IBS Supplement: for cramping and diarrhea

Part 1 (Intestinal Lining Support): contains L-glutamine, N-acetyl D-glucosamine, gamma oryzanol and other ingredients the body needs to build and maintain a healthy mucosal lining in the intestine.

Supplement Facts		
Serving Size: 2 Capsules	Servings per Container: 30	
	Amount per Serving	%DV**
L-Glutamine	835 mg	***
N-Acetyl D-Glucosamine	35 mg	***
Gamma Oryzanol	20 mg	***
Proprietary Herbal Blend	10 mg	
Cranesbill root		***
Ginger root		***
Marigold Extract 5:1 flower		***
Marshmallow root		***

Part 2 (Bowel Support): contains a formulation of Western and Chinese herbs that have been traditionally used to support proper bowel health and function and reduce cramping.

Supplement Facts		
Serving Size: 2 Capsules	Servings per Container: 30	
	Amount per Serving	%DV**
Western Herbal Blend	400 mg	
Slippery Elm bark		***
German Chamomile flower		***
Fenugreek seed		***
Fennel seed		***
Skullcap herb		***
Cranberry Extract 25:1 fruit		***
Peppermint leaf		***
Chinese Herbal 12:1 Extract Blend	300 mg	***
MSM (methylsulfonylmethane)	100 mg	***

L-glutamine with N-acetyl D-glucosamine (NAG) and gamma oryzanol: The amino acid L-glutamine is the primary fuel for the cells of the intestinal tract. It is essential in the repair of the intestinal lining (leaky gut). NAG is the glue that forms the mucosal layer. This mucosal layer acts to protect the underlying intestinal tissue from exposure to enzymes, acid and bacterial assault while providing a selectively absorptive surface. Gamma oryzanol, derived from rice bran oil, is an anti-inflammatory that is effective in a broad range of gastrointestinal disorders such as gastric and duodenal ulcers, gastritis and irritable bowel syndrome. The product should also contain herbs like ginger, cranesbill, and marshmallow. Recommended dosage of L-glutamine ranges from 3,000 mg to 20,000 mg per day based on the severity of the condition. Look for a powder formula.
L-glutamine poultice: Add enough water to the glutamine powder to make a paste, which can be applied topically for rectal conditions.

Supplement Facts		
Serving Size: 1 Level Scoop (5.4 gm)	Servings per Container: About 30	
	Amount per Serving	%DV**
Calories	21	
Protein	5 g	10%
L-Glutamine	5,000 mg	***
N-Acetyl D-Glucosamine	200 mg	***
Gamma Oryzanol	125 mg	***
Proprietary Herbal Blend	75 mg	
Cranesbill root		***
Ginger root		***
Marigold Extract 5:1 flower		***
Marshmallow root		***

Natural Heartburn Formula: A natural antacid formula can be taken short-term to relieve heartburn symptoms. This formula should contain calcium, magnesium and L-glutamine in addition to ingredients like fava bean, aloe vera gel, raspberry and pomegranate (which contain ellagic acid) and apple pectin.

Supplement Facts		
Serving Size: 1 Tablet	Servings per Container: 30	
	Amount per Serving	%DV**
Calories	8	
Sodium (as sodium bicarbonate)	5 mg	<1%
Total Carbohydrate	1 g	<1%
Sugars	1 g	<1%
Calcium (as calcium carbonate)	200 mg	20%
Magnesium (as magnesium carbonate/hydroxide)	100 mg	25%
L-Glutamine	150 mg	***
Proprietary HEARTBURN STOP Blend	130 mg	
Fava Bean		***
Raspberry (contains ellagic acid)		***
Aloe Vera extract gel 200:1		***
Pomegranate extract 35:1 (contains ellagic acid)		***
Apple Pectin		***
Papaya		***
Papain (96,000 PU)		***

Natural Laxative Formula: Bowel cleanse formula can be taken for constipation and will include natural laxatives that promote peristalsis (cape aloe and rhubarb), help to retain water in the colon (magnesium), and soothe the bowel (marshmallow and triphala).

Supplement Facts

Serving Size: 2 Capsules   Servings per Container: 30

	Amount per Serving	%DV**
Magnesium (as magnesium hydroxide)	230 mg	58%
Proprietary Blend	1,200 mg	
Cape Aloe leaf		***
Rhubarb root		***
Slippery Elm bark		***
Marshmallow root		***
Triphala (Blend of Amalaki, Bibhitaki and Haritaki)		***

Vitamins and minerals: A good multivitamin, antioxidant mineral complex would include the following: vitamin A (acetate) 10,000 I.U. (international units); pure ascorbic acid, 1,000 mg.; vitamin D3, 200 I.U.; d-alpha tocopherol succinate (vitamin E), 400 I.U.; thiamine HCl (B1,) 100mg.; riboflavin HCl (B2), 25 mg.; riboflavin 5′ phosphate (activated B2); niacinamide, 100 mg.; inositol hexaniacinate (no flush niacin); pyridoxine HCl (B6); pyridoxal 5′ phosphate (activated B6), folic acid, 800 mcg. (micrograms); hydroxycobalamin (activated B12), 1,000 mcg.; biotin, 800 mcg.; pantothenic acid (calcium pantothenate, B5); calcium (citrate), 300 mg.; magnesium (citrate), 200 mg.; zinc (picolinate), 25 mg.; selenium (selenomethionine), 200 mcg.; manganese (asparate), 20 mg., chromium (picolinate), 200 mcg.; molybdenum (asparate), 100 mcg.; boron (glycinate), 2 mg.; di-potassium (aspartate), 99 mg.; mixed carotenoids, 15,000 I.U., vanadium (aspartate), 200 mcg., and extra antioxidant and liver protection can be added with N-acetyl-cysteine, up to 1,000 mg.

This type of product provides a good baseline since it lacks added iron, copper and iodine—minerals that should be supplemented on an individual basis. The addition of the activated form of B vitamins is important since patients with toxicity problems may not convert their B2, B6 and B12 to the usable forms. In order to get this many nutrients in a capsule form, it would require about eight capsules. Ideally, a hypo-allergenic product with no hidden excipients, binders, fillers, shellacs, artificial colors or fragrance should be selected. In addition, the product should not contain dairy, wheat, yeast, gluten, corn, sugar, starch or preservatives of hydrogenated oils.

Vitamin D: a fat soluble vitamin, also considered a hormone which can be obtained by sun exposure, or through the diet or supplementation. Vitamin D is found naturally in a limited number of foods, but it is added to certain foods such as milk. Through sun exposure, when unprotected skin is exposed to ultraviolet B (UVB) rays, the body manufactures its own vitamin D. It has recently been discovered that much more vitamin D is needed than previously thought. It is also becoming increasingly clear that vitamin D status is involved with many different health processes and conditions in the body. Most notably, vitamin D benefits the immune system, and is protective against cold and flu, many different forms of cancer, cardiovascular disease, insulin resistance, mortality, cognitive decline, depression, kidney disease, asthma, gut integrity and inflammation, as well as having long-known bone health benefits.

Recent studies are finding that most people (70 percent of Americans and 90 percent of Canadians) have insufficient levels of vitamin D in their blood. Optimal blood levels of vitamin D3 should be between 50 and 70 ng/mL. Research is also finding that the recommended allowable intakes are much too low, even though they were recently doubled. Recommendations for dosage of vitamin D3 are 1,000 to 2,000 iu per day are more in line with current research, and some researchers think even those levels are too low.

The best form of supplemental vitamin D is vitamin D3 (cholecalciferol). This form is more easily converted into the active form of vitamin D (calcitriol) in the body. Many vitamin D supplements use D2, however, which is a poorer form of vitamin D. Because vitamin D is a fat-soluble vitamin, it should be taken with a meal that contains fat.

ACID BLOCKER RECOVERY

Long-term use of acid-blocking medications is associated with increased infections such as Clostridium difficile (C. diff), pneumonia, H. pylori and Candida overgrowth. Sudden discontinued use of these medications can have a rebound effect, however, involving increased production of stomach acid that the body is not ready for. Therefore, gradual weaning off the medication is best. The following protocol will help you to regain control of your digestive symptoms so that you can manage your health naturally, without the harmful effects of long-term blockage of stomach acid production.

It takes seven days for the effects of acid-blocking medications to diminish in the body. For this reason, it is best to lower the dosage of the medication before discontinuing use.

First seven days: Take acid-blocking medication at half the normal dose. In addition, take the following: 5,000 to 10,000 mg (5 to 10 g) of L-glutamine powder with gamma oryzanol daily on an empty stomach first thing in the morning; 200 billion culture count probiotic powder daily; High-potency digestive enzyme containing at least 100,000 H.U.T. protease with meals.

*If heartburn is experienced, use a Natural Heartburn Formula. This should be temporary.

Most people who have been on long-term acid blockers will have hypochlorhydria (low stomach acid). If you do not experience any heartburn while following these suggestions, begin taking a digestive enzyme that includes HCl (hydrochloric acid) with meals after you finish the first round of digestive enzymes. Hydrochloric acid is necessary in the stomach for the absorption of key nutrients.

A small percentage of people will have hyperchlorhydria (high stomach acid), often due to stress and excess caffeine consumption. It is best to wait until you are not under stress before beginning this protocol. Addressing the underlying stress with stress-reduction techniques, as well as reducing or eliminating caffeine intake, are essential steps in this healing process.

If you experience uncomfortable symptoms while following this protocol, discontinue the process and consult your doctor. Let him/her know that you are concerned about the harmful effects of long-term acid blocking medications, and are looking for a safer, more natural solution to your health problem.

After seven days of not taking your acid-blocking medications, you can be tested with the Heidelberg pH Diagnostic System in order to determine what your stomach pH is. (See the Alternative Diagnostics section in this Appendix.)

High-potency Digestive Enzyme

Supplement Facts

Serving Size: 1 Capsule

	Amount per Serving	%DV**
Plant-based Enzyme Blend	470 mg	
Protein Digestive Complex with *SmartZYME*		
Protease Blend	100,000 HUT	***
Papain	50,000 PU	***
Fat Digestive Complex with *SmartZYME*		
Lipase Blend	3,750 FIP = 18,750 LU	***
Carbohydrate, Fiber and Sugars Digestive Complex with *SmartZYME*		
Amylase Blend	25,000 DU	***
Cellulase Blend	3,000 CU	***
Lactase	1,200 ALU	***
Invertase	250 SU = 80 INVU	***
Glucoamylase	50 AG	***
Alpha Galactosidase	500 GAL	***
Beta Glucanase	25 BGU	***
Xylanase	550 XU	***
Hemicellulase	30 HCU	***
Pectinase w/Phytase	45 ADJU	***
Phytase	5 U	***

** Percent Daily Values (DV) are based on a 2,000 calorie diet.
*** Daily Value not established

Digestive Enzyme with HCl

Supplement Facts

Serving Size: 2 Capsules

	Amount per Serving	%DV**
Betaine HCl	440 mg	***
	423 mg	
Proprietary Digestive Blend		
Digestive Enzyme	*Activity*	
Protease *SmartZYME*	50,000 HUT	***
Amylase *SmartZYME*	10,000 DU	***
Lipase *SmartZYME*	1,000 FIP	***
Cellulase *SmartZYME*	1,000 CU	***
Proprietary Soothing Blend		
Gentian root		***
Ginger extract (4:1) root		***
Meadowsweet extract (4:1) herb		***
Peppermint leaf		***

** Percent Daily Values (DV) are based on a 2,000 calorie diet. *** Daily Value not established

ENDNOTES

Chapter 1

[1] Steven R. Peikin, MD, *GastroIntestinal Health*, Quill, 1999, p. 17.

[2] M. Sara Rosenthal, *The Gastroinstestinal Sourcebook*, Lowell House, 1997,p. 2.

[3] Tonia Reinhard, MS, RD, *Gastroinstestinal Disorders and Nutrition*, Contemporary Books, 2002, p. 17.

[4] M.A. Schmidt, *Beyond Antibiotics, North Atlantic Books, 2009, p. 20.*

[5] http://nihroadmap.nih.gov/hmp/

[6] http://www.vivo.colostate.edu/hbooks/pathphys/endocrine/gi/overview.html

[7] Michael D. Gershon, MD, *The Second Brain*, Harper Perennial, 1998, p. 70.

[8] Ibid., p.xiii.

[9] Ibid.

Chapter 4

Barrett's Esophagus

[1] A.J. Cameron, et al., "The Incidence of Adenocarcinoma in Columnar-lined (Barrett's) Esophagus," *New England Journal of Medicine*, 1985; 313(14): 857-9.

[2] A.J. Cameron, et al., "Prevalence of Columnar-lined (Barrett's) Esophagus: Comparison of Population-Based Clinical and Autopsy Findings," *Gastroenterology*, 1990; 99(4):918-22

[3] http://digestive.niddk.nih.gov/ddiseases/pubs/barretts/index.htm

[4] E. Hassall, American Journal of Gastroenterology, Barrett's Esophagus: Congenital or Acquired?, 1993; 88(6):819-24.

[5] B. Westhoff, et al., "The Frequency of Barrett's Esophagus in high-risk patients with chronic GERD," *Gastrointestinal Endoscopy*, 2005;61(2):226-31.

[6] www.barrettsinfo.com

[7] Ibid.

[8] www.jamesline.com/output/barrett.htm.

[9] Op cit., http://health.yahoo.com

[10] A.J. Cameron and C.T. Lomboy, "Barrett's Esophagus: Age, Prevalence, Etiology, and Complications." *Gastroenterology*, 1992; 103(4):1241-5.

[11] Ibid.

[12] Op cit., www.jamesline.com.

13 Op cit., www.barrettsinfo.com.

[14] Mark R. Dambro, *Griffith's 5-Minute Clinical Consult*, 2003, p. 430.

[15] Op cit., www.gicare.com

[16] A.K. Musana et al., "The Diagnostic Accuracy of Esophageal Capsule Endoscopy in Patients with Gastroesophageal Reflux Disease and Barrett's Esophagus: a Blinded Prospective Study, 2008; 130(3): 525-532.

[17] R.E. Sampliner, "Practice Guidelines on the Diagnosis, Surveillance, and Therapy of Barrett's Esophagus: The Practice Parameters Committee of the American College of Gastroenterology. *The American Journal of Gastroenterology*, 1998; 93(7):1028-32.

[18] C.N. Foroulis et al., "Photodynamic Therapy (PDT) in Barrett's Esophagus With Dysplasia or Early Cancer," *European Journal of Cardiothoracic Surgery*, 2006; 29(1): 30-4.

[19] http://www.cancer.gov/cancertopics/factsheet/Therapy/photodynamic

[20] N.J. Shaheen, et al., "Radiofrequency ablation in Barrett's esophagus with dysplasia." N Engl J Med. 2009 May 28;360(22):2277-88.

[21] http://www.cancer.gov/cancertopics/factsheet/Therapy/photodynamic

[22] N.J. Shaheen, et al., "Radiofrequency ablation in Barrett's esophagus with dysplasia." *N Engl J Med.* 2009 May 28;360(22):2277-88.

[23] Op cit., www.barrettsinfo.com

Esophagitis

[1] http://gastroresource.com/GITextbook/en/chapter5/5-8-pr.htm

[2] Op cit., http://gastroresource.com

[3] Ibid.

[4] Ibid.

[5] Op cit., Reinhard.

[6] www.intelihealth.com/IH/ihtlH/WSlHW000/8293/25982/187000 /html?d=dmtHealthAZ

[7] Tonia Reinhard, MS, RD, *Gastrointestinal Disorders and Nutrition*, Contemporary Books, 2002, p. 40.

[8] www.digitalnaturopath.com/cond/C341769.html

[9] E. Hoshino, et al., "Role of Proton Pump Inhibitor As a Predisposing Factor of Candida Esophagitis." *Gastro Endosc.* Apr 28;67(5):AB190.

[10] Op cit., http://gastroresource.com

GERD

[1] H. El-Sarag, "The association between obesity and GERD: a review of the epidemiological evidence." *Dig Dis Sci.* 2008 Sep;53(9):2307-12. Epub 2008 Jul 24.

[2] Jonathan V. Wright, MD and Lane Lenard, PhD, *Why Stomach Acid is Good for You*, M. Evans and Company, Inc., 2001, p. 135.

[3] Op cit., Wright, p. 40.

[4] *The Merck Manual*, Eleventh Edition, Merck Sharp & Dohme Research Laboratories, 1966, p.531.

[5] Op cit., Wright Lenard,, p. 16.

[6] Michael Murray, ND & Joseph Pizzorno, ND, *Encyclopedia of Natural Medicine*, Prima Health, 1998, p. 135.

[7] Ibid., p. 130.

[8] Judy Kitchen, "Hypochlorhydria: A Review – Part I," *Townsend Letter for Doctors and Patients*, October 2001, p. 56.

[9] John D. Kirschmann and Lavon J. Dunne, *Nutrition Almanac*, McGraw Hill Book Company, 1984, p. 171.

[10] Dr. John McKenna, *Hard to Stomach*, Newleaf, 2002, p. 78.

[11] Op cit., Wright and Lenard, p. 33.

[12] Raphael Kellman, MD, *Gut Reactions*, Broadway Books, 2002, p. 86.

[13] M. Sara Rosenthal, *The Gastrointestinal Sourcebook*, Lowell House, 1997, p.61.

[14] T.W. Higginbotham, "Effectiveness and safety of proton pump inhibitors in infantile gastroesophageal reflux disease." *Ann Pharmacother.* 2010 Mar;44(3):572-6. Epub 2010 Feb 2.

[15] S. Dial et al., "Proton Pump Inhibitor Use and Risk of Community Acquired Clostridium difficile-associated disease defined by prescription for oral vancomycin therapy," *Canadian Medical Association Journal*, 2006; 175(7):745-8.

[16] M. Aseeri, et al., "Gastric Acid Suppression by Proton Pump Inhibitors as a Risk Factor for Clostridium Difficile-associated Diarrhea in Hospitalized Patients," *American Journal of Gastroenterology*, 2008;103(9):2308-13.

[17] C.A. Martinez et al., "Rick Factors for Esophageal Candidiasis," *European Journal of Clinical Microbiology and Infectious Diseases*, 2000;19(2):96-100.

[18] L.E. Tarqownik et al., "Use of Proton Pump Inhibitors and Risk of Osteoporosis-Related Factors," *Canadian Medical Association Journal*, 2008;179(4):306-7.

[19] T. Schinke, et al., "Impaired gastric acidification negatively affects calcium homeostasis and bone mass." *Nat Med.* 2009 Jun;15(6):674-81.

[20] S.E. Gulmez et al., "Use of Proton Pump Inhibitors anddc the Risk of Community acquired Pneumonia," *Archives of Internal Medicine*, 2007;167(9):950-5.

[21] R.J. Valuck et al., "A Case-control Study on adverse effects: H2 Blocker or Proton Pump Inhibitor use and Risk of Vitamin B12 Deficiency in Older Adults," *Journal of Clinical Epidemiology*, 2004;57(4):422-8.

[22] S. Vakevainen et al., "Hypochlorhydria Induced by a Proton Pump Inhibitor Leads to Intragastric Microbial Production of Acetaldehyde from Ethanol," 2000;14(11):1511-8.

[23] J.M. Mullin, et al., "Esomeprazole induces upper gastrointestinal tract transmucosal permeability increase." *Aliment Pharmacol Ther.* 2008 Dec 1;28(11-12):1317-25. Epub 2008 Aug 4.

[24] Op cit., Vakevainen.

[25] American Gastroenterological Association. "Acid-Reducing Medicines May Lead To Dependency." *ScienceDaily* 2 July 2009. 12 May 2010 <http://www.sciencedaily.com / releases/2009/07/090701082909.htm>.

[26] Op cit., Wright and Lenard, p. 25-30.

[27] Op cit., Murray & Pizzorno, p. 134.

[28] Leonard Smith, "Ease the Burn – Promote Acid Production," *Complementary Therapies in Chronic Care*, January, 2001.

[29] Op cit., Kellas and Dworkin.

[30] Op. cit., Wright and Lenard, p. 95.

[31] P.K. Papasavas et al., "Effectiveness of Laparoscopic Fundoplicationin Relieving the Symptoms of Gastroesophageal Reflux Disease (GERD) and Eliminating Antireflux Medical Therapy," *Surgical Endoscopy*, 2003;17(8):1200-5.

[32] L.O. Jeansonne et al., "Endoluminal Full-Thickness Plication and Radiofrequency Treatments for GERD: an Outcomes Comparison," *Archives of Surgery*, 2009;144(1):19-24.

[33] T.W. Higginbotham, "Effectiveness and safety of proton pump inhibitors in infantile gastroesophageal reflux disease." *Ann Pharmacother.* 2010 Mar;44(3):572-6. Epub 2010 Feb 2.

Heartburn

[1] National Heartburn Alliance, *Get Heartburn Smart*, Chicago, Il (www.heartburnalliance.org),p. 3.

[2] Steven R. Peikin, MD, *Gastrointestinal Health*, Quill, 2001, p. 43.

Hiatal Hernia

[1] Tonia Reinhard, MS, RD, *Gastrointestinal Disorders and Nutrition*, Contemporary Books, 2002, p. 52.

[2] Ibid.

[3] Raphael Kellman, *MD, Gut Reactions*, Broadway Books, 2002, p. 91.

[4] Jonathan V. Wright , MD and Lane Lenard, PhD, *Why Stomach Acid is Good for You*, M. Evans and Company, Inc., 2001, p. 54.

[5] Ibid.

[6] Op cit., Reinhard, p. 54.

[7] Ibid., p. 52.

[8] Ibid.

[9] Ibid.

[10] Ibid.

General Recommendations for all Esophageal Problems

[1] Op cit., Wright and Lenard, p. 142, 143.

[2] Phyllis A. Balch, CNC and James F. Balch, MD, *Prescription for Nutritional Healing*, Third Edition, Avery, 2000, p. 423.

[3] Ibid.

[4] Op cit., Balch and Balch, p. 422.

[5] Op cit., Wright and Lenard, p. 144.

[6] Ibid., p. 152.

Gastritis

[1] Tonia Reinhard, MS, RD, *Gastrointestinal Disorders and Nutrition*, Contemporary Books, 2002, p. 55.

[2] Ibid., p. 59.

[3] T. Matysiak-Budnik, et al., "Helicobacter pylori increases the epithelial permeability to a food antigen in human gastric biopsies." *Am J Gastroenterol.* 2004 Feb;99(2):225-32.

[4] http://www.medscape.com/viewarticle/407970_4

[5] Op cit., Reinhard, p. 57.

[6] Ibid.

[7] Raphael Kellman, MD, *Gut Reactions*, Broadway Books, 2002, p. 84.

[8] Op. Cit., Reinhard, p. 56.

[9] Ibid., p. 58.

[10] Steven R. Peikin, MD, *Gastrointestinal Health*, Quill, 2001, p. 52.

[11] Op. Cit., Reinhard, p.60.

[12] Elizabeth Lipski, MS, CCN, *Digestive Wellness*, Keats Publishing, Inc., 1996, p.204.

[13] Op. Cit., Reinhard, p. 62.

[14] Ibid.

[15] D. Lesbros-Pantoflickova, et al., "Helicobacter pylori and probiotics." *J Nutr.* 2007 Mar;137(3 Suppl 2):812S-8S.

[16] N. Hodgson, et al., "Gastric carcinoids: a temporal increase with proton pump introduction." *Surg Endosc.* 2005 Dec;19(12):1610-2. Epub 2005 Oct 5.

Peptic Ulcers

[1] *Dorland's Pocket Medical Dictionary*, 23rd edition, W. B. Sanders Company, 1982, p. 527.

[2] http://www.gastro.org/patient-center/digestive-conditions/peptic-ulcer-disease

[3] Michael Murray, ND and Joseph Pizzorno, ND, *Encyclopedia of Natural Medicine*, Revised 2nd Edition, Prima Health, 1998, p. 810.

[4] Steven R. Peikin, MD, *Gastrointestinal Health*, Quill, 2001, p. 54.

[5] Ibid.

[6] Henry D. Janowitz, MD, *Indigestion*, Oxford University Press, 1992, p. 62.

[7] Raphael Kellman, MD, *Gut Reactions*, Broadway Books, 2002, p. 101.

[8] Ibid.

[9] Ibid.

[10] Ibid., p. 101-102.

[11] M. Sara Rosenthal, *The Gastrointestinal Sourcebook*, Lowell House, 1998, p.51.

[12] Ibid.

[13] L.M. Brown, "Helicobacter Pylori: Epidemiology and Routes of Transmission," *Epidemiology Review*, 2000;22(2)283-97.

[14] P.M. Sherman, "Appropriate Strategies for Testing and Treating Helicobacter Pylori in Children: When and How?" *American Journal of Medicine*, 2004;117Sup5A:30S-35S.

[15] Op cit., Murray and Pizzorno, p. 811.

[16] Linda M. Ross (editor), *Gastrointestinal Diseases and Disorders Sourcebook*, Volume 16, Omnigraphics, Inc.1996, p. 140.

[17] Op cit., Reinhard, p. 69.

[18] Ibid., p. 812.

[19] Dr. John McKenna, *Hard to Stomach*, Newleaf, 2002, p. 121.

[20] Op cit., Murray and Pizzorno, p. 813.

[21] Ibid.

[22] D. Lindsey Berkson, *Healthy Digestion the Natural Way*, John Wiley and Sons, Inc., 2000, p. 117, 122.

[23] Op cit., Murray and Pizzorno, p. 813.

[24] Ibid.

[25] Ibid., p. 812.

[26] Ibid.

[27] Op cit., Ross, p.139.

[28] Ibid., p. 138.

[29] Op cit., Berkson, p. 114.

[30] Op cit., Peikin, p. 53.

[31] Op cit., Berkson.

[32] Op cit., Janowitz, p. 68.

[33] Op cit., Peikin, p. 57.

[34] M. Otto-von-Guericke et al., "Current Concepts in the Management of Helicobacter Pylori Infection: The Maastricht III Consensus Report," *Gut*, 2007;56(6): 772-81.

[35] Op cit., Berkson, p. 119.

[36] Op cit., Kellman, p. 102

[37] Op cit., Murray and Pizzorno, p. 811.

[38] Op cit., Peikin, p. 63.

Appendicitis

[1] http://www.sciencedaily.com/releases/2007/10/071008102334.htm

[2] *The Merck Manual*, Home Edition, p. 547.

[3] D.S. Nelson et al., "Appendiceal Perforation in Children Diagnosed in a Pediatric Emergency Department," *Pediatric Emergency Care*, 2000; 16(4):233-7.

[4] T.L. Storm et al., "What Have We Learned Over the Past 20 Years About Appendicitis in the Elderly?" *American Journal of Surgery*, 2003;185(3):198-201.

[5] J.A. Story et al., "Denis Parsons Burkitt," *The Journal of Nutrition*, 1994;124:1551-4.

[6] http://www.uptodate.com/patients/content/topic.do?topicKey=gi_dis/20863&linkTitle=INTRODUCTION&source=preview&selectedTitle=3~114&anchor=1#1

[7] Phyllis A. Balch, CNC and James F. Balch, MD, *Prescription for Nutritional Healing*, 3rd edition, Avery, 2000, p. 183.

[8] Radiology, October 2002; 225(1):131-6

[9] http://www.hopkinsmedicine.org/health_information_library/index.html?ArticleID=83643

Candidiasis

[1] D. Lindsey Berkson, *Healthy Digestion the Natural Way*, John Wiley & Sons, Inc., 2000, p. 158.

[2] X.L. Xu et al., "Bacterial Peptidoglycan Triggers Candida albicans Hyphal Growth by Directly Activating the Adenylyl Cyclase Cyr1p, Cell Host Microbe," 2008;4(1):28-39.

[3] F.L. Lorsheider et al., "Mercury Exposure from 'Silver' Tooth Fillings: Emerging Evidence Questions a Traditional Dental Paradigm," *The FASEB Journal*, 1995;9:504-8.

[4] Dr. William R. Kellas and Dr. Andrea Sharon Dworkin, *Surviving the Toxic Crisis*, Professional Preference, 1996, p. 184.

[5] Michael Murray, ND and Joseph Pizzorno, ND, *Encyclopedia of Natural Medicine*, Revised 2nd edition, Prima Health, 1998, p. 300.

[6] Op cit., Kellas and Dworkin, p. 438.

[7] Phyllis A. Balch, CNC and James F. Balch, MD, *Prescription for Nutritional Healing*, Third Edition, Avery, 2000, p. 263.

[8] Op cit., Murray and Pizzorno, p. 301.

[9] Op cit., Kellas and Dworkin, p. 438.

[10] Luc De Schepper, MD, PhD, CA, *Candida*, Second Edition, 1990, p. 6.

[11] Op cit., Kellas and Dworkin, p. 437-438.

[12] Op cit., Balch and Balch.

[13] http://www.drz.org/asp/conditions/candida2.asp#7

[14] J.M. Joneja et al., "Abnormal Gut Fermentation: the 'Auto-Brewery' Syndrome," *Journal of the Canadian Dietetic Association*, 1997;58(2)97-100.

[15] T.J. Rogers et al., "Immunity to Candida albicans," *Microbiol Rev.* 1980 December; 44(4): 660–682.

[16] http://www.sciencedaily.com/releases/2009/05/090528142833.htm

[17] Op cit., Murray and Pizzorno, p. 304.

[18] William Crook, MD, *The Yeast Connection*, Professional Books, Inc., p. 216.

Constipation

[1] Andrew Gaeddert, *Healing Digestive Disorders*, North Atlantic Books, 1998, p. 130.

[2] Linda M. Ross (editor), *Gastrointestinal Diseases and Disorders Sourcebook*, Omnigraphics, Inc., 1996, p.240-241.

[3] Raphael Kellman, MD, *Gut Reactions*, Broadway Books, 2002, p. 74 -75.

[4] Steven R.Peikin, MD, *Gastrointestinal Health*, Revised edition, Quill, 1999, p. 93-94.

[5] Henry D. Janowitz, MD, *Your Gut Feelings*, Consumer's Union, 1987, p. 95-96.

[6] Phyllis A. Balch, CNC and James F. Balch, MD, *Prescription for Nutritional Healing*, Third edition, Avery, 2000, p. 301.

[7] Elizabeth Lipski, MS, CCN, *Digestive Wellness*, Keats Publishing, Inc., 1996, p. 231.

[8] Life Extension Media, *Disease Prevention and Treatment*, Expanded Third Edition, Life Extension Foundation, 2000, p. 213.

[9] D. Lindsay Berkson, *Healthy Digestion the Natural Way*, John Wiley & Sons, Inc. 2000, p. 74.

[10] www.wilsonsthyroidsyndrome.com

[11] Op cit., D. Lindsey Berkson, p. 12. For more information on bowel transit time, visit the following website: http://www.webmd.com/digestive-disorders/bowel-transit-time

[12] Op cit., Kellman, p. 74.

[13] Op cit., Ross, p. 242.

[14] Op cit., Lipski, p. 228.

[15] Op cit., Berkson, p. 69-70.

[16] Op cit., Balch and Balch.

[17] Ibid.

[18] Op cit., Berkson, p. 68.

[19] Ibid., p. 70.

[20] Op cit., Berkson, p. 12-13.

[21] Op cit., Balch and Balch, p. 302.

[22] Tonia Reinhard, MS, RD, *Gastrointestinal Disorders and Nutrition*, Contemporary Books, 2002, p. 104.

[23] Op. Cit., Life Extension Media, p. 212.

[24] https://profreg.medscape.com/px/getlogin.do?urlCache=aHR0cDovL3d3dy5tZWRzY2FwZS5jb20vdmlld2FydGljbGUvNTU0NDA3

[25] http://www.tuftshealthplan.com/providers/pdf/pharmacy_criteria/Zelnorm.pdf

Diarrhea

[1] D. Lindsey Berkson, *Healthy Digestion the Natural Way*, John Wiley & Sons, Inc., 2000, p. 81.

[2] Ibid.

[3] Michael Murray, ND and Joseph Pizzorno, ND, *Encyclopedia of Natural Medicine*, Prima Health, 1998, p.433.

[4] http://www.epa.gov/ogwdw000/crypto.html

[5] Steven R. Peikin, MD, *Gastrointestinal Health*, Quill, 1999, p.108.

[6] W.R. Jarvis, et al., "National point prevalence of Clostridium difficile in US health care facility inpatients, 2008." *Am J Infect Control*. 2009 May;37(4):263-70. Epub 2009 Mar 10.

[7] M. Aseeri, et al., "Gastric acid suppression by proton pump inhibitors as a risk factor for clostridium difficile-associated diarrhea in hospitalized patients." Am J Gastroenterol. 2008 Sep;103(9):2308-13. Epub 2008 Aug 12.

[8] Raphael Kellman, MD, *Gut Reactions*, Broadway Books, 2002, p. 79.

[9] Henry D. Janowitz, MD, *Your Gut Feelings*, Consumer's Union, 1987, p. 83.

[10] Ibid., p. 80.

[11] Ibid.

[12] Linda M. Ross (editor), *Gastrointestinal Diseases and Disorders Sourcebook*, Volume 16, Omnigraphics, Inc., 1996, p. 236.

[13] Michael D. Gershon, MD, *The Second Brain*, Harper Perennial, 1998, p. 150.

Diverticular Disease

[1] D. Lindsey Berkson, *Healthy Digestion the Natural Way*, John Wiley & Sons, Inc., 2000, p. 89.

[2] Andrew Gaeddert, *Healing Digestive Disorders*, North Atlantic Books, 1998, p. 147.

[3] Tonia Reinhard, MS, RD, *Gastrointestinal Disorders and Nutrition*, Contemporary Books, 2002, p. 111.

[4] Phyllis A. Balch, CNC and James F. Balch, MD, *Prescription for Nutritional Healing*, Third Edition, Avery, 2000, p. 328.

[5] A.A. Sheth, et al., "Diverticular disease and diverticulitis." *Am J Gastroenterol.* 2008 Jun;103(6):1550-6. Epub 2008 May 13.

[6] Raphael Kellman, MD, *Gut Reactions*, Broadway Books, 2002, p. 82.

[7] Steven R. Peikin, *Gastrointestinal Health*, Quill, 1999, p.107.

[8] Op. Cit., Balch and Balch.

[9] D.O. Jacobs et al., "Diverticulitis," *New England Journal of Medicine*, 2007;357:2057-66.

[10] Op cit., Peikin, p. 108.

[11] Ibid.

[12] Henry D. Janowitz, MD, *Your Gut Feelings*, Consumer's Union, 1987, p. 139.

[13] Ibid.

[14] Op. Cit., Berkson, p. 92.

[15] Op. Cit., Renihard, p. 114.

[16] Op. Cit., Reinhard.

[17] Op. Cit., Janowitz, p. 139.

[18] Op. Cit., Janowitz, p. 143.

[19] Op. Cit., Sheth.

Gas

[1] D. Lindsey Berkson, *Healthy Digestion the Natural Way*, John Wiley & Sons, Inc., 2000, p. 49.

[2] Henry D. Janowitz, MD, *Your Gut Feelings*, Consumer's Union, 1987, p. 178.

[3] Steven R. Peikin, MD, *Gastrointestinal Health*, Quill, 1999, p. 89.

[4] Op. Cit., Peikin.

[5] Ibid.

[6] M. Pimental, et al., "A link between irritable bowel syndrome and fibromyalgia may be related to findings on lactulose breath testing." *Ann Rheum Dis.* 2004 Apr;63(4):450-2.

Gluten Sensitivity

[1] John H. Dirckx, MD, editor, *Stedman's Concise Medical Dictionary for the Health Professions*, Lippincott Williams & Wilkins, 2001, p. 406.

[2] R. Mc Manus and D. Kelleher, "Celiac disease--the villain unmasked?" *N Engl J Med.* 2003 Jun 19;348(25):2573-4.

[3] Raphael Kellman, MD, *Gut Reactions*, Broadway Books, 2002, p.72.

[4] Michael Murray, ND and Joseph Pizzorno, ND, *Encycopedia of Natural Medicine*, Prima Health, 1998, p. 325.

[5] Op cit., Kellman, p. 73.

[6] Op cit., Murray and Pizzorno, p. 325.

[7] Ibid.

[8] A. Ivarsson et al., "Breast Feeding Protects Against Celiac Disease," *Am Journal of Clin Nutr*, 2002;75(5):914-21.

[9] Elizabeth Lipski, MS, CCN, *Digestive Wellness*, Keats Publishing, Inc., 1996, p. 222.

[10] Ibid.

[11] Phyllis A. Balch, CNC and James F. Balch, MD, *Prescription for Nutritional Healing*, Third Edition, Avery, 2000, p. 279.

[12] Op cit., Lipski.

[13] Op cit., Murray and Pizzorno.

[14] Tursi, A., "Can Histological Damage Influence the Severity of Coeliac Disease? An Unanswered Question," *Digestive and Liver Disease*, 2007;39:30-32.

[15] Op cit., Kellman, p. 73.

[16] Tonia Reinhard, MS, RD, *Gastrointestinal Disorders and Nutrition*, Contemporary Books, 2002, p. 154.

[17] Op cit., Balch and Balch.

[18] Hadjivassiliou M. et al., “Neuromuscular disorder as a presenting feature of coeliac disease,” *Journal of Neurological Neurosurgery*, 1997;36:770-775.

[19] Zelnik N. et al., “Range of Neurologic Disorders in Patients with Celiac Disease,” *Pediatrics*, 2004;113(6):1672-6.

[20] Op cit., Reinhard, p. 156.

[21] Henry D. Janowitz, MD, *Your Gut Feelings*, Consumer's Union, 1987, p. 151.

[22] Op cit., Murray and Pizzorno.

[23] Op cit., Balch and Balch.

[24] M. Sara Rosenthal, *The Gastrointestinal Sourcebook*, Lowell House, 1997, p. 25.

[25] Op. cit., Tursi, A.

[26] https://www.enterolab.com/StaticPages/Faq_Result_Interpretation.htm

[27] P. Brandtzaeq, “Do Salivary Antibodies Reliably Reflect Both Mucosal and Systemic Immunity?” *Annals of NY Academy of Science*, 2007 Mar;1098:288-311.

[28] Op cit., Murray and Pizorno, p. 325.

[29] Op cit., Balch and Balch, p. 281.

Hemmorrhoids

[1] Michael Murray, ND and Joseph Pizzorno, ND, *Encyclopedia of Natural Medicine*, Revised 2nd edition, Prima Health, 1998, p. 507.

[2] Ibid.

[3] www.hemorrhoid.net

[4] Phyllis A. Balch, CNC and James F. Balch, MD, *Prescription for Nutritional Healing*, Third Edition, Avery, 2000, p. 427.

[5] Ibid., p. 429.

[6] J.P. Arnaud, et al., “Treatment of hemorrhoids with circular stapler, a new alternative to conventional methods: a prospective study of 140 patients.” *J Am Coll Surg*. 2001 Aug;193(2):161-5.

Crohn's

[1] Tonia Reinhard, MS, RD, *Gastrointestinal Disorders and Nutrition*, Contemporary Books, 2002, p. 129.

[2] James Scala, PhD., *The New Eating Right for A Bad Gut*, A Plume Book, 2000, p. 11.

[3] J. Wehkamp et al., “NOD2(CARD15) Mutations in Crohn's Disease are Associated with Diminished Mucosal Alpha-Defensin Expression,” *Gut*, 2004;53(11):1658-64.

[4] Phyllis A. Balch, CNC and James F. Balch, MD, *Prescription for Nutritional Healing*, Third Edition, Avery, 2000, p. 307.

[5] S. Nuding, et al., “Reduced mucosal antimicrobial activity in Crohn's disease of the colon.” *Gut*. 2007 Sep;56(9):1240-7. Epub 2007 Apr 24.

[6] M. Sara Rosenthal, *The Gastrointestinal Sourcebook*, Lowell House, 1997, p. 106-107.

[7] Carol Nacy PhD and Mary Buckley PhD, Mycobacterium Avium Paratuberculosis: Infrequent Human Pathogen or Public Health Threat? Report from the American Academy of Microbiology, 2007, p. 8.

[8] http://www.medscape.com/viewarticle/549397_4

[9] Elizabeth Lipski, MS, CCN, *Digestive Wellness*, Keats Publishing, Inc., 1996, p. 244.

[10] Ibid.

[11] Ibid.

[12] D. Lindsey Berkson, *Healthy Digestion the Natural Way*, John Wiley & Sons, Inc., 2000, p. 103.

[13] Dr. John McKenna, *Hard to Stomach*, Newleaf, 2002, p. 133.

[14] Op. Cit., Reinhard, p. 130.

[15] Ibid.

[16] Michael Murray, ND and Joseph Pizzorno, ND, *Encyclopedia of Natural Medicine*, Revised Second Edition, Prima Health, 1998, p. 589.

[17] Ibid.

[18] Op. Cit., Lipski.

[19] J. Wyatt, et al., “Intestinal permeability and the prediction of relapse in Crohn's disease.” *Lancet*. 1993 Jun 5;341(8858):1437-9.

[20] Ibid., p. 245

[21] Op cit., Murray and Pizzorno, p. 593.

[22] Ibid.

[23] Ibid.

[24] S.M. Cohen, et al.,“A Critical Review of the Toxicological Effects of Carrageenan and Processed Eucheuma Seaweed on the Gastrointestinal Tract,” *Critical Review of Toxicology*, 2002;32(5):413-44.

[25] Op cit., Murray and Pizzorno, p. 592.

[26] Op cit., Renihard, p. 135.

[27] E.V. Loftus et al., “The Epidemiology and Natural History of Crohn's Disease in Population-Based Patient Cohorts from North America: A Systematic Rreview,” *Alimentary Pharmacology Therapy*, 2002;16(1):51-60.

[28] Henry D. Janowitz, *Your Gut Feelings*, Consumer's Union, 197, p. 40.

[29] Op cit., Balch and Balch, p. 309.

[30] Raphael Kellman, MD, *Gut Reactions*, Broadway Books, 2002, p. 78.

[31] Op cit., Reinhard

[32] Steven R. Peikin, *Gastrointestinal Health*, Quill, 2001, p. 112.

[33] Op cit., Murray and Pizzorno, p. 593.

[34] Ibid., p. 594.

[35] Ibid.

[36] Op cit., Balch and Balch, p. 309.

[37] Ibid.

[38] Op cit., Rosenthal, p. 113.

[39] Op cit., Scala, p. 85.

[40] Op cit., Reinhard, p. 138 & 141.

[41] Ibid., p. 134.

[42] http://www.google.com/webhp?sourceid=navclient&ie=UTF-8&rlz=1T4GGHP_enUS364

Ulcerative Colitis

[1] Henry D. Janowitz, MD, *Your Gut Feelings*, Consumer's Union, 1987, p. 39.

[2] Phylllis A. Balch, CNC and James F. Balch, MD, *Prescription for Nutritional Healing*, Third Edition, Avery, 2000, p. 666.

[3] Ibid.

[4] Michael Murray, ND and Joseph Pizzorno, ND, *Encyclopedia of Natural Medicine*, Revised Second Edition, Prima Health, 1998, p. 590.

[5] Tonia Reinhard, MS, RD, *Gastrointestinal Disorders and Nutrition*, Contemporary Books, 2002, p. 146.

[6] Op. cit., Murray and Pizzorno, p.588.

[7] http://emedicine.medscape.com/article/183084-overview

[8] Tonia Reinhard, MS, RD, *Gastrointestinal Disorders and Nutrition*, Contemporary Books, 2002, p. 148.

[9] Linda M. Ross, editor, *Gastrointestinal Diseases and Disorders Sourcebook*, Omnigraphics, Inc., 1996, p. 206.

[10] Op. cit., Peikin, p. 122.

[11] Ibid., p. 120.

[12] Ibid.

[13] Op. cit., Ross, p. 208.

[14] R.W. Summers, et al., “Trichuris suis therapy for active ulcerative colitis: a randomized controlled trial.” *Gastroenterology*. 2005 Apr;128(4):825-32.

[15] D.E. Elliot, “Does the failure to acquire helminthic parasites predispose to Crohn's disease?” *FASEB J*. 2000 Sep;14(13):1848-55.

[16] Frank DN, St. Amand AL, Feldman RA, et al., “Molecular-phylogenetic characterization of microbial community imbalances in human inflammatory bowel diseases.” *Proc Natl Acad Sci U S A* 2007; 104:13780.

[17] T.J. Borody, et al., “Bacteriotherapy using fecal flora: toying with human motions.” *J Clin Gastroenterol*. 2004 Jul;38(6):475-83.

[18] L. Langmead, et al., “Randomized, double-blind, placebo-controlled trial of oral aloe vera gel for active ulcerative colitis.” *Aliment Pharmacol Ther*. 2004 Apr 1;19(7):739-47.

Irritable Bowel Syndrome

[1] Steven R. Peikin, MD, *Gastrointestinal Health*, Quill, 1999, p. 81.

[2] Raphael Kellman, MD, *Gut Reactions*, Broadway Books, 2002, p. 92.

[3] H.C. Lin MD, “Small Intestinal Bacterial Overgrowth, a Framework for Understanding Irritable Bowel Syndrome,” *JAMA*, 2004;292(7):852-8.

[4] Ibid.

[5] Ibid.

[6] Ibid.

[7] Ibid.

[8] B. M. Speigel et al., “Bacterial Overgrowth and Irritable Bowel Syndrome: Unifying Hypothesis or a Spurious Consequence of Proton Pump Inhibitors?” *American Journal of Gastroenterology*, 2008;103:2972-6.

[9] Phyllis A. Balch, CNC and James F. Balch, MD, *Prescription for Nutritional Healing*, Third Edition, Avery, 2000, p.476-477.

[10] Elizabeth Lipski, *Digestive Wellness*, Keats Publishing, Inc., 1996, p. 238.

[11] Ibid.

[12] Michael Murray, ND and Joseph Pizzorno, ND, *Encyclopedia of Natural Medicine*, Revised Second Edition, Prima Health, 1998, p. 611.

[13] Op cit., Lipski, p. 239.

[14] A. Tungtrongchitr, et al., “Blastocystis hominis infection in irritable bowel syndrome patients.” *Southeast Asian J Trop Med Public Health*. 2004 Sep;35(3):705-10.

[15] H. Santelmann and J.M. Howard, “Yeast metabolic products, yeast antigens and yeasts as possible triggers for irritable bowel syndrome.” *Eur J Gastroenterol Hepatol*. 2005 Jan;17(1):21-6.

[16] Op cit., Balch and Balch, p. 476.

[17] Op cit., Peikin, p. 82.

[18] Op cit, Balch and Balch

[19] Michael D. Gershon, MD, *The Second Brain*, Harper Perennial, 1998, p. 180.

[20] Ibid., p.179-180.

[21] Tonia Reinhard, MS, RD, *Gastrointestinal Disorders and Nutrition*, Contemporary Books, 2002, p. 117.

[22] Op cit., Gershon.

[23] Ibid., p. 181.

[24] Henry D. Janowitz, MD, *Your Gut Feelings*, Consumer's Union, 1987, p. 18.

[25] Op cit., Peikin, p. 83.

[26] Linda M. Ross, editor, *Gastrointestinal Diseases and Disorders Sourcebook*, Omnigraphics, Inc., 1996, p. 233.

[27] Op cit., Peikin, p. 84.

[28] M. Pimental, et al., “Normalization of lactulose breath testing correlates with symptom improvement in irritable bowel syndrome. a double-blind, randomized, placebo-controlled study.” *Am J Gastroenterol*. 2003 Feb;98(2):412-9.

[29] M.H. Pittler and E. Ernst, “Peppermint oil for irritable bowel syndrome: a critical review and metaanalysis.” *Am J Gastroenterol*. 1998 Jul;93(7):1131-5.

Lactose Intolerance

[1] http://www.vivo.colostate.edu/hbooks/pathphys/digestion/smallgut/lactose_intol.html

[2] Phyllis A. Balch, CNC and James F. Balch, MD, *Prescription for Nutritional Healing*, Third Edition, Avery, 2000, p. 486.

[3] James Scala, Ph.D., *The New Eating Right for a Bad Gut*, A Plume Book, 2000, p. 51.

[4] Tonia Reinhard, MS, RD, *Gastrointestinal Disorders and Nutrition*, Contemporary Books, 2002, p. 90.

[5] Raphael Kellman, MD, *Gut Reactions*, Broadway Books, 2002, p. 94.

[6] Ibid.

[7] Michael Murray, ND and Joseph Pizzorno, ND, *Encyclopedia of Natural Medicine*, Revised Second Edition, Prima Health, 1998, p. 435.

[8] Op cit., Kellman

[9] Op cit., Balch and Balch.

[10] Ibid, p. 487.

[11] Ibid.

[12] Op cit., Kellman.

[13] Op cit., Scala.

[14] Op cit., Reinhard, p. 94.

[15] Linda M. Ross, editor, *Gastrointestinal Diseases and Disorders Sourcebook*, Ominigraphics, Inc., 1996, p. 271.

[16] Ibid.

[17] Ibid.

[18] Op cit., Balch and Balch, p. 487.

[19] Op cit., Ross.

Leaky Gut Syndrome

[1] Elizabeth Lipski, MS, CCN, *Digestive Wellness*, Keats Publishing, Inc., 1996, p. 78.

[2] Wendy Marson, “Gut Reactions,” *Newsweek*, November 17, 1997, p. 95-99.

[3] http://www.health-n-energy.com/ronagut.htm

[4] Lynn Toohey, MS, PhD, “Leaky Gut – Detoxification,” *Nutri Notes*, Vol. 5, #2, March-April, 1998.

[5] Dr. John McKenna, *Hard to Stomach*, NewLeaf, 2002, p. 10.

Parasitic Disease

[1] Timothy Kuss, Ph.D., *A Guidebook to Clinical Nutrition for the Health Professional*, Institute of Bioenergetic Research, 1992, p. 17.

[2] Ibid, p. 17-18

[3] M.E. Scott and K.G. Koski, "Zinc deficiency impairs immune responses against parasitic nematode infections at intestinal and systemic sites." *J Nutr*. 2000 May;130 (5S Suppl):1412S-20S.

[3] O.M. Amin, "Seasonal prevalence of intestinal parasites in the United States during 2000." *Am J Trop Med Hyg*. 2002;66(6):799-803.

[5] http://www.cdc.gov/Ncidod/dpd/public/geninfo_statistics_avail.htm

[6] W.R. Mac Kenzie et al., "A Massive Outbreak in Milwuakee of Cryptosporidium Infection Transmitted Through the Public Water Supply," *New England Journal of Medicine*, 1994;331(3):161-7.

[7] Center for Disease Control and Prevention, "Community Wide Cryptosporidiosis Outbreak-Utah 2007," 2008;300(15):1754-6.

[8] Dr. William R. Kellas and Dr. Andrea Sharon Dworkin, *Surviving the Toxic Crisis*, Professional Preference, 1996, p. 347, 359, 368 and 371.

[9] A. Tungtrongchitr, et al., "Blastocystis hominis infection in irritable bowel syndrome patients." *Southeast Asian J Trop Med Public Health*. 2004 Sep;35(3):705-10.

[10] Ibid., p. 363.

[11] Ibid., p. 366.

[12] Op cit., Amin.

[13] Op cit., Kellas, p. 369.

[14] Op cit., Amin.

[15] Ann Louise Gittleman, *Guess What Came to Dinner*, Avery Publishing Group, Inc., 1993, p. 97.

[16] Op cit., Kellas, p. 357.

[17] Op cit., Gittleman, p. 97-100.

Cirrhosis

[1] *Disease Prevention and Treatment*, Expanded Fourth Edition, Life Extension Media, 2003, p. 993.

[2] Linda M. Ross, editor, *Gastrointestinal Diseases and Disorders Handbook*, Omnigraphics, Inc., 1996, p. 332.

[3] Dr. William R. Kellas and Dr. Andrea Sharon Dworkin, *Surviving the Toxic Crisis*, Professional Preference, 1996, p. 54, 55.

[4] Ibid., p. 217 and 228.

[5] Rosenthal, M. Sara, *The Gastrointestinal Sourcebook*, Lowell House, 1997, p. 122.

[6] C. Pande et al., "Small-intestinal bacterial Overgrowth in Cirrhosis is Related to the Severity of Liver Disease," *Aliment Pharmacol & Ther*, 2009, 29(12), p. 1273-81.

[7] http:// www.liverfoundation.org/about/news/33

[8] Op cit., Ross.

[9] Op cit., *Disease Prevention and Treatment*.

[10] Op cit., Ross, p. 331.

[11] Op cit., *Disease Prevention and Treatment*, p. 991.

[12] Ibid.

[13] Ibid., p. 994.

[14] Ibid., p. 996.

Gallstones

[1] http://www.uptodate.com/patients/content/topic.do?topicKey=~OOIIricadskc9/

[2] Henry D. Janowitz, MD, *Indigestion*, Oxford University Press, 1992, p. 117.

[3] Ibid.

[4] Steven R. Peikin, MD, *Gastrointestinal Health*, Quill, 1999, p. 76-77,

[5] Linda M. Ross, *Gastrointestinal Diseases and Disorders Sourcebook*, Omnigraphics, Inc., 1996, p. 365.

[6] Dr. William R. Kellas and Dr. Andrea Sharon Dworkin, *Surviving the Toxic Crisis*, Professional Preference, 1996, p. 66.

[7] Op cit., Peikin, p. 77.

[8] M.A. Cahan et al., "Proton Pump Inhibitors Reduce Gallbladder Function," *Surgical Endoscopy*, 2006;20(9):1364-7.

[9] Op. cit., Ross.

[10] D. Lindsey Berkson, *Healthy Digestion the Natural Way*, John Wiley & Sons, Inc., 2000. p. 128.

[11] Michael Murray, ND and Joseph Pizzorno, ND, *Encyclopedia of Natural Mediicine*, revised 2nd edition, Prima Health, 1998, p. 480.

[12] Phyllis A. Balch, CNC and James F. Balch, MD, *Prescription for Nutritional Healing*, third edition, Avery, 2000, p. 390.

[13] Op cit., Berkson, p. 127.

[14] Elizabeth Lipski, MS, CCN, *Digestive Wellness*, Keats Publishing, Inc., 1996, p. 210.

[15] Op cit., Janowitz, p. 116.

[16] Op cit., Peikin, p. 76.

[17] Op cit., Murray and Pizzorno, p. 479.

[18] Op cit., Lipski, p. 210.

[19] Op cit., Murray and Pizzorno, p. 476-477.

[20] Op cit., Ross, p. 366.

[21] Op cit., Peikin, p. 33.

[22] http://digestive.niddk.nih.gov/ddiseases/pubs/ercp

[23] Ibid., p. 79

[24] Op cit., Janowitz, p. 131.

[25] Ibid.

[26] Andrew Gaeddert, *Healing Digestive Disorders*, North Atlantic Books, 1998, p.151.

[27] Op cit., Janowitz, p. 125-126.

[28] Ibid., p. 127.

[29] Ibid., p. 128.

[30] *The Merck Manual*, Centennial Edition, Merck & Co., Inc., 1999, p. 402.

[31] Op cit., uptodate.

[32] Op cit., Janowitz, p. 122.

[33] Op cit., Lipski, p. 212.

Hepatitis

[1] Melissa Palmer, MD, *Hepatitis Liver Disease*, Avery Publishing Group, 2000, p. 72.

[2] Ibid., p. 73.

[3] http://www.medicinenet.com/fatty_liver/page3.htm

[4] Op cit., Palmer, p. 78.

[5] D. Villalta et al., "High Prevalence of Celiac Disease in Autoimmune Hepatitis Detected by Anti-Tissue Transglutaminase Auto-Antibodies," *Journal of Clinical Laboratory Analysis*, 2005;19(1):6-10.

[6] Op cit., Palmer, p. 381.

[7] Ibid., p. 382.

[8] Phyllis A. Balch, CNC and James F. Balch, MD, *Prescription for Nutritional Healing*, Avery, 2000, p. 430.

[9] Ibid.

[10] www.mercola.com, "Hepatitis B Vaccine Continues to Kill Infants," #444.

[11] Michael Murray, ND and Joseph Pizzorno, ND, *Encyclopedia of Natural Medicine*, Revised 2nd Edition, Prima Health, 1998, p. 513.

[12] Ibid.

NAFLD/NASH

[1] E. Bugianesi et al., "Expanding the natural history of nonalcoholic steatohepatitis: from cryptogenic cirrhosis to hepatocellular carcinoma." *Gastroenterology*. 2002 Jul;123(1):134-40.

[2] P. Hamil, "The 'Hidden' Liver Disease." *Life Extension Magazine*. 2004, February.

[3] P. Loria, et al., "Is liver fat detrimental to vessels?: intersections in the pathogenesis of NAFLD and atherosclerosis." *Clin Sci* (Lond). 2008 Jul;115(1):1-12.

[4] http://www.mayoclinic.com/health/nonalcoholic-fatty-liver-disease/DS00577

[5] http://www.uptodate.com/patients/content/topic.do?topicKey=~FXYFR93Lol53pY&selectedTitle=3%7E28&source=search_result

[6] Op cit., Hamil.

[7] A.E. Feldstein and M.H. Kay, "Fatty Liver Disease." American College of Gastroenterology. Cleveland Clinic Foundation, Department of Pediatric Gastroenterology and Nutrition and Department of Cell Biology.

[8] P. Angulo and K.D. Lindor, "Non-alcoholic fatty liver disease." *J Gastroenterol Hepatol*. 2002 Feb;17 Suppl:S186-90.

[9] E.E. Powell et al., "Dangerous liaisons: the metabolic syndrome and nonalcoholic fatty liver disease." *Ann Intern Med*. 2005 Nov 15;143(10):753-4.

[10] G. Farrell, "Is bacterial ash the flash that ignites NASH?" *Gut*. 2001 February; 48(2): 148–149.

[11] D.S. Jones, M.D. (editor), *Textbook of Functional Medicine*, The Institute for Funtional Medicine, 2005, p. 567.

[12] Op cit., Angulo Lindor.

[13] Ibid.

[14] A.J. Wigg, et al., "The role of small intestinal bacterial overgrowth, intestinal permeability, endotoxaemia, and tumour necrosis factor alpha in the pathogenesis of non-alcoholic steatohepatitis." Gut. 2001 Feb;48(2):206-11.

[15] Op cit., Jones.

[16] Op cit., Wigg.

[17] Op cit., Jones.

[18] Wiley-Blackwell. "Intestinal Bacteria Associated With Non-Alcoholic Fatty Liver Disease." ScienceDaily 31 May 2009. 26 January 2010.

[19] H. Tilg and A.M. Diehl, "Cytokines in alcoholic and nonalcoholic steatohepatitis." N Engl J Med. 2000 Nov 16;343(20):1467-76.

[20] J.M. Joneaja and E.A. Ayre, "Abnormal gut fermentation: the "auto-brewery" syndrome." J-Can-Diet-Assoc. Toronto, Ontario : Dietitians of Canada. Summer 1997. v. 58 (2) p. 97-100.

[21] Op cit., Wigg.

[22] Op cit., Jones, p. 568.

[23] S. Nair, et al., "Obesity and female gender increase breath ethanol concentration: potential implications for the pathogenesis of nonalcoholic steatohepatitis." Am J Gastroenterol. 2001 Apr;96(4):1200-4.

[24] A. Rubio-Tapia and J.A. Murray. "The liver in celiac disease." Hepatology. 2007 Nov;46(5):1650-8.

[25] M.T. Bardella, et al., "Prevalence of hypertransaminasemia in adult celiac patients and effect of gluten-free diet." Hepatology. 1995 Sep;22(3):833-6.

[26] Ibid., Rubio-Tapia

[27] K. Kaukinen, et al., "Celiac disease in patients with severe liver disease: gluten-free diet may reverse hepatic failure." Gastroenterology. 2002 Apr;122(4):881-8.

[28] Op cit., Jones, p. 568.

[29] S. Zelber-Sagi, et al., "Long term nutritional intake and the risk for non-alcoholic fatty liver disease (NAFLD): a population based study." J Hepatol. 2007 Nov;47(5):711-7. Epub 2007 Aug 14.

[30] Op cit., Angulo.

[31] N.M. Wilfred de Alwis and C.P. Day, "Genes and nonalcoholic fatty liver disease." Current Diabetes Rep. 2008 Apr;8(2):156-63.

[32] Op cit., Feldstein.

[33] Ibid., Hamil.

[34] J.M. Clark and A.M. Diehl, "Nonalcoholic fatty liver disease: an underrecognized cause of cryptogenic cirrhosis." JAMA. 2003 Jun 11;289(22):3000-4.

[35] Op cit., Hamil.

[36] Op cit., Uptodate.

[37] Ibid.

[38] Op cit., Angulo.

[39] B. Garait, et al., "Fat intake reverses the beneficial effects of low caloric intake on skeletal muscle mitochondrial H(2)O(2) production." Free Radic Biol Med. 2005 Nov 1;39(9):1249-61. Epub 2005 Aug 8.

[40] J.M. Weinberg, "Lipotoxicity." Kidney Int. 2006 Nov;70(9):1560-6. Epub 2006 Sep 6.

[41] Ibid.

[42] Z. Li, et al., "Probiotics and antibodies to TNF inhibit inflammatory activity and improve nonalcoholic fatty liver disease." Hepatology. 2003 Feb;37(2):343-50.

Pancreatitis

[1] Michael D. Gershon, MD, *The Second Brain*, HarperPerennial, 1998, p. 123.

[2] Henry D. Janowitz, MD, *Your Gut Feelings*, Consumer's Union, 1987, p. 140.

[3] www.nlm.nih.gov/medlineplus/ency/article/001144.htm#visualContent

[4] Phyllis A. Balch, CNC and James F. Balch, MD, *Prescription for Nutritional Healing*, Third Edition, Avery, 2000, p. 556.

[5] Op cit., www.nlm.nih.gov

[6] Op cit., Janowitz, p. 138.

[7] Linda A. Ross, editor, *Gastrointestinal Diseases and Disorders Sourcebook*, Omnigraphics, Inc., 1996, p. 360.

[8] Ibid.

[9] B.J Ammori, "Early increase in intestinal permeability in patients with severe acute pancreatitis: correlation with endotoxemia, organ failure, and mortality." *J Gastrointest Surg*. 1999 May-Jun;3(3):252-62.

[10] Op cit., www.nlm.nih.gov

[11] Ibid.

Appendix

[1] www.gsdl.com/assessments/finsystems/metabolic. html

[2] Jonathan V. Wright, MD and Lane Lenard, PhD, *Why Stomach Acid is Good for You*, M. Evans and Company, Inc., 2001, p. 133.

[3] Elizabeth Lipski, MS, CNN, *Digestive Wellness*, Keats Publishing, Inc., 1996, p. 118.

[4] Omar M. Amin, "Seasonal Prevalence of Intestinal Parasites in the United Sates During 2002," *Am J. Trop Med. Hyg.*, 66(6), 2002, p. 799.

INDEX

A

B

C

D

H

N

O

T

U

V

W

Y

Z

PHOTO CREDITS

Cover & Intro

1 Shutterstock 2263503, **2** Shutterstock 18223555, **3** Photo Researchers C003/3222, **4** Shutterstock 13949599, **5** Shutterstock 33673117, **6** Shutterstock 54772381, **7** Shutterstock 53394925, **8** Shutterstock 23091934, **9** Wolter's Kluwer 9859H, **10** Wolter's Kluwer 9861AB

Basics of Digestion

1 Shutterstock 41097238, **2** Shutterstock 23723875, **3** Shutterstock 51079348, **4** Shutterstock 46900594, **5** Photo Researchers C003/3222, **6** Shutterstock 54173683, **7** Shutterstock 56998466, **8** Shutterstock 59890912, **9** Shutterstock 60166105

Digestive System

1 Shutterstock 33673195, **2** Renew Life Formulas, **3** Photo Researchers SL9332, **4** Photo Researchers BH6767, **5** Shutterstock 12165187, **6** Shutterstock 25940518, **7** Renew Life Formulas, **8** Renew Life Formulas, **9** Photo Researchers BC6570, **10** Photo Researchers SA8871, **11** Photo Researchers E07441, **12** Shutterstock 17113172, **13** Shutterstock 57190135, **14** Shutterstock 46841284, **15** Wolter's Kluwer Images 9965b, **16** Shutterstock 33673117, **17** Shutterstock 46601353, **18** Photo Researchers SC9922, **19** Shutterstock 10067413, **20** Shutterstock 2332480, **21-23** Renew Life formulas, **24** Shutterstock 40330843, **25&26** Renew Life Formulas, **27** Shutterstock 20664115, **28&29** Netter Images 23989, **30** Shutterstock 9355402, **31** Photo Researchers SB7875, **32** Shutterstock 16327189, **33** Shutterstock 17307, **34** John Stuart Photography, **35** Shutterstock 16695568, **36** Netter Images 2986, **37** Shutterstock 42388171, **38** Photo Researchers SE0346, **39** Shutterstock 21476713, **40** Photo Researchers MRF_30299, **41** Shutterstock 34447892, **42** Renew Life Formulas, **43** Netter Images #39791, **44** Shutterstock 20910016, **45** Shutterstock 54416914, **46** Shutterstock 56026987, **47** Shutterstock 60188491, **48** Shutterstock 16209130, **49** Shutterstock 8871772, **50** Renew Life Formulas, **51** Photo Researchers BC6570, **52** Shutterstock 57374719, **53&54** Renew Life Formulas, **55** Shutterstock 1464382, **56** Shutterstock 59598688, **57** Shutterstock 60124258, **58** Shutterstock 55456801, **59** Renew Life Formulas, **60** Shutterstock 13643545, **61** Shutterstock 2263503, **62** Shutterstock 25524850, **63** Shutterstock 51891274, **64** Shutterstock 18223576, **65** Shutterstock 54203587, **66** Shutterstock 1329359, **67** Shutterstock 40073206, **68** Shutterstock 56180668, **69** Renew Life Formulas, **70** Shutterstock 24737392, **71** Renew Life Formulas, **72** Photo Researchers SB7755, **73** Shutterstock 19706080, **74** Shutterstock 9759598, **75** Michael Black Photo-Black Sun, **76** Shutterstock 11943016, **77** Shutterstock 59075992, **78** Shutterstock 56999630, **79** Shutterstock 60365377, **80** Shutterstock 41097235, **81** Shutterstock 26490754, **82** Shutterstock 6481264, **83** Shutterstock 55777618, **84&85** Renew Life Formulas, **86** Shutterstock 50802868, **87** Nature: American Journal of Gastrology, **88** Shutterstock 2139435, **89** Renew Life Formulas, **90** Photo Researchers SB7878, **91** Photo Researchers BC1951, **92** Shutterstock 22166761, **93** Shutterstock 18198067, **94** Shutterstock 12162256, **95** Renew Life Formulas, **96** Photo Researchers C001/2922, **97** Shutterstock 53621455, **98** Shutterstock 17583976,99 Shutterstock 17103874, **100** Shutterstock 50518060, **101** Netter Images 22176, **102** Shutterstock 60212959, **103** Renew Life Formulas, **104** Photo Researchers SH1443, **105** Shutterstock 54664579, **106** Shutterstock 5327335, **107** Netter Images 6733, **108** Shutterstock 1787729, **109** Shutterstock 53457175, **110** Shutterstock, **111&112** Renew Life Formulas, **113** Shutterstock 28887322, **114** Shutterstock 27729736, **115** Shutterstock 52471888, **116-120** Renew Life Formulas, **121** Shutterstock 52614928, **122&123** Renew Life Formulas, **124** Photo Researchers SL9039, **125** Shutterstock 14214418, **126** Shutterstock 14313940, **127** Shutterstock 54070438, **128** Shutterstock 33140836, **129** Shutterstock 32022751, **130** Shutterstock 24408601, **131** Renew Life Formulas, **132** Shutterstock 47176669, **133** Shutterstock 40294330, **134** Shutterstock 11322163, **135** Shutterstock 56928736, **136** Shutterstock 17583973, **137** Shutterstock 42085507, **138** Shutterstock 53644528, **139** Shutterstock 58145728, **140** Renew Life Formulas, **141** Photo Researchers M165/245, **142** Photo Researchers M165/141, **143** Shutterstock 5341537, **144** Shutterstock 16062436, **145** Shutterstock 56319280, **146** Shutterstock 23905972, **147** Shutterstock 44302405, **148** Renew Life Formulas, **149** Photo Researchers BQ2620, **150** Shutterstock 53664055, **151** Shutterstock 50680078, **152** Shutterstock 57485323, **153** Wolter's Kluwer Images 9992D, **154** Renew Life Formulas, **155** Shutterstock 47176672, **156** Shutterstock 14214499, **157** Shutterstock 47541235, **158** Shutterstock 46952047, **159** Shutterstock 21638278, **160** Shutterstock 28660328, **161** Shutterstock 22809769, **162** Renew Life Formulas, **163** Photo Researchers SM1784, **164** Shutterstock 56754211, **165** Shutterstock 52824478, **166** Shutterstock 60427912, **167** Shutterstock 56558938, **168** Shutterstock 40943353, **169** Shutterstock 2676544

Appendix

1 Shutterstock 57910114, **2** Shutterstock 26302414, **3&4** Renew Life Formulas, **5** Shutterstock 14314000, **6** Shutterstock 55481185, **7** Shutterstock 58384366, **8** Shutterstock 55648906, **9** Shutterstock 55648906, **10** Heidelberg, **11** Shutterstock 1909905, **12** Shutterstock 5341768, **12** Michael Black Photo-Black Sun, **13** Shutterstock 54444748, **14&15** Michael Black Photo-Black Sun, **16** Renew Life Formulas, **17** Shutterstock 37126294, **18** Shutterstock 62269855, **19** Shutterstock 45747331, **20&21** thecandidadiet.com, **22** Shutterstock 904623, **23** thecandidadiet.com, **24-27** Renew Life Formulas, **28** Shutterstock 53690905, **29** Shutterstock 7724206, **30** Shutterstock 18489850, **31**Shutterstock 59839630, **32** Renew Life Formulas, **33** I-ACT, **34** Renew Life Formulas, **35** Shutterstock 14703724, **36** Renew Life Formulas, **37** Shutterstock 24284092, **38&39** Renew Life Formulas, **40** IFOS, **41-53** Renew Life Formulas